THE PATIENT'S GUIDE TO MEDICAL TESTS

THE PATIENT'S GUIDE TO MEDICAL TESTS

Cathey Pinckney
and
Edward R. Pinckney, M.D.

THIRD EDITION

Facts On File Publications
460 Park Avenue South
New York, N.Y. 10016

The nature of medical testing is that it is constantly evolving and subject to interpretation. Therefore, while the authors of this book have made their best efforts to ensure the accuracy and completeness of the material presented, the reader is advised that no claim can be made that all relevant information concerning the medical tests described in this book is included here. Additionally, the reader is advised that this book is not a manual for self-diagnosis or self-treatment, and is further advised to consult with his or her physician in search of answers or treatment for any medical problems.

THE PATIENT'S GUIDE TO MEDICAL TESTS

Copyright © 1978, 1982, 1986 by Cathey Pinckney and Edward R. Pinckney, M.D.

All rights reserved. No part of this book may be reproduced or utilized in any form or by any means, electronic or mechanical, including photocopying, recording or by any information storage and retrieval systems, without permission in writing from the Publisher.

Library of Congress Cataloging-in-Publication Data

Pinckney, Cathey.
   The patient's guide to medical tests.

   Rev. ed. of: The encyclopedia of medical tests. 1982.
   1. Diagnosis—Dictionaries.   2. Diagnosis, Laboratory
—Dictionaries.   I. Pinckney, Edward R. (Edward Robert),
1924–   .   II. Title.   [DNLM: 1. Diagnosis, Laboratory
—Dictionaries.   2. Diagnostic tests, Routine—
Dictionaries. QY 13 P647p]
RC71.P56   1983   616.07′5   82-21129
ISBN 0-8160-1292-X
ISBN 0-8160-1593-7 (pbk.)

Printed in the United States of America

10 9 8 7 6 5 4 3 2 1

For *Cathey Lee*
Health Sciences Librarian *Extraordinaire*

CONTENTS

Preface to the Third Edition ix
Introduction xi
    Your Rights in Medical Testing xiv
    Why Many Medical Tests Are Performed xviii
    Defensive Medicine xix
    On Being a Participatory Patient xx
    Risks vs. Benefits xxii
    Invasive vs. Noninvasive Tests xxii
    Consequences and Alternatives xxii
    Costs xxiv
    Testing for Profit xxv
    Where Tests Are Performed xxvii
    Patient-Related Causes of Inaccurate Test Results xxvii
        Medications xxvii
        Diet xxviii
        Routine Activities xxviii
        Attitude xxviii
        Physical Factors xxviii
    If the Test You Want to Know About Is Not
      in the Book xxix
    Two Caveats xxxi
How to Use This Book xxxiii
    When Performed xxxiii
    Normal Values xxxiii
    Abnormal Values xxxiv
    Risk Factors xxxv
    General Risk Factors xxxv
        Blood Testing xxxv
        Catheter and Needle Insertion xxxv
        Contrast Substance (Dye) Use xxxvi

    X-Ray and Radioactive Substance Application xxxvii
    Electrical Instrument Use........................ xxxvii
General Pain/Discomfort Factors xxxviii
    Blood Testing xxxix
    Catheter and Needle Insertion xxxix
Cost xxxix
Where Performed xli
Accuracy and Significance xli
Tests (alphabetically) 1
Measurements: Equivalency Chart 383
About the Authors 384

PREFACE TO THE THIRD EDITION

In the four-year interval between the printing of the second and third editions of this book, three major medical test phenomena took place. First, there was the extraordinary introduction of more than 500 new, albeit not always totally different, tests into the medical milieu. Compare this to the fact that in the four-year period of time between the first and second editions of the book (1978 to 1982), fewer than 100 new tests became part of a physician's armamentarium. There are now over 1,500 medical tests being performed on patients, with nearly 900 different analyses on blood alone. Despite the evident increase in the quantity of medical testing, it seems fair to say that the quality of such testing has made very little progress. True, there are some improvements in existing techniques: computerized tomography has become a bit more precise; magnetic resonance imaging may, in some instances, reveal more than computerized tomography, and the application of more sophisticated skills to the mechanical performance of laboratory tests has been able to reduce the time needed to reveal the result of a few blood examinations. But all in all, there has been no relative improvement in the doctor's ability to arrive at a diagnosis. The medical test that, by itself, can make a diagnosis is still unavailable, and doctors, not tests, still must come to the ultimate conclusion upon which therapy is based.

The second revelation concerning medical testing has been the surprising disclosure of the known—but heretofore hidden—dangers related to undergoing a medical test. No doubt this has come about as more and more patients, as well as doctors, have become aware of, and adhered to, the law of "informed consent," wherein doctors are required to tell patients of all the risks—as opposed to the benefits—related to every medical test. Now patients know, or at least can become aware of, the fact that 800 people die each year during X-ray testing that uses injected contrast media such as dyes as part of the procedure or that for every 10,000 stress electrocardiogram tests performed, 4 people will have a heart attack—and 1 will die—during the testing. In addition, patients are now required to be told of less dangerous, alternative tests that can provide similar information.

The third thing that has occurred over the past few years has been the exposé of the accuracy—or rather, *lack* of accuracy—of most medical tests. Despite the fact that more than half of all tests have an accuracy rating of only 80 percent or less, most patients—and even well people—still have a blind faith that virtually all tests are perfect and will reveal a vast store of knowledge about them to the doctor. A test with an accuracy rating of 80 percent or less is considered to be a "poor" test by those who specialize in this aspect of medical practice. Here are two striking examples: X-rays of the gallbladder, in which the patient swallows a dye-containing pill, to detect gallstones are reported to have an accuracy range from only 13 to 30 percent (compared to gallbladder ultrasound testing, which is 97 percent accurate). The stress electrocardiogram test, especially when performed on healthy people to evaluate the heart's condition, has been reported to be accurate only 16 to 21 percent of the time; after taking this test, the chances of being told you have heart disease when you do not is well over 50 percent.

But in spite of all this new information, most patients still consider medical tests as infallible. Whether this is because they really do not trust their doctors as much as they trust a mechanical process and a printed, numbered conclusion (as some surveys have indicated) or whether they relish the attention that accompanies being stabbed by a needle, photographed by X-rays or having a very private orifice invaded and explored (as other surveys have revealed) is still not known. What is known, however, is that most patients throw caution to the wind with their ridiculous worship of—and demand for—medical testing; the end result being that medical tests now make up about half of the cost of all medical care (nearly $225 billion in 1985) and comprise a greater overall risk to life and limb than any other medical procedure.

Thus it is that the major changes in this third edition consist, first, of 345 new tests in addition to the 718 in the last edition. The vast majority of the new tests were suggested for inclusion by doctors throughout the country. Not all the proposed tests could be included, if not for limitations of space then because many are simply a regular part of a routine physical examination (e.g., the "cough" test to help detect a hernia; coughing exerts pressure inside the abdomen that can force a hernia to reveal itself). When it comes to psychological tests, there is one book alone that describes more than 3,500 of these; virtually all are in use. Second, there is increased emphasis on the risks and dangers related to a test. The section on risk factors in general in the Introduction has been expanded to offer additional information to be considered before undergoing any medical test. Third, data on a test's accuracy and significance have been amplified where possible. The estimated accuracy of virtually every medical test has, at one time or another, been published in medical books and journals; true, there are disagreements among physicians, mostly depending on whether the doctor performs or orders the particular test or not, but where there might be some discrepancy, averages were used. Other changes include cost increases (on the average, medical test costs increased 15 percent each year, while all other medical costs rose only 10 percent) and new uses that have been claimed for old tests; and where appropriate, more extensive information is provided in the introductory section of each test. Normal and abnormal values have remained fairly constant, and the pain/discomfort factors have not, in most cases, been lessened.

If nothing else, should the reader demand to know the accuracy and risk factors of each test ordered or performed by a doctor prior to undergoing that test, the book will have served a useful purpose. If the reader learns to insist on the reason for a medical test (ask what will happen if the test result is positive, or abnormal, and what will happen if the test result is negative, or normal, and if the answers are the same, insist on knowing just why the test is even being performed) and gains the courage to refuse any medical test without a basis in fact and personal benefit, the book will have made a valuable contribution to the saving of lives, limbs, and money. If the reader becomes aware of the risks versus the benefits of medical tests and weighs both factors prior to submitting to any test—or any medical procedure, for that matter—rejecting those that can cause more harm than good, the book will have performed a miracle.

January 1, 1986

INTRODUCTION

Four years ago, to begin the Introduction to the second edition of this book, the 10 most commonly asked questions concerning medical tests were listed—along with the answers appropriate for that time. Four years later, not only are the 10 questions still the same, but somewhat surprisingly, so are the answers. Despite the profusion of new medical tests and the technological advances that either spawned those tests or accompanied their introduction, not that much has changed when it comes to what medical tests can reveal. Here are the questions and their answers:

- "Is there any test that will tell me if I have cancer?"

Some medical tests can hint that cancer might be present; there are a few tests that might even help locate where a cancer might be lurking. But there is no test, at this time, that can guarantee a definite answer for everyone.

- "Can a doctor predict whether I will have a heart attack?"

It is not possible to predict future heart disease in healthy people. There are, however, medical tests that can offer early warnings sufficient to prompt preventive measures.

- "I think my son is taking drugs; is there any way to be sure?"

There are simple tests a doctor can perform in his office that can expose the use of illegal drugs and narcotics. But not all dangerous drugs are readily detected; LSD, for example, is almost impossible to spot.

- "Can I find out whether my baby will be born all right?"

While there are several different ways of discerning congenital abnormalities and potentially tragic metabolic disturbances in an unborn baby, not all inherited disabilities can be detected at present. In addition, neither a positive nor a negative test is always accurate.

- "My memory seems to be going; is it possible to determine whether something is wrong and do something about it.?"

There are ways to test for most kinds of memory defects. Some tests can reveal the specific cause of a loss of memory, which, when determined, may be quickly reversible.

- "We just came back from a trip abroad and have been sick ever since. Could we have picked up a strange bug?"

It is not difficult to uncover the germ—or, more likely, the parasite—that is causing repeated bouts of fever, stomach and intestinal problems, and even joint aches. The tests take a great deal of patience and uninhibited participation by those who are afflicted. And some forms of hepatitis from exotic countries still cannot be unmasked.

- "I can't get pregnant; isn't there some way to prove it's not my fault?"

It is possible to determine, through a series of tests, whether a man is sterile, or so deficient in the production of normal sperm as to be functionally sterile. It is sometimes possible to learn exactly why a woman cannot conceive.

- "It seems that medical tests are not always precise. How much can I rely upon a test result?"

Very few medical tests are infallible; most are subject to endless sorts of error; while occasional tests are disease-specific (that is, positive or abnormal results strongly suggest the presence of a specific disease), most can show positive results in the presence of a wide variety of conditions; most tests can also show negative (normal) results even when a specific illness is known to be present. Never depend on the results of one test. Whenever a test you have taken shows a positive or abnormal test value, be sure to have that test repeated two or three times, preferably at different laboratories or in a different doctor's office.

• "If that's the case, how can I ever trust any medical test? More important, how can I be sure I have all the information necessary to understand a test's results?"

You can never be sure that the result of any single medical test, or even of a single battery of medical tests, is reliable. A test should never be regarded as anything more than a means of confirming other clinical observations; your symptoms, the physical signs you exhibit, your family's medical history, and your doctor's impressions. If a test result corresponds with everything else, fine; if it does not, you must neither forego proper therapy nor undergo potentially dangerous treatments on the basis of the test alone. Once you are aware that most medical tests are not absolutely reliable, you are well on your way to understanding test results as your doctor does. Your doctor also has an obligation to tell you everything you need to know about any test before you undergo it.

• "But what if my doctor won't discuss the details of medical tests with me?"

You have the moral right—and ultimately, the legal right—to be told all medical facts about yourself, including medical test results and their meanings. Most states now have a law or regulation that allows patients to review their medical records and even obtain copies for a fee. Fourteen states actually require doctors and hospitals to give patients copies of records on request; others may require a formal written demand or even a court order. Ohio courts have ruled that patients have a property right to their records, because the records can help determine the course of future treatments. In California, doctors are required to give patients copies of their records, although they may keep the originals from their patients' eyes. Florida law requires physicians, but not hospitals, to show patients their records; in Connecticut, Louisiana, and Massachusetts, hospitals must show patients the information on their charts, but doctors are not required to do so. Oklahoma law permits a patient to see physical health records, but records concerning mental illness may be restricted if a psychiatrist so demands. Anyone who was once a patient in a hospital or other medical facility operated by the United States government may review all original health records or obtain copies of them. If direct requests fail, you can always obtain a subpoena (court order) forcing the doctor or hospital to provide you with your records; these are almost always granted, unless your doctor can prove to the judge that the information would harm you more than it would help. States change their laws concerning access to medical records periodically, so find out what your state's laws provide so that you can use them in your own behalf.

And you can use this book. When you are told that you should have a specific medical test, or several different tests, you can look each test up and find why it is usually performed; what it is supposed to reveal; whether it is performed on your blood, your urine, some other secretion or excretion, or directly on your body; normal and abnormal values and what they might signify; and a reasonable assessment of the test's accuracy. You will also be made aware of any risk factors involved and the degree of pain or discomfort that might be endured by the average person. In several instances, you may be surprised to learn that some of your normal daily activities, some of the foods you eat, and some of the medicines you take could have an adverse effect on the test's results, producing a false value. Your doctor, or whoever performs a test on you, should inquire about anything that might interfere with testing—but this is not always done, and the consequences could be disastrous for you.

It may seem at times that medical tests can result in miracles. To the parents whose newborn baby is tested for phenylketonuria (PKU), found to have the enzyme deficiency, and put on a diet in time to prevent mental retardation, the test is a miracle. And imagine the feelings of a family whose father collapses with what seems to be a heart attack when, within an hour, medical tests prove that he does not suffer from a heart problem at all and that he will recover completely by the next day.

Yet medical tests may also have other, wholly nonmiraculous results. Take the case of one 45-year-old automobile dealer. He had experienced slight chest pains off and on for several years, but his doctor had never been able to make a precise diagnosis; his electrocardiogram results were always normal. Finally, the man was referred to a specialist who performed a vectorcardiogram, a variation on the standard electrocardiogram in which subjective rather than objective interpretation of test results plays an important role. The heart specialist thought he detected evidence of a previous heart attack (also known as a myocardial infarction or coronary thrombosis) and told the patient that he had to move immediately from his two-story home to a one-story home so that he would not have to climb stairs; that he could never physically exert himself again; that he had to abandon his ethnic diet for one abhorrent to his taste and incompatible with his way of life; that he had to give up his job because of the constant emotional involvement it required; and finally, that he had to forego any and all excitement if he wanted simply to stay alive. All this on the basis of one medical test and one doctor's blind belief in that test. The man followed the doctor's recommendations for two miserable years.

Now for the good news. On an impulse, the invalid auto dealer sought out a new doctor. The tests, including the vectorcardiogram, were repeated by a different specialist, and no evidence of any heart disease was found. A third physician was called upon; he confirmed the absence of any disability. The patient was then told that he could return to his former life-style without fear. He has since lived happily for 10 years. With the help of his new doctor, he sued the doctor who had caused him to alter his life-style so severely. In court, the doctor could not offer any tangible proof (other than his subjective interpretation of the vectorcardiogram) that heart muscle pathology was, indeed, present; the patient collected a tidy sum to help compensate for the years of misery he had endured.

Never, under any circumstances, rely upon the good or bad results of a single medical test. Any medical test report that could change your life must be repeated at least twice— and in different settings, such as another laboratory or another doctor's office—before it can be considered a valid part of your medical record. What is more, it is a rare medical test whose results cannot be confirmed, supported, or substantiated by several other, entirely different medical tests. Equally important, should a test seem to indicate the absence of disease whose presence you or your doctor strongly suspects, that test, too, must be duplicated and triplicated by others before its results are accepted.

If you think this warning is superfluous, you should know that when medical laboratories were tested for accuracy in government surveys, more than one out of every seven tests results were found to be either in error or totally unreliable—and that means that the results of at least 4.5 million tests every day are inaccurate. Defective testing reagents (chemicals) cause many of these erroneous test results. The Food and Drug Administration reports weekly that test chemicals found to be out of date, contaminated, or mislabeled have been seized or recalled.

In 1985, the Centers for Disease Control (CDC) of the Public Health Service disclosed that after one commercial medical laboratory reported a great many patients having amebiasis (an intestinal disease caused by a parasite), a recheck of those patients by other laboratories showed that only 5 percent of the so-called positive test patients actually had the disease; the results of 95 percent of those so diagnosed were erroneous.

When a biochemist at the Memorial Sloan-Kettering Cancer Center in New York City wanted to assess the proficiency of commercial medical laboratories, he sent slides of fecal occult blood around the country. He reported that only 50 percent of the laboratories produced correct results; one out of every two would have reported erroneous results to the doctor.

When thousands of sphygmomanometers (blood pressure measuring devices) were evaluated, one out of every two was found to give wrong readings—mostly on the high side. Similar surveys showed that thousands of electrocardiograph machines were improperly calibrated and that numerous X-ray machines, often operated by inadequately trained technicians, produced ineffective or faulty X-ray pictures. Again, do not become overly concerned about an initial test that seems to indicate the presence of a medical problem; have the test verified and keep in mind that the odds are more with you than against you.

In the event a laboratory or other test proves erroneous, you have strong legal recourse, since the courts have held that a mistake in medical testing is negligence on the part of the testing facility or doctor. This applies both to medical tests that falsely indicate the presence of a disease and to tests that fail to recognize signs of an existing or impending affliction.

Your rights in medical testing. When you undergo any medical test, you have the right to expect absolute accuracy. You also have the right to know and understand just what each medical test is supposed to detect; how well it should perform; what extraneous information it might show; what, if any, dangers or possible complications it might involve; and most of all, just what its results mean to you.

First and foremost, whenever you have a medical test—whether it requires the use of some machine such as an X-ray, electrocardiograph, spirometer (a device for measuring lung function) or audiometer (an instrument for evaluating hearing thresholds), or the microscopic or chemical examination of one or more of your secretions, excretions, blood, or other body fluids—you have the right to assume that every phase of the test will be performed correctly by trained people using properly maintained, precisely calibrated equipment. This amounts to an implied warranty offered to you by the doctor who orders the test and who ultimately interprets the results, as well as the testing facility and the manufacturer of any equipment, chemicals, or other products involved in the test. Any error, no matter how slight, is not to be tolerated and should be compensated for, usually by some monetary award.

Just imagine being told you have a high blood sugar, and the subsequent grief that could cause, all because a laboratory technician left the tourniquet on your arm too long just prior to drawing a blood sample; the abnormal concentration of blood in your lower arm would cause almost all evaluations of your blood chemistry to be erroneously high. Or imagine your doctor failing to diagnose diabetes because the laboratory technician left your blood sample standing around for a few hours before analyzing it; as a result, your blood-sugar level would be mistakenly reported as low and your metabolic disease might then progress to dangerous and even irreversible levels.

Almost every clinical laboratory will repeat any medical test, without charge, should you or your doctor feel the test result does not complement your complaints or symptoms or your doctor's suspicions. Although this may help weed out a technical or human error, it is often better to have the test repeated at a totally different facility.

Another of your rights is that you be informed just how precise a test can be, assuming all technical criteria have been met and human error has been eliminated. For even when a test is performed correctly, its results are not necessarily conclusive proof of the existence or nonexistence of a medical problem. Virtually every medical test can be evaluated by three parameters: sensitivity, specificity, and predictive value or relative accuracy.

Sensitivity reflects the ability of a medical test to show a positive (abnormal) result, indicating the presence of the disease being searched for when that disease actually exists in the individual being tested—or in other words, how often the test is right. A test with 100 percent sensitivity is never wrong—but there are very few of these. As a test's sensitivity rating decreases, the lowered percentage figure denotes how often it will fail to show its expected positive, or abnormal, result even though the disease being tested for exists in the person being tested. For example, a test with an 80 percent sensitivity rating will fail to diagnose its disease in 20 out of every 100 cases. The vast majority of medical tests do not always reveal the presence of the disease they are intended to detect. One example, mentioned briefly in the Preface, is the stress electrocardiogram, which is administered while the patient walks or runs on a treadmill, climbs a few steps, or exercises vigorously. The test is designed to show potential heart damage as well as to reveal previously undetected minimal heart damage; patients with the latter condition are considered more susceptible to future heart attacks. Experience has shown, however, that a stress electrocardiogram fails to show potential abnormalities or identify existing heart disease in more than half of all patients who undergo the test.

The second basic determinant of a test's accuracy is called *specificity*. This percentage figure reflects the test's ability to show a negative (normal) result when the disease being tested for does not exist in the individual being tested. The lower the percentage rating of a test's specificity, the greater the chance the test will wrongly show the presence of a disease when that disease does not exist. A test with an 80 percent specificity will give a false-positive result in 20 out of every 100 cases, erroneously implying a healthy individual is suffering from a disease that really does not exist. A test with 100 percent specificity would never give a false-positive result—but there are none of these. When the values of both sensitivity and specificity are combined, they give a reasonable indication of a test's accuracy. A test with a 50 percent accuracy rating will be wrong—and give a false result—once for every two times it is performed. Again, the stress electrocardiogram provides a good example; of the people who have taken this test, more than half of those with no known heart disease have gotten results that falsely indicated existing pathology.

As with all medical tests, even sensitivity and specificity are relative. They may vary with the quality controls in different laboratories as well as with the doctor's or laboratory's criteria for normal values.

The third parameter for measuring a test's precision is *predictive value*, or relative accuracy. Predictive value is determined by a mathematical formula that weighs the ratio of true positives (how often the test is right) against false positives (how often the test is wrong) and arrives at an overall figure that indicates the probability of the existence of a disease should a medical test show a positive result for that disease.

Before you submit to any medical test, your doctor should make you aware of the sensitivity, specificity, and predictive value of that test.

Obviously, there is much more to sensitivity, specificity, and predictive value. For instance, these parameters may be affected by the prevalence of the particular disease for which a patient is being tested. When a disease is very prevalent, a great many people may show a positive test result without having any symptoms; in contrast, when a disease is rare, a positive test may have much greater significance. Your doctor should take such factors into account when explaining a test's value in your particular case. He might also simply summarize sensitivity, specificity, and predictive value by describing the test's *marginal benefit* to you; that is, just how much more knowledge about you and the suspected diagnosis will the doctor have after the test is performed?

While accuracy, based on sensitivity and specificity, is the primary factor to be considered when assessing the true value of a medical test, a secondary, quite different factor called *significance* is almost as important—especially when comparing a test's worth to its cost. A test's significance indicates how precise it is for a particular disease; a test with little significance can be 95 percent accurate technically but also be positive in 95 different diseases. A highly significant test will show a positive or abnormal result in only a very few different—and not necessarily related—diseases. The most significant test will be positive in only one condition, the particular one being tested for—but there are few, if any, of these. Unfortunately, most medical tests can show a positive (abnormal) result in the presence of many diseases—and they can even give false-positive results as a consequence of physical activity or even the body's position (sitting vs. standing), to mention just a few variables.

The variation in the accuracy and significance of medical tests can be shown by comparing the stress electrocardiogram test to one of the newer tests for diagnosing syphilis. Because the stress electrocardiogram fails to detect heart problems in a great many patients (poor sensitivity) and falsely indicates heart problems in many other people (poor specificity), it is considered to have a very low predictive value, or a relatively low accuracy rating. In contrast, most of today's direct tests for syphilis have a predictive value close to 100 percent; that is, they almost always show a positive result for someone who has the disease (excellent sensitivity) and rarely show a positive result for someone who does not have the disease (excellent specificity). Of incidental interest, many of the older, now out-of-date tests for syphilis, while detecting most cases of the disease (good sensitivity), also showed a positive result for people who had cold sores, jaundice, infectious mononucleosis, bronchitis, pneumonia, childhood diseases (mumps, measles, chicken pox), and some forms of arthritis, and even for women experiencing a normal pregnancy (very poor specificity). Consequently, the older tests—such as the Wassermann, Kline, Kahn, and VDRL—had a low accuracy rating and were of very low significance. In fact, most of the usual blood tests can show a positive (abnormal) result—indicating from dozens to hundreds of different diseases—in essentially healthy people. The typical enzyme evaluations that are part of most routine blood tests can show a false-positive, or abnormal, result in a healthy person for days, simply because the person did nothing more than exercise moderately.

Because so many medical tests are not very significant—and rarely point to any one specific disease—they can cause a great deal of anxiety and even physical problems if their results are accepted at face value or uncritically. If both doctor and patient are unaware of the significance of the medical test being performed, two extremely dangerous outcomes can occur. First, there are all the catastrophic consequences of undergoing more and more tests while trying to find some explanation for the initial false-positive test result. Second, treatment—even surgery—could be implemented for a condition that does not really exist; the latter could be considered the ultimate danger of medical testing.

One particular hazard—quite unique to medical testing—while published in a major medical journal, has not been brought to the public's attention. As a preface to this peril, it seems necessary to mention *iatrogenic disease*. You may have heard the term; it means that the real cause of the patient's illness or suffering came directly from the doctor's actions or words—not from a germ, improper living, or genetic defect. More often than not, such an illness is secondary to the doctor's therapy, whether the treatment be a wrong drug, unnecessary surgery, or even improper counsel. But how many people have heard of "Ulysses syndrome"? This appellation was devised by Dr. Mercer Rang of Canada and should be considered a most formidable warning to all patients. Remember the Greek warrior Ulysses? He spent nearly a dozen years searching for trouble, and with each new, unexpected adventure, he also endured greater and greater hazards. When a doctor goes searching for some—any—sort of disease through literally endless medical testing, a patient is very apt to suffer from "Ulysses syndrome"; in this instance, all the physical, mental, and even monetary hazards so disastrously associated with a doctor's "adventurous" medical investigation. Being a victim of "Ulysses syndrome" leaves the patient even more exposed to iatrogenic disease later on when some superfluous or erroneous treatment is applied as a result of all the gratuitous testing.

Every necessary medical test puts you in some degree of jeopardy; every unnecessary medical test—while your doctor plays Ulysses—puts you in that much more needless jeopardy. And your vulnerability is not limited to side effects, accidents, and injuries; it has been shown that for every seven tests you have, you are assured of at least one false-positive result, with all the subsequent calamities that can come from that fictitious verdict.

And it has been said, by physicians considered by their peers to be the best in the country, that someone who has a false-positive medical test—indicating illness when none exists—suffers the greatest harm of all: all the risks and expense of a patient who really has the disease along with the possibility of being killed by the treatment for a nonexistent disease.

Bearing all this in mind, do not be surprised if your doctor insists that you undergo a not-too-accurate stress electrocardiogram test. He probably has spent anywhere from $5,000 to $25,000 for his stress electrocardiogram equipment (treadmill, monitoring machines, and related instruments), and at anywhere from a $100 to $500 charge for each stress test, he must do at least one test a week for a year in order to recoup his initial investment and allow the gadget to start making its expected profit.

Before you submit to any medical test, your doctor should make you aware of the commonly accepted accuracy and significance of that test as well as his own interpretation of the test's true value. Only when you know how accurate a test is, as well as your chances of coming up with a false result, can you judge the relative worth of that test for you—and your money.

Why many medical tests are performed. Medical tests are sometimes ordered for reasons over which you have little or no control. On occasion, a test may be demanded by a school, by an employer, by some governmental agency (such as the military or health department), or by a hospital, whose "routine" admission requirements often wastefully duplicate previous tests, primarily for profit. Most often, however, such tests are for the protection and benefit of the community, health facility, or business and not primarily for your personal welfare. As but one example of the success of a legally mandated test program, the state of California has detected 412 cases of hypothyroidism, 74 cases of phenylketonuria, and 19 cases of galactosemia since it began required newborn screening.

A great many tests are, in reality, nothing more than "fishing" expeditions. True, often a patient has so many vague complaints that a doctor will order a battery of tests, hoping that at least one will lead to a more circumscribed diagnosis. Younger doctors are trained to practice medicine in this manner, substituting the findings of medical tests for the observations of experience. It used to be that doctors questioned and examined their patients far more carefully and applied testing to confirm their suspicions; today, the tests usually come first and it is the test results, more than the patient's complaints, that guide the doctor's ultimate application of therapy.

Another vivid illustration of why medical tests are performed came from a 1984 study of the number of tests ordered by British vs. American doctors on patients who had an identical illness—high blood pressure. The United States physicians—in this case from Boston, Massachusetts—performed up to 40 times as many tests, during a two-week period, as did their London colleagues. The most commonly exploited test was the electrocardiogram; American doctors performed this test several times on each patient, despite the fact no contributory data were obtained. Eight times as many

X-rays were taken by the American doctors, and most of these were of parts of the body essentially unrelated to high blood pressure, such as of the gallbladder and barium enemas; not one of these was ordered by a British doctor. The major reason for the difference in the number of tests turned out to be the fee-for-service system in America, where doctors here are paid extra for each and every procedure; British doctors receive no reimbursement for ordering, or performing, medical tests. Of particular interest, no difference was detected in the quality of care provided by either group. The study's other conclusion was: American patients seem to prefer testing, regardless of its need or effect. An American doctor, quoted in *The New Yorker* magazine, confirmed that observation when he said: "Patients, for their part, never protest charges for tests. The public seems to value tests and procedures to an extent not justified by their relative scientific value."*

A good example of the blind love for tests can be found in health fairs. People seem to flock to such opportunities to undergo multiple screening tests—especially when such tests are offered without the need to visit a doctor's office. In 1985, more than 2 million supposedly "well" individuals visited nearly 1,000 health fairs and underwent more than 20 million tests. What they really received has been published in medical journals. Two out of every 5 had at least one false-abnormal test result. The consequence was more than simply a great deal of money wasted on follow-up testing to confirm or refute the false-positive test value; there was significant evidence of physical and mental harm associated with subsequent, albeit unnecessary, test procedures. When you volunteer to undergo medical tests, such as at health fairs, you are not required to be informed of any related risks as you would be in your doctor's office. No medical test is without risk, be it some devastating side effect such as an allergic reaction, an infection, or excruciating anxiety wondering just how long you have left to live based on a false-test death sentence. The least dangerous side effect is the useless expense of disproving a wrong test result. When medical tests are performed for this reason—nothing more than your desire to have them—you have only yourself to blame. Out of all this potential agony, a condition previously unknown to the person was discovered in just over 1 percent of all those tested, and not even all of those findings turned out to be of benefit to the individual.

Defensive medicine. At this point, it is important to bring up the matter of "defensive medicine." The term *defensive medicine* describes how doctors perform all sorts of totally uncalled-for, dubious, and dangerous tests, ostensibly to protect themselves against the possibility of losing a malpractice lawsuit should a patient take them to court for alleged negligence at some future date. In 1977, the American Medical Association surveyed doctors and revealed that at least 75 percent of them admitted they regularly practiced defensive medicine (an AMA official has since said that he feels a more reliable figure for that time, based on subsequent studies, would be only 70 percent). The most recent survey, in 1985, showed that 42 percent of those doctors *increased* the amount of defensive medicine they practiced and an additional number of doctors adopted defensive medicine for the first time. It now seems fair to say that over 80 percent of all doctors order far more medical tests than can be medically

*July 23, 1984.

justified; one doctor in the survey added the comment: "I am no longer willing to take *any* chances based on my considered professional judgement." The former president of the Los Angeles County Medical Association goes so far as to say that this superfluous testing unnecessarily raises the cost of medical care by at least $20 billion a year. Doctors, of course, blame lawyers, and our litigious society, for this incongruous situation. And doctors go on to say that they are afraid to appear in front of a jury without records that show they performed every conceivable test that might be brought up by a lawyer as possibly—just possibly—being relevant, no matter how remotely, to the patient's complaint. Unfortunately, it has been shown that lawyers can easily convince a jury that a doctor who failed to perform some esoteric test—even if medically unjustified—is guilty of negligence and should be punished. But if everyone would begin to question the accuracy and significance of all medical tests and the true value of each test in question were made known to jury members, lawyers would no longer be able to impress those juries with not-too-accurate, insignificant, and even irrelevant tests. As a most serendipitous consequence, doctors could not feel they have to order redundant, risky tests solely on a lawyer's behalf rather than a patient's. Think of the savings in life, limb, and money that would bring.

A physician practicing in the state of Washington examined a patient who had stomach problems. As part of his medical testing, he performed a chest X-ray, a standard electrocardiograph, and even some of the enzyme tests. The same tests were repeated two weeks later, and although the enzyme tests were slightly abnormal, the patient had no complaints relative to his heart. Eight years later, after the patient had died of heart disease, the patient's wife sued the doctor for not having given her husband a stress electrocardiogram. The court found the doctor guilty of not having performed the additional diagnostic test and said it was his duty to disclose to the patient every test available to help diagnose all theoretically possible non-life-threatening causes of stomach pain. Thus, the doctor was found guilty of malpractice for not performing a medical test with an accuracy rating of less than 50 percent.

Because of defensive medicine, a patient with a common cold has a 90 percent chance of having his blood tested for 20 or more different substances. A study in New York state showed that a patient complaining of a sprained ankle will have *both* ankles, legs, and feet X-rayed (primarily to show any difference between the two ankles, legs, or feet) along with nearly a dozen chemical tests that could indicate bone pathology, a bone metabolism defect (such as gout), rheumatic disease, anemia, and even chronic alcoholism. This is true even in cases where the doctor is 99 percent sure it is nothing more than a sprain. More than any other reason, including the increased ability to diagnose disease, the existing legal process is responsible for the growth of medical testing.

On being a participatory patient. One way you can participate in test evaluation is to ask your doctor what the reason is for the test.

By fully understanding the need for a test and its purpose and knowing your past medical history and, especially, that of your family, you may come up with the answer to some obscure medical problem. You could even avoid a great deal of supplementary, possibly painful, and irrelevant testing. For instance, if diabetes runs in your family, there is a better-than-average chance the condition will afflict you; consequently, you should inform your doctor of such a potentially inherited trait so that he can first concentrate on the obvious rather than spread his testing far and wide for the cause of your symptoms. Since many forms of anemia, heart and kidney problems, eye and ear difficulties, and even skin disorders are genetic in origin, information on your family's illnesses could be particularly relevant to your medical problem.

Another reason for you to know why your doctor is ordering one or more tests for you is to prevent duplication of testing. It is not unusual for one doctor to follow the same line of reasoning as another doctor, based on your complaints, and repeat tests that you have already had. Your symptoms, for example, may make a doctor think the problem is related to your kidneys; if you tell your doctor you have had kidney tests repeatedly without any abnormal findings, you might avoid possible complications resulting from needless testing. Unless your doctor can justify repeating tests that were done in the past, you should not subject yourself to such a waste of time and money and an unnecessary hazard.

The obvious concern arises, "But what if my doctor won't tell me why he is ordering a test and what if he says that I wouldn't understand the results anyway?"

Nonsense! It is not difficult for a patient to understand that a doctor is looking for some sort of problem—a thyroid condition, for example—and that the tests ordered are to determine the specific nature of the problem. (Of course, if you feel cold when others around you are warm, or if you always seem to be hot in a cool environment, you are already more than halfway to your diagnosis.) Furthermore, how complicated can a thyroid problem be? To be sure, there are always a very few people who have some rare and exotic type of illness, but the vast majority of thyroid gland dysfunctions are common, easily diagnosed, and even more easily treated.

Again, assuming you learn that your doctor is searching for a suspected thyroid condition, you should find out just what other information the tests might, rightly or wrongly, reveal. It is all too common for a particular test to hint at another, totally different condition that may or may not exist. Unfortunately, thousands of people are treated needlessly for essentially fictitious diseases simply on the basis of some random test finding totally unrelated to the original search. It is even sadder that much of this seeming misfeasance is due more to the patient's ignorance of or lack of interest in his condition than to incompetence or greed on the part of the doctor. By becoming a participatory patient, you will assure yourself of the best possible care.

"That's fine," you say, "but what if my doctor still won't tell me anything?" You have a legal right to know what your doctor has decided about your condition and how he came to his decisions. Do not be put off by the idea that the jargon is similar to a foreign language or that the terms will be too difficult to understand. In almost all instances, the information a doctor writes in a patient's chart is in plain English, and a medical dictionary can be consulted for any terms that are not explained. The information is about your physical well-being and may have a direct bearing on your life. You must make the decision to use it in your best interests.

When your doctor orders you to undergo any medical tests, one of the best examples of patient participation is to ask: "What will you do if the test value is abnormal? What will you do if the test value is normal?" If the doctor gives the same answer to both questions, you should then ask, "Why do the test?"

Risks vs. benefits. Every medical tests carries some degree of risk that must always be weighed against the expected benefits. Your doctor is legally required to warn you about all possible risks before you undergo any test. Only then can you make an informed decision about whether the possible information to be derived from the test is worth the possible dangers that might accompany the procedure. The doctrine of "informed consent" protects you from being forced to make a decision without first being offered all relevant information in plain English.

Unfortunately, the law also assumes that your submission to a medical test—especially the simpler ones, such as blood examination—implies your consent. In many courts, the very fact that you willingly let your blood be taken, or exposed your body to an electrocardiogram or X-ray, or allowed your doctor or a technician to look inside of you with some sort of observation device has been considered sufficient evidence that you had the opportunity to question your doctor or the technician about all prospective dangers and either did so or deliberately avoided doing so. In such cases, it can be very difficult to prove that potential risk factors were purposely hidden from you. Therefore, never assume a medical test is relatively harmless until you feel you have had that test procedure explained to your satisfaction.

Invasive vs. noninvasive tests. When considering risk factors, a distinction must be made between invasive and noninvasive tests. Any test that involves penetration of the body is, literally, an invasive test. An invasive test normally poses a much greater risk than a test that does not penetrate the skin or an orifice of the body. The use of a plethysmograph to detect thrombosis of the leg is noninvasive; the injection of dyes or nuclear radioactive substances into the leg is not only invasive but carries a greater degree of risk without always offering a greater significance for diagnosis. While some doctors feel that the simple sticking of a needle into the arm to draw blood should not be considered invasive, in truth it is, as is the insertion of a sigmoidoscope, a bronchoscope, or a catheter; even ultrasound and X-rays "invade" the body with their invisible forms of energy. Recent research has revealed that the use of an invasive test itself is sufficient to produce a false-abnormal test result where no abnormality exists and where an equally productive noninvasive test would show a normal result. Whenever an invasive procedure is ordered, ask if there is a noninvasive test that would be just as efficient.

Consequences and alternatives. Of course, there is another aspect to the risk factor of testing: knowing and understanding just what the consequences may be both in having the test and, equally important, in *not* having the test. Forgoing a proposed medical test might be much more dangerous than any possible risk associated with the test. If you are told to have a Pap test to look for early signs of cancer and you hesitate, you may hesitate for too long and your cancer, assuming it exists, may grow to an incurable stage. For years, a woman refused her doctor's advice to have a Pap test. When she died of cancer, her family sued the doctor, claiming the physician had failed to impress her sufficiently about the dangers of not having the test. A doctor is required to disclose all information relevant to a meaningful decision by the patient, generally including the nature of the proposed medical test or procedure, its purpose, the risks involved, *and* the alternatives to it. Only in this way can the patient's decision not to have the test be considered an "informed refusal."

Alternatives may include different but related tests. The use of an echocardiogram in place of angiography is a good example. An echocardiogram entails no invasion of the body (no needles, no catheter, no dyes, no radioactive chemicals) and, consequently, no pain or discomfort. Angiography, however, is a prolonged, painful procedure that poses dangers. Many cardiologists feel that an echocardiogram can provide sufficient data for a diagnosis in the vast majority of cases where the two tests could be used.

And there are a great many alternatives to various radiographic tests that are potentially far less harmful. Computerized tomography (CT or CAT scanning) is a painless, noninvasive technique that provides a more efficient means for studying the brain than pneumoencephalography, an X-ray test in which air is injected through the spinal cord into the brain. CAT scanning may also eliminate the need for a myelogram, a potentially dangerous procedure in which dye is injected into the spinal canal to study the vertebrae and their spacing; if some of the dye remains in the canal, leg paralysis can result. Plethysmography, the application of a blood pressure cuff around the leg attached to recording instruments, can often reveal a thrombosis (blood clot) as efficiently and with far less risk than the injection of a dye into the supposedly clogged vein to make it stand out on an X-ray (the dye itself can cause thrombosis). Magnetic resonance imaging, unlike machines that use X-rays, emits no dangerous ionizing radiation and can, in many instances, offer the same —and sometimes better—information.

In attempting to detect developing physical defects, as opposed to inherited metabolic disorders, the use of a sonogram (a picture produced by sound waves) may offer as much information about a fetus as an amniocentesis test, which has inherent dangers for both mother and child. Ultrasound, while a form of an invasive test, is, at the present time, considered relatively less dangerous than X-rays or the insertion of a needle or other medical device. Chorionic villi sampling is said to offer as much information as amniocentesis, at a much earlier time after pregnancy has begun, and at less risk to the mother and child. Ultrasound testing can replace many other potentially harmful tests used for diagnosing liver, gallbladder, kidney, and other gland problems. It can also differentiate cysts, clots, abscesses, and other masses from solid growths, thereby eliminating the need for a great deal of unnecessary exploratory surgery. In addition, many new tests utilizing radioimmunoassay techniques (which examine blood samples for minute chemical imbalances) can be substituted for some risky and uncomfortable poking and digging around in your body in the search for cancers.

But unless you are made aware of the alternatives, you cannot make an informed decision about whether or not to undergo a test or battery of tests. While one doctor may well prefer and even insist on a more hazardous test approach, you are entitled to know the reasons for his choice and just why he considers the alternatives inappropriate.

Your final, ultimate right in medical testing is to be made aware of any existing test that might make a difference in your way of life. After a 38-year-old woman gave birth to a child with a congenital defect, she sued her doctor for not informing her that there was a practical test (amniocentesis) that could have warned of the possibility of a birth defect. The court not only awarded the woman a cash settlement but forced the doctor to pay the cost of her daughter's medical care for life. In another, somewhat similar case, a woman who was not tested for rubella (German measles) when she became pregnant gave birth to a defective child; she sued her doctor, who was then required to make financial restitution for not informing the woman that the rubella test existed and should be performed on all pregnant women.

While knowledge of existing medical tests is not the primary responsibility of the patient, you should be made aware of all available tests relevant to any medical problem or condition you may have.

Should any test, whether performed as a screening panel or as an individual test in the privacy of your doctor's office, indicate a reportable disease, your doctor *must* notify the proper government authorities. In addition to infectious illnesses such as AIDS, tuberculosis, typhoid, and sexually transmitted diseases (venereal diseases), diabetes, epilepsy, heart ailments, senility, alcoholism, and any other affliction that could affect your ability to drive a car must also be reported.

Costs. The vast majority of patients do not pay for medical testing directly but have it paid for through health insurance plans. Although most people do not care about the cost of testing, they are wrong in assuming that someone else is paying for it. Employers' payments for workers' health care are reflected in the cost of merchandise; so, indirectly, you are still paying for the increasing cost of medical tests. As noted in the Preface, the cost of medical testing, when all direct and indirect charges are included, came to nearly $225 billion in 1985, out of $450 billion expended for all health care. Although there are no absolute figures for the cost of specific medical testing, studies that report on the numbers and kinds of tests performed annually indicate that the cost of laboratory testing alone came to $55 billion; X-rays and other radiological test techniques amounted to $35 billion, $2 billion of which went for coronary angiography alone; electrocardiography, endoscopy, biopsy, eye, ear, and other instrumental tests added up to $65 billion; and the additional required expense of hospitalization or office visits solely for testing purposes was $70 billion. While hospital bills seem to be the greatest single health cost item, medical testing accounts for the largest portion of a hospital bill—even larger than the separate costs for a patient's room, nursing care, use of operating rooms, and maintenance. At the same time, medical tests provide the greatest source of income for hospitals, which is why many hospitals demand that every patient undergo a battery of tests upon admission—even though they may have been performed the day before in a doctor's office or a laboratory.

Duplication of tests that have recently been performed, and the results confirmed, generally has more financial than patient value. One departure from the practice of repetitive hospital testing has come about as a consequence of DRGs (diagnostic related groups, used as a basis for payment from the government for Medicare patients, where the hospital receives a scheduled lump sum depending solely on the patient's diagnosis, no matter how long the patient stays in the hospital or what tests and procedures are provided). In this unique situation, the hospitals request the doctors to perform all the tests in their offices, prior to admission to the hospital, since specific reimbursement for testing is paid only to the doctors.

But the cost, duplication, and application of medical tests are not half as surprising as some other observations made by researchers who attempted to assess the value of medical tests. One study showed that in spite of the expense of medical testing, only 5 percent of all laboratory tests actually resulted in altered patient care or had any impact on a patient's diagnosis or treatment. And there have been several studies revealing that a great many doctors never even look at the reported results of medical tests after they have been recorded on their patients' hospital chart. One recent medical article, from the Cleveland Clinic, described how out of 2,912 patients admitted to the hospital, 75 had a positive test result for syphilis. But 43 of those patients were never evaluated for the disease; the doctors simply ignored the reported test results.

In a 1985 evaluation of 2,000 patients who received an extensive battery of "routine" medical tests prior to undergoing surgery, it was revealed that more than 60 percent of those tests could not be justified medically. And out of every 1,000 tests performed (well over 20,000 total), only 2 offered some information that could affect the need for, or outcome from, the operation; yet the majority of those extremely rare positive findings were completely ignored by all the professionals involved.

Testing for profit. Although medical tests have always been a steady source of income for doctors, what has been called the "new entrepreneurial fever" is now in vogue. That is where doctors have financial interests in laboratories, X-ray facilities, and other commercial ventures where the profit comes primarily from testing. Although doctors are ethically—and even legally in some states—required to inform their patients of any financial interest they may have in any resource they refer their patients to, this code is not always followed. Although this inherent conflict of interest can cost the patient (or the third-party payer of the bills) a great deal of money that may not be medically justified, even the American Medical Association draws certain illogical distinctions, thereby permitting this essentially unethical practice. The practice of medicine for profit—regardless of how much—does more to abuse and exploit patients than make them well.

Ethics aside, doctors are constantly being reminded of the profit to be made from medical testing by salesmen at medical meetings and by articles in medical journals. An advertisement for an electrocardiograph machine in a major scientific publication was headlined: "Buy the EK-8 now and receive enough ECG supplies to reward you with $3,000 potential income." The ad went on to say that if a doctor purchased the machine, the company would then furnish, free, enough supplies to produce 150 electrocardiograms, which, at a minimum fee of $20 per ECG, would cover the entire cost of the machine. A doctor performing no more than 5 electrocardiograms a day would have his money back in 30 days and well over $20,000 profit before the year was over. (Most physicians and hospitals charge far more than $20 for an electrocardiogram; in 1985, the average fee throughout the country was $40.)

Lest you think that doctors must invest a great deal of time and money learning how to read and interpret electrocardiograms, there are many services that read ECGs for doctors and charge from $1 to $2 per reading, depending on the volume of business. Some even transmit the ECG and its analysis over the telephone while it is being performed, and certain new machines have built-in computers that give the doctor the interpretation as the ECG is recorded.

It has become extremely profitable for a physician to perform most blood and urine tests in his own office. Machines that perform dozens of routine examinations, at a minimum cost to the patient of $5 per test, are now available to doctors for less than $1,000. A doctor who performs tests in his office can charge a health insurance plan or governmental health program or agency several hundred dollars for the same number of tests a clinical laboratory, using automated equipment, will perform for a fraction of the cost. He can also perform 10 different urine tests by simply dipping a 25-cent strip of chemically coated plastic into his patient's urine specimen and charge up to $50 for those tests. In actuality, when a doctor performs a laboratory test in his office, the cost to him rarely exceeds $1 for each test. One company advertises a machine that will perform 12 different tests at a cost to the doctor of only 84 cents for all 12.

There are commercial clinical laboratories that charge doctors $6.95 to carry out up to 27 different chemical analyses of a patient's blood; some will even perform 42 tests for $16. Incidentally, the quality of work performed by a laboratory in a doctor's office is not always under direct supervision, evaluation, inspection, or control by governmental or professional agencies, as is the case with most commercial laboratories, which must demonstrate their competence regularly.

An article in a medical journal described how any physician could easily triple his income by performing most medical tests in his office. It was estimated that such testing would add at least $60,000 in net income to a doctor's earnings annually.

Thus, medical testing has far more of an economic than scientific impact on a patient's care. At the same time, doctors admit that the present fee system for medical care far better rewards physicians who rely on medical tests and testing apparatus than those who use cognitive skills—a doctor's reasoning and judgment based on training and experience. As one doctor put it: "Why not gastroscope [perform an examination of the walls of the esophagus, the stomach, and at times, the first part of the small intestine] every patient at five hundred dollars for fifteen minutes' work, when an hour's time devoted to listening to and examining a patient will only bring in eighty-five dollars at best?" Backing up this philosophy, a study by the Congressional Office of Technology Assessment, called "The Cost-Effectiveness of Upper Gastrointestinal Endoscopy," concluded: "Current financial incentives undoubtedly encourage physicians to perform many more endoscopies than are clinically justified at this time. Steps should be taken to discourage the unnecessary use of this procedure and to lessen the financial incentive by lowering reimbursement to doctors who perform such tests."

The same doctor, quoted earlier from *The New Yorker* magazine concerning patients' blind love for tests, also said: "The money in medicine these days is in tests and procedures, and this leads to a conflict in interests—to tests that are not necessary." It is easy to see why X-rays and other tests that require expensive instruments or machines are much more in vogue than in necessary service.

Of course, there is the other side of the coin. As one internist put it: "Try and limit a patient's testing to one or two evaluations; he'll got right out and find another doctor who will perform an endless barrage of tests. It seems as if you can never test a patient enough—and relevance is never considered by either party."

While health insurance plans and government-sponsored medical care programs actually reward doctors in proportion to their use of medical tests, and while fear of malpractice has forced an increase in testing, the patient's faith in medical tests is an equally important factor in their increasing use. Patients mistakenly believe that having as many tests as possible ensures better medical care.

In most instances, if you are a member of a health insurance plan and your doctor is also part of that plan, the total cost of medical testing is paid to the doctor, with no extra charge to you. If, however, your doctor is not a member of your insurance plan and has not agreed to accept the insurance fee as total payment, you may have to make up the difference. Depending on the number of tests performed, this could amount to hundreds of dollars. Before you undergo a test, check with your doctor to see if there will be any additional costs to you.

Where tests are performed. Most medical tests are performed in a doctor's office, at a commercial laboratory or in a hospital. A sample for a blood test can be obtained anywhere—even at home—and then analyzed at any one of the three usual places. Almost all tests that involve X-rays, including those that use dyes or radionuclear substances as well as computerized tomography, can be performed in a doctor's office, although the latter is most often carried out in a radiologist's office or a hospital. Heart function examinations, including exercise testing, usually take place in a physician's office. A few tests, such as cardiac catheterization as part of angiography, and some endoscopy procedures, are more likely to be performed in a hospital setting; doctors prefer to have a patient check into the hospital the night before a test so as to control his activities and environment prior to testing. Some physicians like to keep their patients in the hospital an extra day after certain complicated or extensive examinations, such as angiography, or dilatation and curettage. Where a test is done may depend as much on who the referring doctor feels is the best qualified to perform the test and interpret the results as where the equipment is located. There are no hard and fast rules about where a test should be performed; the doctor's convenience, not the patient's, may well be the deciding factor.

With the recent advent of inexpensive office testing equipment, more and more tests are being performed in doctors' offices, as much for the income they produce— perhaps more—as for the alleged patient convenience. But keep in a mind, a 1984 study published in a leading medical magazine concluded that laboratory tests conducted in physicians' offices were far less accurate than those performed in licensed commercial laboratories.

Patient-related causes of inaccurate test results. The more tests that you undergo, the greater the possibility that some false hint of a nonexistent disease process will arise. While test results may make it appear that you have incipient diabetes, heart or kidney trouble, a hormone deficiency, a hidden infection, or even cancer, the cause may well be something you ate, drank, or did the night or day before. Although you really have no control over the ineffective chemicals, inefficient machines, and other sources of error in a laboratory, you can reduce the possibility of a faulty test result caused by your own activities.

Here is a list of things that can affect the results of medical tests.

Medications. Aspirin, laxatives, cold pills, cough preparations, sleeping aids, vitamins, nose drops, pain relievers, and especially, stomach antacids can markedly alter a test value. Prescription drugs have an even greater influence on medical testing. In 1972, the American Association of Clinical Chemists published a list of over 9,000 different adverse effects on laboratory tests caused by drugs alone, and the list has been growing ever since.

Birth control pills (oral contraceptives), which many women do not regard as a medicine, can greatly alter the value of more than 60 medical tests, including 15 of those most frequently performed. Alcohol, too, can affect test values; a very small amount will distort blood pressure testing, lipid tests (such as for cholesterol and triglycerides), the prothrombin time test, and any form of diabetes testing (glucose, insulin, etc.).

Before you undergo any test, inform your doctor and/or laboratory performing the test about every medication you are taking; the doctor can then decide whether to have the medication discontinued prior to the test or taken into account when the test results are evaluated.

Diet. A great many food substances can alter test results. For example, iodine from table salt, fish, hot dogs, or other foods can totally disrupt the outcome of certain thyroid function tests. Foods containing large amounts of vitamin K (green leafy vegetables or fish) may cause abnormal values in prothrombin time tests; some of the chemicals in commercial French-fried potatoes will adversely affect prothrombin time for a week. Drinking milk before a calcium or phosphorus test will lead to inaccurate results. Coffee can cause a false-positive uric acid test. Even water can affect test results; there are times when water should be avoided prior to testing, just as there are times when a specified amount must be consumed. Consumption of bone meal tablets as a food supplement can cause cancerlike abnormalities on X-rays.

Routine activities. A patient's daily routine, including his sleeping habits, can have a direct effect on certain tests, especially hormone evaluations. If a patient works all night and sleeps during the day, the physician should be informed of this. Physical activity or lack of it can influence the results of a great many tests. Many routine blood tests will have different results depending on whether a patient has been lying down or standing up just before blood is taken. Excessive exercise, including running, can produce what seem to be abnormal values even though there is no disease process.

Work-related factors, such as indirect contact with certain chemicals on the job, can alter many test results. The amount of noise in a work location and even the lighting conditions can change the body's hormone production, which, in turn, can distort certain test results.

Attitude. If a patient experiences stress or anxiety a few days before a test or at the time the test is performed, the altered mental attitude can produce an abnormal test value. A patient who is kept waiting a long time for a test appointment may have a false-abnormal result, especially if waiting causes him to miss another important appointment. The test values for a blood sample from a male patient can be altered by the fact that the sample was taken by an attractive female technician.

Physical factors. Sex, age, height, weight, and body surface area must be taken into account when interpreting the results of a medical test. It is perfectly normal for a woman to have a sedimentation rate twice as high as that of a man. Most pulmonary function tests and some hormone tests are dependent on size and physical build. Test results may even vary because of changes in the weather. Some families have genetic traits that produce abnormal test values even though no true disease condition is present. More than 100 million people have an inherited glucose-6 phosphate dehydrogenase enzyme deficiency (rare in central European Caucasians), which causes a hemolytic type of anemia (destruction of red blood cells) in reaction to certain drugs and false-abnormal test values in testing for certain other types of anemia.

More recently, particular attention has been given to the changes in test results as a consequence of normal aging. What would indicate a disease in a person under 50 years of age could be quite normal for someone over 65. In some instances, an elevated laboratory test value is quite normal in elderly persons; in other cases, a lower test result is just as normal. For example, alkaline phosphatase values usually increase with age, while blood calcium levels decrease. Some hormone levels decrease after the age of 40 (testosterone in men), while others may increase after the age of 50 (gonadotropin in women). The point is that normal values for young people may not be appropriate for the healthy elderly, and if this factor is not taken into consideration, treatment—even surgery—that is totally uncalled for could be undertaken in older persons.

If the test you want to know about is not in the book . . . The medical tests listed in this book are those in regular, if not always frequent, use. Some tests are utilized only by specialists; other tests are almost routine with a visit to the doctor. Although new medical tests are introduced to doctors every day, most of these are experimental and will never gain professional acceptance. Such tests, often without any proven scientific value, are most frequently performed in hospital settings where research and teaching predominate. Other tests may become outmoded, either because newer, more specific, easier, less complicated, or less expensive substitutes come along, or simply because the tests never really proved their worth in spite of their common use.

But most old, outmoded tests do not die; they rarely—regardless of their cost or value—even fade away. While a majority of doctors now consider the basal metabolic rate (BMR) test to be one of the least accurate means of measuring thyroid function, it is still used relatively frequently. This may be because many antiquated but profitable BMR measuring machines are still around, or because some doctors feel more comfortable employing this once-standard test as a confirmation of nuclear age techniques. Should your doctor order this test for you, the chances are quite slim that your health insurance company will pay for it. Nor will most insurance companies reimburse you or your doctor for a cephalin flocculation test to help diagnose liver disease; yet many laboratories still receive requests for, and perform, this particular test.

As a matter of fact, over the past 12 years, a great many different tests have been declared outmoded or obsolete—some because they are now considered unreliable, some because they have been shown to be worthless. Certain health insurance programs, while at times allowing reimbursement for an obsolete test, may insist that the doctor justify the need for the test prior to its being performed. And some insurers no longer pay for tests when performed in the hospital. In spite of these efforts at cost saving, there are a great many doctors who still order outmoded tests (requiring the patient to pay for them out of pocket) solely to protect themselves from a possible malpractice suit. What provokes this essentially useless—to the patient—testing is a statement from the American Bar Association's Commission on Professional Liability: "If the doctor doesn't request some test that he should have, there is a potential for liability." That "some test" is not decided on medically but legally. Furthermore, the spokesman went on to tell lawyers that if a patient were subsequently to come down with a condition—even if completely unrelated to what the doctor was treating the patient for—that just might have been detected with the help of a medical test, no matter how outmoded or obscure, the patient's lawyer could use this "oversight" to justify awarding money to the patient. A medical test does not have to be of any value to the patient; all the lawyer has to do is convince a jury that the test *might* have been of value to someone for the doctor to be found negligent.

You should know which medical tests have been classified as outmoded, whether by medical associations, insurance companies, or government agencies. When such tests are ordered for you, most likely you will have to pay for them yourself, unless your doctor can convince a medical review board of the absolute necessity of that test under your specific circumstances.

But the fact that one state insurance company may consider a medical test outmoded does not necessarily mean that reimbursement will be refused in another state. Each insurance plan sets up its own rules, and only your doctor knows which medical tests are covered.

Outmoded or obsolete tests, at present, include:

Adrenocorticotrophin hormone
Amylase isoenzymes
Angiography (certain techniques)
Arthroscopy (a form of endoscopy)
Ballistocardiography
Basal metabolism
Bendien's (for cancer)
Biopsy of certain organs and tissues
Blood pressure monitoring (portable)
Bolen (for cancer)
Calcium clotting time
Capillary fragility
Cardiac blood pool imaging
Cephalin flocculation
Chromium
Chymotrypsin (intestinal)
Circulation time
Computerized tomography (certain applications)
Congo red
Diagnex blue (for stomach acid)
Drug-abuse screening (body tissue)
Drug monitoring (for certain drugs)

Endoscopy (with contrast dyes in the lungs)
Gastric analysis for pepsin
Gonadotropic hormones
Guanase
Hair analysis
Icteric index
Impotence (various techniques)
Leucine aminopeptidase
Mucoprotein (seromucoid)
Nonprotein nitrogen
Pesticide poisoning
Phonocardiogram
Plethysmography (lung function)
Pneumoencephalography
Pregnancy (employing animals)
Protein-bound iodine
Pulmonary function (screening)
Red blood cell indices
Rehfuss (stomach acid secretions)
Skin reactions for actinomycosis, brucellosis, cat-scratch fever, leptospirosis, Frei, psittacosis, trichinosis
Streptococcal agglutination
Syphilis using colloidal gold
Thymol turbidity
Upper gastrointestinal endoscopy
X-rays for fetal age and in many instances where air and other contrast media are included

With each passing year, more and more medical tests will undoubtedly be labeled as superfluous—or possibly unprofitable—but do not be surprised if you are ordered to undergo an antiquated test; be even less surprised when it turns out that you must pay for the test directly in spite of your health insurance coverage.

Again, the tests listed in this book are in actual use regardless of any controversy over their value. Where possible, their significance and value are stated. To many physicians, the value of certain tests is relative; one doctor may swear by a particular test that another doctor abhors. Yet it is the ultimate diagnosis that counts, and every doctor is entitled to utilize the procedures that he feels will result in successful diagnosis and treatment. Tests in themselves cannot and do not make diagnoses; they assist, amplify and confirm a doctor's thought processes—nothing more.

Two caveats. If, after reading this introduction, you are still not sure of the need to participate actively in your medical testing, remember that in several recent studies, anywhere from 25 to 50 percent of abnormal test results reported to doctors were *not* followed up by those doctors. Surprisingly, some doctors simply ignored test reports that indicated the possibility of pathology—even when the tests were ordered by the doctors themselves and were not required as part of a hospital admission program. If you go through the trouble of having a test performed, you should see to it that the results of that test are not simply made known but fully explained to you. It is your body and your life.

Finally, it must be stressed that this book is not a manual for self-diagnosis. Although some tests may be indicative of specific disease processes, no test or battery of tests can be considered conclusive in determining the cause, presence, or absence of illness. Even when an abnormal test value is consistent, it alone may not be considered diagnostic. A medical test must always be interpreted in the context of the patient's symptoms and the doctor's other findings. A test in itself is relatively meaningless; it is only one of many guides to a patient's health.

HOW TO USE THIS BOOK

Tests are listed in alphabetical order under the name most commonly used by doctors. Where a test is known by other names or terms, the most customary alternative references are also listed. For example, the most common name for a thyroid function test is T_4. Some doctors use the term *thyroxin*, and others may order a hyperthyroid test. Yet all these terms refer to the same test. In addition, there are more than a dozen other thyroid tests, all of which assess the functioning of the thyroid gland.

This does not mean that a test, by virtue of its inclusion in the book, is necessarily valuable or even useful; it simply means it is in regular, if not very common, use. The tests selected for inclusion in the book were drawn from a survey of those tests regularly, even if infrequently, performed at several hospitals, many different commercial laboratories, and in the offices of 50 physicians representing all the various specialties in medical practice.

If there are different but closely related tests that might reveal similar information, such tests are noted. Tests that appear in **boldface type** are described separately under their own names.

When performed. Medical tests are performed primarily to confirm a doctor's diagnosis. Because so many medical tests do not have a specific purpose, the same test may be performed to help diagnose many different diseases. Physicians also order medical tests when their suspicions do not coincide with a patient's symptoms or complaints. In such cases, it is not unusual for a doctor to order a battery of different tests with the hope that one or more test results will raise a red flag and help narrow the focus toward a precise diagnosis.

Then, of course, there are the tests required by a law or regulation, such as by an employer, the military or school, or simply for screening or checkup purposes.

Normal values. The normal values cited for a test are those commonly accepted by most of the medical profession. Lately, doctors have come to use the term *reference value* when relating a patient's test findings to what would be considered normal—ostensibly indicating the absence of disease. So-called normal values have been changing recently; as but one example, take the cholesterol test. Although blood cholesterol values for Americans are reported to be higher than for people in some other countries, some doctors no longer consider the typical or usual American values as being "normal." Thus, the "normal" blood cholesterol level of around 300 may be considered to be abnormal by those doctors who insist on treating their patients with any cholesterol value greater than 200. And as with cholesterol test values, there are doctors who have narrowed the range of many other tests' normal or reference values; such an interpretation can lead to a greater test indication of disease suspicion, since so-called abnormal values will become more frequent. Thus, it becomes quite important for you to know your own doctor's concept of "normal" test values and how much they differ from accepted standards, or you may find yourself being treated for some nonexistent disease or a condition that a different doctor, based on his interpretation of the test result, would feel precludes any therapy. For the purposes of this book, however, virtually all instances of normal values reflect the test results found in 95 percent of supposedly healthy people. In the case of laboratory test results, normal values may vary from laboratory to laboratory, primarily because of different technical procedures employed; a normal value obtained by one laboratory may well be considered abnormal by a different laboratory. In the case of nonlaboratory tests, such as X-rays, electrocardiograms, reflex tests, or nuclear scanning observations, a doctor usually draws his own conclusions on the basis of training, knowledge, and experience, with a large measure of subjective evaluation. Thus, all normal values should be considered primarily as reference points and are sometimes called "reference range." Some medical tests have such a wide range of values within normal limits that it takes a significant deviation from the normal to indicate the possible presence of a medical problem.

A test result that is within normal limits does not guarantee that the disease being tested for is not present. Sometimes a shift in test values, even within the limits considered normal, can be as much an indicator of illness as an abnormal value. It is the clinical interpretation of a test value by a doctor, taking into account all other related facts, that ultimately determines whether a test result is normal or abnormal. Where laboratory test results are reported in numerical form, a patient need not understand the exact meaning of the measurement associated with that numerical value (mg per 100 ml, mMol, mEq—see Measurements: Equivalency Chart), but he should be able to note whether the reported value of a test lies within or outside the normal values for that test. Some doctors have recently begun reporting certain blood values as so many mg per dl, or deciliter; this is simply another way of saying 100 ml (milliliters)—the equivalent of a dl. And it seems more and more laboratory test results are being reported as SIs, or in international system units—a form of metrics used primarily outside the United States. Chemistry values are usually given in moles (abbreviated mol) or millimoles (abbreviated mMol) to mean an amount of substance. Thus, a cholesterol value of 200 mg per 100 ml (or dl) would read 52 mMol per liter (or mMol/L).

Abnormal values. Depending on the type of test, abnormal values are either expressed in numerical terms or described. Since in numerous medical tests, an abnormal value could be caused by any of a hundred different diseases, only the most common conditions reflected by an abnormal value are listed.

It must be reiterated that a single abnormal test value does not necessarily signify the presence of a disease. Because of the likelihood of error in medical testing, any test with an abnormal result must be repeated, preferably by a different physician or laboratory. When a reported abnormal test value is critical, most doctors will insist on a third evaluation before attributing significance to the results. Consideration must also be given to those daily activities of a patient that may directly affect medical test results and cause false-abnormal values (diet, drugs, smoking, etc.).

There are a great many tests that, in essence, do not have an absolute normal or abnormal value; the result is more a subjective interpretation by the doctor. And as previously noted, a positive, or abnormal, test result in one person may well be considered negative, or normal, in another individual. Different tests can also have different meanings for different patients; as but one example, a particular test to help diagnose heart disease in an individual under 30 years of age can be totally worthless in someone past 60 and could result in a false-positive result. Thus, before an abnormal test value can be applied to a patient, it must be deciphered within all the possible related environmental, mental, physical, and individual characteristics that apply. An abnormal test value only has meaning when it can be applied to a patient's problem and indicate a definite course of action. When a test's result has no real effect on the doctor's decision making, it has been a waste of time and money—not to mention the risks entailed.

Risk factors. Almost every medical procedure, be it a test or a treatment, involves some risk. The hazard posed by sticking a needle into a vein, while negligible, does exist. General risk factors for blood testing, the insertion of catheters and needles, the use of contrast substances (dyes), the application of X-rays and radioactive substances, and the employment of electrical instruments, which comprise the vast majority of tests, are listed here and simply noted in each appropriate test. Where a specific medical test involves greater risk factors, the dangers are described under the test heading.

General risk factors.

Blood testing. Blood is normally taken from a vein in the antecubital area (inside the arm, in front of the elbow, where the arm bends); samples are also drawn from arteries or veins in the groin area, the neck, the back of the hand, the fingertip, the earlobe, and from the heel. In the case of infants, blood is commonly obtained from veins along the side of the head.

Toward the latter part of 1985, test machines were being marketed that performed identical tests on fingertip blood in adults; virtually any test that once needed a blood specimen from a vein can now be done with one drop of whole blood from anywhere in the body (e.g., earlobe, heel).

Although the dangers related to the insertion of a small needle through the skin are relatively minimal, there are a few possible complications. The most notable hazard is called hematoma, which usually occurs when the needle goes through the vein to the opposite side of the intended vein puncture site or when the technician makes several unsuccessful attempts to find the vein. Blood then extravasates (leaks) into the surrounding areas, swelling the adjacent tissue and usually turning the skin black and blue. A hematoma is rarely dangerous and usually disappears within a few weeks. More often than not, this occurs in a patient who has been taking large amounts of aspirin or a drug prescribed to keep the blood from clotting; it may also occur in a patient who has high blood pressure. Although the reported incidence is extremely rare, there is the remote possibility that a severe hematoma could cause destruction of any tissues affected. Another extremely rare risk is the breakage of the needle within the body; although this problem is not necessarily serious, a subsequent surgical procedure might be required to locate and remove the needle. When needles and glass syringes are cleaned and reused, as opposed to utilizing disposable ones, there is always the risk of infection, especially hepatitis, depending on the effectiveness of resterilization And there have been reports in the medical literature that reveal the possibility of acquiring an infectious disease even from brand-new, previously unused blood collection equipment. In these cases, bacteria were found in allegedly sterile tubes furnished by the manufacturers. It would not be out of place to request that brand-new blood collection tubes be properly resterilized before use.

Catheter and needle insertion. A catheter is a thin rubber or plastic tube that is inserted into the body, most commonly in the arm, groin area, or neck, to pass through to a specific location (guided by X-rays) in order to deliver test materials to a precise spot (heart chambers, arteries of the heart, kidneys, or particular areas of the brain). At times, depending on the area to be tested, a rigid metal needle is used in place of a catheter.

Although the dangers are almost as remote as using a needle to obtain blood for testing, they do exist. Needles are usually used to guide a catheter into the body. Catheters sometimes break off in the body, necessitating surgery to effect their removal. The risk of infection from catheters increases proportionately with the amount of time they remain in the body, which is almost always a prolonged period.

Needles and/or catheters are also inserted into the bladder to obtain sterile urine samples; into joint spaces, where the risk of bone infection is not uncommon, even when meticulous antiseptic techniques are observed; and into the ducts of various body glands, such as the salivary glands, to obtain test material. Whenever ducts are probed, in addition to the risk of infection and catheter breakage, there is always the scant but real possibility of tearing or rupturing the duct, causing a condition that usually requires surgery and is difficult to repair.

In the past few years, there have been frequent reports of needles and syringes manufactured strictly for one-time use (called disposables) having been resterilized and reused. One study revealed that 40 percent of physicians who perform skin reaction testing reuse the same syringe—even if they do change the needle—and this practice could spread hepatitis or even AIDS. Hospitals are said to be even greater offenders in reusing so-called disposable equipment and supplies. For your own sake, insist on assurance that test material used on you has never been used on anyone else.

Contrast substance (dye) use. Many tests involving organs of the body depend on the use of a contrast dye, either swallowed, inserted by catheter or enema, or injected into the bloodstream. The dye, no matter what its chemical name, is resistant to X-rays and thus markedly enhances an organ's image on an X-ray picture. When swallowed, the dye, usually a barium mixture, fills the gastrointestinal tract from the esophagus through the stomach to the intestines, outlining each portion of the bowel much more than if the intestines contained nothing but food or air. The failure of the dye to outline a portion of the organ being studied usually indicates a "filling defect," or abnormal area. Different chemical dyes are used to study different organs of the body.

New evidence indicates that some contrast dyes, especially those used in angiography, may cause damage to chromosomes; this is in addition to the damage caused by prolonged X-ray exposure. The subsequent offspring of young people on whom the contrast substance is used could consequently be affected. Otherwise, the risk attending the use of any contrast dye is primarily one of allergy, although other adverse reactions have been reported. In general, at least 1 out of every 20 people who take a test where contrast dyes are used has some sort of dangerous side effect, such as a severe breathing problem, kidney failure, heartbeat irregularities, and even mental aberrations. From 200 to 800 patients die every year as a consequence of some related allergic-type reaction to the dye. This means that for every 10,000 to 40,000 times a test using a contrast dye is performed, a patient dies as a direct result of the test. The risk factors increase dramatically with patients who have any sort of allergy, and those with known allergies must be pretested meticulously for the slightest sensitivity to contrast dye prior to undergoing such a test.

X-ray and radioactive substance application. The application of X-rays and radioactive chemicals to the body is not innocuous, no matter how minimal their use or how common the procedures. X-ray dosage can be cumulative and not show any evidence of damage until many years later. Some of the risks of excessive X-ray exposure include hair loss, skin changes that may lead to cancerous lesions, and even organ changes.

Some other, lesser or more remote risk factors include loss of elasticity in the skin (this makes the skin look much older than it is, particularly the facial area) and possible deleterious effects on the reproductive organs. Whenever X-rays are taken, even such small pictures as dental X-rays, a lead shield should be placed over the lower abdomen to protect the ovaries or testicles.

Electrical instrument use. Any time a testing machine utilizes electricity, there is always the risk, although minute, of electric shock and even electrocution. While such instruments are usually kept in proper working order, there have been enough instances of faulty equipment or operator carelessness to warrant mention of this hazard. In addition, it is also dangerous to use electrical instruments in the vicinity of explosive gases or chemicals, such as anesthetic gases, including even ether.

Failure of electrical equipment presents another risk factor. In many tests, such as computer tomography or nuclear scanning, television cameras or cathode ray tubes are used to visualize internal organs. In several different X-ray examinations involving contrast dyes, television is used to watch the dye disbursement. It is not unusual for a television screen to go dead or for some highly integrated electrical circuit to fail at the precise moment it is needed. While the electrical mishap is not directly harmful, it may necessitate a prolonged delay of the testing procedure, which—in the case of a catheter inside the heart, a dye inside the knee, or injected radioactive material—can be dangerous. Electrical failures may thus force repeat testing, indirectly doubling or tripling any of the test's original inherent risk factors.

Patients over 60 years of age who undergo medical tests that include laxatives, enemas, and fluid or diet restrictions are exposed to special risks; they may suffer blood pressure changes, metabolic abnormalities, and even mental status changes as a consequence of test preparation procedures. All patients, regardless of age, would do well to inquire about such pretest requirements, how they might cause complications, and what can be done to avoid such risks.

But in addition to the many technically associated dangers that accompany medical testing, there are what some doctors consider even greater risks related to taking a test. As noted in the Introduction, a false-positive test result—where a medical test wrongly portends the patient has a disease—might well be listed as the greatest liability of all. A false-positive medical test result is bad enough, but when it leads to additional tests, especially far more dangerous ones, for no other reason than to attempt to justify the erroneous test result, the aftermath can be catastrophic. *Never trust the positive, or abnormal, result of a medical test until it has been repeated—preferably by another doctor or a different laboratory.*

Medical tests are not innocuous. They can cause as much, if not more, suffering by what they falsely imply as the disease whose presence they help to verify. If used properly, the tests can have value; when used improperly, they can carry with them a far greater risk than the most serious diseases. If nothing else, do not insist on a medical test you really do not need. Always keep in mind that there are no governmental regulations or professional standards for medical tests—as there are for drugs, automobile tires, and even sports equipment such as tennis balls. At the present time, a medical test does not have to prove itself accurate, or even useful, to be ordered or performed by a doctor and paid for by whomever is responsible for the bill. No matter how risky or dangerous a test may be, other than that those risks must be told to you, there are no legal restrictions on medical tests.

General pain/discomfort factors. In describing the amount of pain or discomfort a person might feel in undergoing various tests, it is difficult to be specific. Every individual perceives and tolerates pain differently. The quantity and quality of pain is so subjective that it is impossible to say one kind of pain is minimal while another is excruciating. The prick of a needle in the arm and the subsequent drawing of blood may be a negligible annoyance for one person and agony for another. Only you can really know the extent to which you feel and react to pain and other forms of discomfort. There are patients who feel tormented when forced to lie motionless on a hard table, as is often required for many different X-ray examinations, nuclear scanning procedures, and ultrasound observations and even for an electrocardiogram and an electroencephalogram.

For some people embarrassment can be far more uncomfortable than pain. Having to urinate on command may be quite a trial. The necessary exposure and probing of the body can also cause distress. More than a few people are mortified when they have to furnish a stool specimen for a feces examination; yet even that experience may not be as bad as having to undergo a semipublic enema or other rectal survey. And in spite of the so-called new sexual freedom, there are still many women who feel embarrassed when they have a gynecologic examination, just as there are many men who become unsettled when tested for impotence, fertility, or sexually transmitted diseases. For a patient who is claustrophobic, pulmonary function tests conducted in small, sealed chambers can be insufferable.

Fear or anxious anticipation of a test procedure or test result is fairly common. The time required for a test, including waiting time, can cause apprehension. For example, a glucose tolerance test requires at least five hours, during which time blood and urine samples are collected every hour, or even every half-hour. Almost all X-ray tests that utilize dyes require you to lie still for one to two hours after the tests are completed so that you can be treated immediately for any allergic reaction. Any test that involves physical activity should be explained so that you will not be shocked when you find you have to exert yourself—for example, walking uphill on a treadmill for several minutes.

You also should be alerted to all consequent physical reactions to tests. After certain eye examinations, the drops in your eyes may blur your vision for hours—even to the point where it would be dangerous to drive a car. If skin tests are to be performed, you may want to wear long-sleeved clothing to avoid feeling self-conscious about the many conspicuous red blotches on your arms after leaving the doctor's office. All potential invasions of body areas in the course of an examination should be explained to you ahead of time. Other conceivable vexations such as repeated feces collection should never come as a surprise. Thus, the more you know about the details of any test, the less anxiety you may experience.

Blood testing. Most people rate needle puncture as a momentary, slight pain. The amount of discomfort, of course, depends to a large extent on the technician (usually called a phlebotomist) who draws the blood—be it from the arm, fingertip, or elsewhere. For a number of people, the apprehension of the needle coming toward them is more distressing than the actual pain of the insertion. Some people (usually children) automatically scream throughout the process. An experienced technician who can locate the best vein and insert the needle into the vein without hesitation will automatically reduce the level of perceptible pain. If, however, you find needle puncture particularly painful, there are ways to alleviate the pain. A local anesthetic (a cream, ointment, liquid, or even a freezing spray) can be applied to the test area a moment or two beforehand. Injections of nerve-end-numbing drugs under the skin are sometimes used, but many people feel the burning from the drug insertion is as painful as the needle itself. In most instances, a smaller-size needle is less traumatic; the large needles so commonly used are primarily for the technician's convenience to hasten the procedure. Disposable-type needles are always much sharper and therefore less irritating than needles that are resterilized and reused—most often without being resharpened.

Catheter and needle insertion. The insertion of a catheter or needle other than to take blood can be very uncomfortable, even quite painful. Much depends on the skill of the person doing the insertion. Where the devices are inserted into blood vessels, missing the artery or vein, or causing more than one hole, can allow blood to leak into surrounding tissue, making the area painful for several days. Usually, where pain is a probable consequence, the area around and under the insertion site is anesthetized. The needle used to extract cerebrospinal fluid (spinal tap) is rarely painful—and needs no anesthesia—if performed properly. Thin rubber catheters that are inserted into body orifices (such as in the urethra to collect urine from the bladder) may be uncomfortable but are rarely painful.

Most other tests may well cause discomfort, but should any test have an inherent ability to cause pain, a doctor or technician can usually alleviate the pain by one or more methods.

Cost. While the cost shown for each test was derived from a survey of doctors' offices, commercial clinical laboratories, and hospitals representing all geographical areas of the country, the actual price paid can vary widely (e.g., a test for AIDS can cost anywhere from $3 to more than $300). The list, or stated, price of a medical test may be quite different from the actual amount paid by a health insurer—especially a governmental one. The full price may be charged to a private patient paying his own bills, or the difference between the full price and the remuneration paid by an insurance company may, or may not, be billed to the patient at the doctor's discretion. The particular fee for a medical test may vary considerably from one geographic area to another, from a rural to an urban area, and even from one doctor to another in the same location. For example, a routine electrocardiogram (ECG) can cost anywhere from $15 to $100, the average price being $40 in 1985. Since the advent of Medicare, the federal government has surveyed all of the United States regularly and has come up with the prevailing rate for medical tests for 1984—the prevailing rate being the reimbursement more than half of all physicians in a particular locality would supposedly find acceptable for the test. This is the maximum payment Medicare will make, although the usual payment is 60 percent of the prevailing rate (this percentage applies only to laboratory tests; doctors usually receive 80 percent of the prevailing rate for other than laboratory tests such as ECGs, lung testing, or eye examinations). At present, Congress is considering a plan to reimburse doctors and laboratories on a uniform, countrywide basis rather than pay under the 243 different locality fee schedules as the government now does; there is, of course, an objection to this concept by most of the medical profession, but in fact, the plan may become effective by the end of 1986. A few examples of the present payment schedule might be of interest: In rural Kentucky, the prevailing rate for an electrocardiogram is $19.20, while in Kern County, California, it is $49.51. A blood cholesterol test's prevailing rate is $5 in Virginia but $15 in Nevada, and the identical test is $23 in Alaska. A hemoglobin test (for anemia) has a prevailing rate of $2 in upstate New York, while it costs $8 in Beverly Hills, California (a typical hospital charge for that same test is $38). A colonoscopy (an endoscopy of the entire large intestine or large bowel) averaged from $100 to $500 until the President of the United States underwent the procedure; now some doctors are charging $1,000 for that same test.* Yet another indication of the irrationality that can go into the payment for medical tests is the fact that the federal government will reimburse a specialist much more money than it will pay a family practitioner for simply ordering—not necessarily performing—the identical medical tests. For example, if a surgeon orders a cholesterol test, regardless of whether it is directly related to treatment, he may be paid $25, while a general practitioner ordering the same test—directly related to his patient's care—may receive only $5. There are no controls or regulations governing the cost of medical tests, albeit some insurance companies and governmental agencies may limit the amount of money they will pay a doctor, laboratory, or hospital for performing a test, but even those restrictions are not absolute. It is not unusual for the cost of a medical test to match whatever the traffic will bear. And it has been reliably reported that as the number of doctors increases and the number of patients per doctor decreases, the doctors are turning more and more to performing as many tests as possible as a means of supplementing their incomes.

In general, commercial laboratories charge the lowest fees and hospitals the highest. It is not unusual for tests performed in a hospital to cost two or three times as much as when the same tests are performed in a clinical laboratory or doctor's office. Hospitals justify their higher fees by claiming the profits from testing make up for losses in other departments and help support charitable work. While the fees in this

---

*For anyone particularly interested in the prevailing charges for more than 100 (out of the 6,000) different medical services, including 44 tests, a copy of the "Medicare Directory of Prevailing Charges—1984" can be obtained from the Superintendent of Documents, Government Printing Office, Washington, DC 20402; there is a $9 charge.

book were in effect as of the first part of 1986, they may change overnight as a result of newer techniques, more expensive equipment, higher labor costs, and the state of the economy. Where there is a wide discrepancy between the least and most expensive charge for a test—such as what Medicare or some other insurance plan will pay and what a doctor or hospital charges a self-paying patient—both extremes are listed.

Where performed (included also in section on *Cost*). The cost of a test may depend more on where that test is done than on the simplicity or difficulty of performing it. Over 90 percent of all tests can be and are performed in a doctor's office, assuming the office has the necessary laboratory facilities, instruments, or equipment such as an operating room, an X-ray machine, or an electrocardiograph. In the case of blood tests, some doctors, or their assistants, draw the patient's blood and then send it to a commercial laboratory. Other test specimens—such as urine, feces, biopsies, or material for culture—may also be obtained in a doctor's office and then sent out for evaluation. Where special or unique equipment is required, patients may be referred to a hospital or teaching center. Should a test require careful observation afterward, it is almost always performed in a hospital. There are times when a doctor will send a patient to a hospital for a test more as a matter of the doctor's—as opposed to the patient's—convenience. On the other hand, in some cases, health insurance companies will reimburse the doctor or the patient for the cost of the test only if it is performed in a hospital, regardless of the necessity for hospitalization.

Unless otherwise noted, tests are performed in the doctor's office, or the patient (or the specimen or tissue to be tested) is referred to a commercial laboratory.

Accuracy and significance. The interpretation of the accuracy and significance of any medical test is relative. The conclusions arrived at came from a review of the current medical literature and a consensus of physicians who most often utilize the tests. Even though some tests may seem indicative of specific disease processes, no test or even a battery of tests can be considered absolutely conclusive in determining the cause, presence, or absence of illness. The significance of any medical test must always be interpreted within the context of a patient's medical history and symptoms and the doctor's observations from physical examination of the patient. A medical test in and by itself is relatively meaningless; it is only one of many clues to a patient's condition. Doctors do not always agree on the accuracy or the significance of a test. Many doctors swear by a test that their colleagues deem virtually worthless. Much of a test's significance depends on how a physician applies the result of that test to his patient's condition. And the so-called accuracy of a great many tests can depend on the selection of the patient to be tested. As but one example, there are doctors who extol the stress electrocardiogram test by reporting how accurate it is on patients with *known* heart disease. Obviously, if a diagnosis is known prior to testing, the test cannot help but be close to 100 percent accurate. Unfortunately, most medical tests are performed on patients without a specific diagnosis, and the accuracy rates in the book reflect this aspect of testing.

As but one example of the relativity of a test's accuracy and significance, in the same issue of a medical journal, one doctor reported that the accuracy of the occult blood test for colon cancer was 92 percent—more than twice as accurate as a direct sigmoidoscopy examination—while another doctor wrote about how most medical articles cite the same test as yielding almost 60 percent false-negative reactions—where the pathology was not detected by the test.

At least be aware that clinical pathologists—doctors who specialize in the mechanics of medical testing—consider a test to be excellent when it is accurate 97 percent of the time; a good test is right at least 95 percent of the time. A test with an 80 percent accuracy rate is considered to be a poor test; as an example, if a pregnancy test had an 80 percent accuracy rate, it would give false results in 2 out of every 10 women (actually, today's pregnancy test, when properly performed, is close to 99 percent accurate). And consider, too, a test's significance; if it can show a positive, or abnormal, result in more than five different conditions (let alone dozens), insist on some assurance that its lack of significance will still be meaningful to your doctor in your circumstance. You could save yourself a great deal of grief—and money—if you ascertain the accuracy, and significance, of every test you are about to undergo; if you question the need for any medical test less than 80 percent accurate and refuse such a test until it can be justified to your need and satisfaction, you could even save your life. Much of a test's accuracy depends on the skill of the physician performing it—especially when it comes to obtaining a specimen for a more technical examination. In other instances, a test can range from 0 to 98 percent accurate, depending on the doctor's education, past experience, and present ability; this includes the ability to detect the right area to test and the ability to discern possible pathology. Thus, the figures given for the accuracy of the tests in this book reflect what a good doctor should be able to see, do, and interpret. Of necessity, the accuracy rate of a test must also reflect the chance of error by technical personnel as well as the use of outdated chemicals and miscalibrated equipment, not forgetting the many things a patient can do to interfere with a test's results (these extraneous factors are cited in the Introduction). All this is to say that should there be a disagreement about the book's stated accuracy for a test, consider all the many variables that enter into arriving at a test's value and the relativity of any medical test's accuracy will be far better understood.

Probably the most precise evaluation of medical tests—and in particular, the newest and most technologically advanced tests—comes from a 1985 study comparing autopsy results with that of diagnoses made by physicians dependent on those test results. One out of every five diagnoses was wrong; even worse, it was postulated that 1 of every 10 who died might have lived had the correct diagnosis been made. One of the doctors involved in the study commented: "Figures indicate that despite advances in diagnostic technology [computerized tomography, magnetic resonance imaging, etc.], we're only about 80 percent accurate."

The percentage of accuracy attributed to a test in this book may be limited to that test's application to only one disease or condition. A test that is 90 percent accurate for a particular disease may be relatively worthless for some other illness, albeit the procedure may well be ordered by the doctor. For example, lymphocyte typing is considered 90 percent accurate in differentiating lymph cell diseases; when it is used to diagnose other conditions, such as immunity problems, its accuracy rating may be well below 80 percent. For almost all stipulated test accuracy values, the percentage figure applies mainly to the test's primary purpose.

The American College of Physicians, a group of specialists whose members are primarily internists, cardiologists, and experts in metabolic and endocrine diseases, has been studying the relative value of medical tests for many years. Its finding thus far is: "Unfortunately, there exists no unambiguous method for evaluating medical technology, and the many studies lead to confusing conclusions." In other words, at the present time, there are no absolute standards for the accuracy and significance of medical tests.

THE PATIENT'S GUIDE TO MEDICAL TESTS

Note: Test names that appear in **boldface type** (not italics) are discussed in detail under their own heading (or under a related **boldface type** heading).

A

AAT, see *Albumin/Globulin*

ABDOMINAL ENDOSCOPY, see *Endoscopy*

ABDOMINAL SCANNING, see *Nuclear Scanning*

ABORTION WARNING, see *Placental Lactogen*

ABSCESS CULTURE, see *Culture*

ACCOMMODATION, see *Visual Acuity*

ACETALDEHYDE, see *Alcoholism*

ACETONE, see *Ketones*

ACETYLCHOLINE RECEPTOR ANTIBODY, see *Edrophonium*

ACETYLCHOLINESTERASE, see *Cholinesterase*

ACG, see *Apexcardiogram*

ACHIEVEMENT, see *Learning Disability*

ACHILLES REFLEX, see *Thyroid Function*

ACID-BASE BALANCE, see *pH*

ACID-FAST STAIN, see *Culture*

ACID HEMOLYSIS, see *HAM*

ACID-LABILE INTERFERON-ALPHA, see *Acquired Immunodeficiency Syndrome*

ACIDOSIS, see *Carbon Dioxide; Ketones; pH*

ACID PHOSPHATASE

Acid phosphatase is an enzyme found primarily in the prostate gland. The male hormone testosterone causes the prostate to secrete acid phosphatase into the bloodstream. Blood is taken from an arm vein for serum examination. Urine and prostatic secretion are occasionally tested. Direct aspiration of the prostate by needle is also used to test for prostate disease. There are several new improvements in the technique of measuring acid phosphatase; they allow smaller amounts of the prostate-specific enzyme to be detected — hopefully, to allow an even earlier diagnosis of prostatic cancer. But it should be noted that one-sixth of all prostate cancers exist in men without causing any difficulty (these are found at autopsy).

When performed: If there is a suspected abnormality of the prostate gland; to help identify metastasizing carcinomas (spreading cancers).

In suspected rape, the vaginal fluid may be tested for prostatic acid phosphatase to prove sexual intercourse took place. Many rapists have abnormal sex gland functioning and do not produce sperm; a woman who has been raped may not show a positive sperm test but will usually show a positive acid phosphatase test. In addition, sperm usually disappear after a day or two, but the acid phosphatase remains for at least 72 hours. (Sperm have, however, been found up to seven days after intercourse. See Semen.)

Normal values: Several different methods are used to measure acid phosphatase; the values vary with the method used. The most common values are 0 to 2.0 Bodansky units; 0 to 0.65 Bessey-Lowry units; 0 to 5.0 King-Armstrong units; and 1 to 1.9 IU per liter.

Abnormal values: Acid phosphatase is elevated with metastatic carcinoma (spreading cancer) of the prostate and the spread of some other cancers (a normal acid phosphatase is not an assurance of no cancer), Paget's disease (thickening and softening of the bones), and a form of bone cancer called multiple myeloma. The King-Armstrong method can detect moderate rises in cases of pneumonia and hepatitis, as well as with certain cancers. The Bodansky method is more specific for prostatic cancer. Prostatic examination or massage will also elevate serum acid phosphatase levels, as will the taking of the drug clofibrate (Atromid-S).

The newer radioimmunoassay technique to detect prostatic acid phosphatase (RIA-PAP) is more sensitive and should make it possible to obtain an earlier diagnosis of prostate cancer.

Risk factors: Negligible (see general risk factors for blood testing).

Pain/discomfort: Minimal (see general pain/discomfort factors for blood testing).

Cost: The standard techniques average from $6 to $40 per test. Radioimmunoassay evaluations cost from $10 to $60.

Accuracy and significance: This is considered the best laboratory test for detecting prostate disease in its early stages although only 50 to 75 percent accurate. Radioimmunoassay testing is considered 83 percent accurate. A negative RIA-PAP test is considered about 85 percent accurate in indicating the absence of prostate cancer. A positive test can be caused by conditions other than prostate cancer (anemia, severe infections, hormone diseases that affect bones, thrombophlebitis, heart attack, diabetes, kidney disease, and other forms of cancer). Most doctors regard a rectal examination as the most accurate test for prostate cancer.

Note: There is an experimental, more specific test to detect semen in the vaginal fluid of alleged rape victims. It is called semen glycoprotein p30. It can be found more than 24 hours following rape and can be positive when prostatic acid phosphatase is undetectable.

ACID REFLUX, see *Gastroesophageal Reflux*

ACQUIRED IMMUNODEFICIENCY SYNDROME (AIDS)

The word *syndrome* in this condition refers to a particular group of symptoms (subjective complaints) and signs (objective findings) that are consistent in patients who have the same disability. AIDS, therefore, is not a distinctive disease. An immunodeficiency is, in essence, any lack of immunity or the partial or total inability to fight off an infection, an allergy, or even a cancer (see **Immunoglobulin; Immunology**); most often, it means the body is incapable of producing antibodies (see **Agglutination**), which are the body's primary defense against a disease. An immunodeficiency can, however, also be induced deliberately, as when certain drugs are used to prevent the body's natural attempt to fight off, or reject, a body tissue or organ transplant. The word *acquired* indicates the condition usually comes from contact with someone or something carrying the causative organism.

AIDS, then, is a contagious illness that, when present, manifests itself by a patient's sudden development of a severe infection—usually a form of pneumonia—and/or a type of cancer; either, or both, have been ultimately fatal within from one to five years after the first outward manifestations appeared. The "official" definition of AIDS, as reported by the Public Health Service, has changed or been altered almost yearly and now encompasses a host of various signs and symptoms that include: an unexplained illness accompanied by swollen lymph glands, fever, fatigue, and **Fungus** infections of the mouth and throat called candidiasis or thrush; doctors have reported that virtually all AIDS patients have oral candidiasis or raised white spots on the tongue prior to the more deadly signs of the condition. Fever is also common, usually with no immediate discernible cause; there may be night sweats, and weight loss accompanying the fever. Other outward signs of AIDS are various forms of skin lesions, from black-and-blue blotches to "shingles" (see **Herpes**); an enlarged liver and spleen; and indications of other sexually transmitted diseases. A physical examination usually reveals rales (abnormal lung sounds heard through the stethoscope), pathological lesions on the retina (see **Fundoscopy**), and Kaposi's sarcoma (blisterlike sores and cancerous growths named after the man who first described them).

AIDS was first formally recognized as a syndrome in 1981; at that time, it was initially thought to be limited to homosexual men and Haitians; later, it was found in drug abusers who injected themselves intravenously—particularly those who used common, unsterilized needles—and in individuals who received blood transfusions and blood products (certain vaccines and treatments for hemophilia or other blood-related conditions). Although the syndrome has since been reported in heterosexuals and women prostitutes, worldwide about 78 percent of all cases occur in homosexuals or bisexuals (in Los Angeles, homosexuals are reported to make up 93 percent of all known cases), while 17 percent occur in drug abusers, and the remaining 10 percent occur in those who received blood products, those from Haiti, and alleged heterosexuals. Prior to 1983, less than 1,400 cases were diagnosed; since then, more than 5,000 cases a year are being reported, and it has been estimated that this number will double annually by 1986. By the end of 1985, there were over 16,000 known cases in the United States (in excess of 5,000 cases in New York City alone), and it was also reported that more than 2 million people had been infected with the suspected causative virus—and that was considered to be a conservative estimate. In contrast, less than 3,000 cases of AIDS had been reported in Europe from 1982 through 1985, with Belgium, Denmark, and Switzerland having the highest rates per population. But here, too, the death rate was also 50 percent of those afflicted. Japan had only 4 cases up to May 1985; since that time, Japanese authorities have reported 4 more, with half of all the cases in hemophiliacs who received blood products. China has had 1 case to date, a tourist from Argentina. The Arab world countries have reported only 2 cases, both of whom received transfusions of blood imported from the United States.

The AIDS-causing virus can remain infectious for as long as 10 days in either dry or liquid form and it is believed that live AIDS virus can be transmitted through body secretions or excretions—such as saliva, semen, tears, and vaginal secretions—in addition to blood and blood products and by contact with cuts, bruises, or other bleeding wounds of someone harboring the suspected virus (even through mosquito bites); medical and dental procedures on such individuals are suspected of being particularly risky. It is also thought that those who perform such procedures may pass the virus on to their next patient if proper precautions are not observed. Eye doctors have been warned to pay particular attention to sterilizing trial contact lenses used in fitting their patients. The motion picture industry has indicted open-mouth kissing as a possible route of transmission, and a Pentagon official has admitted he was not confident that the condition could not be spread in an airplane, a tank, or a tent. AIDS has also been shown to pass from an infected mother to her child through breast milk. And in one study, the Public Health Service reported that living in a household with someone who has AIDS triples the chance of acquiring the condition.

There are several tests that are now used to help identify AIDS victims; at this time, however, there is no one specific test that will lead to an unquestionable diagnosis. The primary test being employed at the beginning of 1986 is one that detects antibodies to human T-lymphocyte virus type III (commonly designated as HTLV-III). It is believed—but it has not been definitely proved—that this is the organism that causes the body to lose its immunity. At present, the most common technique used is the ELISA method (see **Agglutination**); an indirect immunofluorescent antibody method is under study that is claimed to be more accurate. Yet another technique, called the Western blot test,* is more difficult to perform but is considered the most accurate of all available tests. The ELISA test alone is used to screen blood as a means of assuring that the virus will not be passed to a transfusion recipient. When an individual is tested, if the ELISA test is positive, it is usually repeated (there are a great many false positives). If the second ELISA is positive, a Western blot test is per-

---

*The Western blot is a form of electrophoresis (see **Albumin/Globulin**); a method of testing rather than a specific test; its name has nothing to do with the "west" but follows a somewhat whimsical pattern. The first test of its kind, called the Southern blot, was devised by a Dr. E.M. Southern; when a colleague reversed Dr. Southern's technique for a different test, he called it the Northern blot. The Western blot's name came about when yet another physician named his, somewhat similar, technique as a tribute to Dr. Southern. The Western blot is also applied to diagnosing other conditions such as brain tissue degenerative diseases.

formed, and only if that test is positive is the person considered to be a possible—but not definite—carrier of the virus.

The name *HTLV-III* came about because the suspected virus is the third member of a family of viruses that are known to cause lymph disorders such as leukemia and other cancers of T lymphocyte cells (see **Lymphocyte Typing**); these are the same **White Blood Cells** that contribute to the body's immunity by producing antibodies against disease. Because the virus is thought to be of the retrovirus family (different virus families have unique physical and growth characteristics), some doctors call the HTLV-III virus the AIDS-associated retrovirus (ARV). And yet another term for the virus is *lymphadenopathy-associated virus* (LAV); any one, or a combination, of these terms may be used for the AIDS antibody test. While there are some doctors who feel all three viruses may be identical, there are others who feel the African swine fever virus (a species from a different family of viruses called iridoviruses) is the real cause of AIDS, and tests to reveal these antibodies are under investigation. And there are those who feel AIDS may come from several different viruses rather than just one as a means of explaining the variation of signs and symptoms in different patients.

There are other tests that can indicate AIDS—either past exposure or present involvement. A particular indication of immunity loss is called cutaneous anergy, where **Skin Reactions** to previous exposure to disease such as fungus infections fail to show the expected response, or if there is a response, it is delayed for several days. Testing for **Cytomegalovirus** and Epstein-Barr virus (see **Herpes** and **Mononucleosis**) as well as for **Immunoglobulin, Hepatitis** antigens and antibodies, **Lysozyme, Syphilis, Gonorrhea,** and serum proteins (see **Albumin/Globulin**) are performed by many doctors to help verify AIDS. Precise measurements of T and B lymphocytes (see **Lymphocyte Typing**), measuring the amount of thymosin (a hormone from the thymus gland), evaluating phytohemagglutin (PHA), which can indicate T lymphocyte cell response, and performing **Blood Cell Differential** and **Platelet Count** tests are all indirect ways of assessing if immunity is lost—possibly due to AIDS. Specific blood proteins called p41 and p24 (believed to be the outer covering of the suspected virus) can be searched for and, if found, are supposed to help distinguish true- from false-positive HTLV-III tests. The presence of these proteins is also thought to be an early warning sign that full-blown AIDS is imminent. A deficiency of **Immunoglobulin** A is thought to be indicative of a susceptibility to AIDS, and an increase in acid-labile interferon-alpha in the blood is supposed to mean the syndrome has a bad prognosis (is worsening). The ultimate test is to **Culture** a body fluid or tissue (see **Biopsy**) and isolate the HTLV-III virus (also see **Parasite**).

Because a large percentage of AIDS patients have signs of brain pathology (usually a form of encephalitis), many doctors recommend that an **Electroencephalogram** (EEG) be performed on everyone suspected of having the syndrome. And because AIDS patients are showing an increased incidence of tuberculosis, they should be skin tested for this disease (see **Skin Reaction**) frequently—as should all those in contact with suspected AIDS victims. Again, it must be emphasized that despite the many different tests now in use, there is still no one test—including the HTLV-III—that is specific; all that is revealed is the presence or absence of antibodies to the virus believed to be the causative agent. A positive test does not mean an individual necessarily has an active or transmissible infection; it only means that the suspected virus was, or possibly is, present in the body. A positive culture, assuming the HTLV-III virus is at fault, would mean infectivity. Other than the skin tests, biopsy, and culture, the tests are usually performed on blood taken from a vein.

When performed: The primary use of the HTLV-III/LAV/ARV tests is for screening blood — especially that of blood donors — with the hope of eliminating this means of transmitting the syndrome. This test and many of the others are also being used on patients with unexplained illnesses — especially those with multiple skin lesions, pneumonias that do not respond to antibiotics, and lymph gland enlargement. Some insurance companies require tests for AIDS prior to issuing policies; some employers — especially those whose work involves food handling — insist on such tests even after employment; the military performs the test on all recruits and those on active duty; and the Public Health Service has strongly recommended that all donors of organs, tissues, and semen be tested prior to donation. A few states have made donor testing a legal requirement. And there are public health agencies that offer the test to anyone requesting it.

Normal values: There should be no test result that indicates the presence of antibodies to any of the suspected AIDS viruses. However, a negative test result is not a guarantee that an AIDS-causing virus and/or its antibodies are not present; a great many false-negative tests have been reported.

Abnormal values: Any test that indicates HTLV-III/LAV/ARV antibodies are present is considered a positive test (abnormal value). The absence of normal skin reactions along with abnormal values for all the other indirect tests that show a loss or lack of immunity is considered to be suspicious of AIDS until proved otherwise; they are — when evaluated along with the patient's history, exposure, and physical evidence — considered to be more confirmatory than specific. An increase in thymosin hormone, especially certain fractions of the hormone, is said to help differentiate between AIDS and other forms of immunodeficiency. False-positive test responses have been reported in patients with systemic lupus erythematosis, arthritis, and other related connective tissue diseases (see **Antinuclear Antibodies**).

Risk factors: The risks are primarily related to the method of testing; with blood testing, they are minimal (see general risk factors for blood testing) to the person being tested but could be dangerous to the person obtaining the blood sample. Biopsy, culture, EEG, and skin-testing risks are described under their separate entries. Aside from the physical risks, there is also the risk of being labeled with the syndrome — rightfully or not. A positive HTLV-III/LAV/ARV test result is required to be reported to most health authorities and could have catastrophic consequences for one's life — be it school, business, or social — especially if the test result is false and since a positive test is not absolute proof that AIDS exists in the individual.

Pain/discomfort: These, too, are related to the method of testing and are described under each test's separate entry. The pain and discomfort from a breach of confidentiality cannot be minimized.

Cost: Blood testing for HTLV-III and related viruses runs from free to $300; much depends on where the test is performed (the cost of ELISA testing to a laboratory is from $1 to $3). The Western blot technique can cost from $90 to $300. Thymosin testing is about $50; other test costs are described under their separate entries.

Accuracy and significance: Again, it must be stressed that all the present tests are not specific for AIDS; they are, at this time, only suggestive. The natural history of the disease itself is not completely understood at present, and a positive test without appropriate signs and symptoms may not be medically significant. So many false-positive and false-negative results are being reported that the accuracy of the tests is still in question—despite their profuse application. ELISA tests are the least accurate; the Western blot is thought to be the most accurate. During the initial phase of testing blood for AIDS antibodies, after all "positive" tests were repeated, less than one out of five were positive on the second testing. Thus, present thinking is that no conclusion should be drawn from one positive test. And for some as yet unexplained reason, women seem to have ten times as many false-positive tests as do men. For the results to have significance, an individual should show two positive ELISA tests—preferably from different laboratories—and a positive Western blot test. And present statistics show that of those who do test positive, only from 9 to 20 percent ultimately develop full-blown AIDS. Of particular interest, at the end of 1985, lawmakers, not doctors, in two states—California and Wisconsin—have declared the tests to be of no diagnostic value.

Practical significance of any AIDS test will be shown when its application results in a decreased incidence of the syndrome at least in those who receive blood or blood products. Eighty-five percent of patients who have shown positive results in all three AIDS tests have also shown live HTLV-III virus in one or more body fluids. A few have had live virus with a negative AIDS test; it is thought that this reflects an early infection—too new to produce antibodies.

Note: AIDS-related complex (ARC) is a diagnosis sometimes given to patients who show many, but not all, of the signs and symptoms designated by the Public Health Service's Centers for Disease Control as the present criteria for AIDS. Some ARC patients do go on to develop AIDS; one out of every five male homosexuals with ARC ultimately develops full-blown AIDS. ARC patients usually have positive HTLV-III and related tests. Although ARC is now considered to be 20 times as common as AIDS, ARC cases are not counted when totaling AIDS cases and victims.

ACROMEGALY, see *Growth Hormone*

ACTH STIMULATION, see *Cortisol*

ACTIVATED CLOTTING TIME, see *Partial Thromboplastin Time*

ACTIVATED PARTIAL THROMBOPLASTIN TIME, see *Partial Thromboplastin Time*

ADDIS COUNT, see *Urine Examination*

ADENOVIRUS, see *Virus Disease*

ADH, see *Vasopressin*

ADRENAL CORTICAL, see *Cortisol*

ADRENAL FUNCTION EOSINOPHIL COUNT, see *Cortisol*

ADRENALIN, see *Catecholamines*

ADRENALIN MEDULLA, see *Catecholamines*

ADRENAL SUPPRESSION, see *Cortisol*

ADVANCE, see *Pregnancy*

AEM, see *Electrocardiogram*

AFP, see *Alpha Fetoprotein*

AGGLUTINATION

Agglutination means the clumping or gathering together of cells (usually red blood cells) into a mass; normally, each cell exists separately. This phenomenon can easily be seen under the microscope; in many instances, it can also be viewed with the naked eye when the lumps settle into the bottom of a test tube or clump together on a glass slide.

Agglutination occurs as a reaction against various diseases, primarily infections. Whenever the body is exposed to bacteria, viruses, fungus, or a toxin that contains antigens (the agents that cause disease), it reacts by producing antibodies. These antibodies then attempt to fight off the specific organism that has invaded the body. Antibodies found in a patient's blood indicate that the patient has already been exposed to a particular infection. The exposure may have occurred many years previously, or it may be of very recent origin.

The principle behind agglutination testing is always the same: to see if antigens of a known condition have already caused a defensive (antibody) reaction against that condition. If antibodies are present and clump with the known antigen, the test is called positive. Some antigens combine with antibodies only in cold temperatures, some need warm temperatures, some clump better when exposed to latex particles, and some show clumping best when sheep red blood cells previously exposed to the disease are used. Sometimes the cells flocculate, or fall like snowflakes, clumping at the bottom of the tube.

A single positive agglutination test is not usually sufficient to make a diagnosis. To determine if the disease is recent enough to be the cause of a patient's symptoms, two or three agglutination tests are performed within a few weeks. The serum is diluted first with equal parts of an innocuous solution and then progressively down to one part serum to well over a thousand parts of diluent (e.g., 1:1,064). The result is reported by titer (the highest titer represents the weakest solution in which agglutination occurs). A noticeable rise in titer with each test usually indicates an active disease with more and more antibodies being formed daily. Blood is taken from a vein, and the serum is tested. Thus, sometimes the test is called "serology."

A related test, **Complement Fixation,** is also used to diagnose mysterious infections. The two tests may be given together. At times, the same disease will give a positive reaction to the agglutination test as well as the complement fixation test. At other times, a particular disease will respond only to one of them.

Some agglutination tests carry the name(s) of the doctor(s) who first described them. The Widal test is one example; it was once almost routinely used to detect typhoid fever. The Weil-Felix test is used to detect rickettsial diseases such as Rocky Mountain Spotted Fever. These tests are sometimes referred to as febrile agglutination tests.

The Coombs' test for agglutination (there is a direct Coombs' and an indirect Coombs'; the direct Coombs' test is performed on red blood cells, while the indirect Coombs' test is performed on serum) is a form of agglutination test to detect antibodies related to blood diseases. The direct Coombs' test is sometimes called an antiglobulin test and is commonly performed on newborn babies to see if the antibodies that could indicate a hemolytic anemia were passed from mother to child during the pregnancy. Usually, the baby's blood is obtained from the umbilical cord, and, if positive, allows immediate treatment. A positive direct Coombs' usually signifies erythroblastosis fetalis (the Rh anemia of newborns) and hemolytic anemia (where a person's own antibodies destroy his red blood cells). The indirect Coombs' is used to detect Rh blood-type factors and to help avoid blood transfusion reactions (see **Typing and Cross-Matching**). The indirect Coombs' is sometimes called Rh testing, the Rh factor being one of the many blood groups (in essence, they are unique characteristics of **Red Blood Cells**) that can cause serious, at times fatal, **Immunology** reactions during blood transfusions, and especially during pregnancy. An awareness of one's Rh factor (as with other common blood types) can prevent many related diseases. Unfortunately, a great many drugs, including penicillin, can also cause a positive direct Coombs'.

There are a number of new adaptations of agglutination and **Complement Fixation** tests. The fluorescent antibody study (FA) is one such adaptation. It is a technique that treats a specific disease antigen with a fluorescent dye that attaches itself to a patient's antibodies—if they are present in the patient's blood—thereby signifying the presence of the disease. This test also provides quantitative results that indicate the progress of the disease. Some doctors designate the particular procedure to be used and refer to a direct fluorescent antibody test (DFA) and an indirect fluorescent antibody test (IFA).

Another recent adaptation is the enzyme-linked immunosorbent assay (ELISA); it, too, is used to detect antibodies to bacteria, parasites, some viruses, and certain antigens. Although the methods are similar to those used in radioimmunoassay (see **Nuclear Scanning**), this procedure employs an enzyme rather than radioactive chemicals to bind the antibodies. Far more rapid results are possible with these two adaptations (some report results the same day) than with standard agglutination techniques.

Countercurrent immunoelectrophoresis also can determine the presence of antigens and antibodies related to infections by applying an electric current and having them migrate toward opposite poles of that current. This test has the advantage of detecting dead microorganisms as the cause of an infection.

Monoclonal antibodies, while not specific tests in themselves, are the newest technique to utilize the antigen-antibody test mechanism. In a sense, they are manufactured antibodies (see **Immunoglobulin**)—as opposed to natural, body-produced, antibodies—grown by combining **White Blood Cells** and special myeloma (cancer) cells to make them quite specific for a disease or a condition under consideration by the doctor. They can be attached to radioactive substances (see **Nuclear Scanning**), used to detect cancers (see **Cancer**), reveal **Pregnancy,** and identify the specific cause of an infection or poisoning within minutes.

The latest technological approach to testing for a specific disease—again, a technique rather than a specific test in itself—is called nonisotopic immunoassay, using magnetic immunochemistry separation; it is also referred to as chemiluminescence. As with radioimmunoassay, the new procedures should provide more precise detection of disease-revealing substances.

When performed: The test is used most often when there is a persistent fever, such as occurs with an infection that cannot be diagnosed. Specific infections for which different forms of agglutination tests are conducted include:

Acquired immunodeficiency syndrome
Amebiasis
American trypanosomiasis
(Chagas' disease; heart muscle infection and facial edema)
Aspergillus
(a *Fungus*-caused, allergic-type lung disease becoming more commonly recognized)
Brucellosis
(undulant fever, usually resulting from association with cows, sheep, or goats and their unpasteurized milk)
Candidiasis
(a *Fungus* disease called "thrush" when it occurs in the mouth, "vaginitis" when it produces signs and symptoms in the vagina—and now considered a sexually transmitted disease; it can also cause pneumonia, gastrointestinal tract destruction, heart, brain, and kidney disease, and severe skin lesions)
Cryptococcosis
(a fungus-caused meningitis)
Cysticercosis
(a tapeworm infestation mostly affecting the eye and brain)
Echinococcosis
(another form of tapeworm infestation that causes large cysts to form in body organs)
Filariasis
(a mosquito-borne parasitic disease that causes elephantiasis—blocked lymph channels that most commonly cause the legs and testicles to swell to gigantic size)
German measles or **Rubella**
(an agglutination test is required by law in some states at the time of marriage or pregnancy to determine if a woman has had the disease and to immunize her if not); see **Rubella.**
Histoplasmosis
(a fungus-caused lung infection)

Infectious **mononucleosis**
Legionnaires' disease
>(a type of pneumonia, first diagnosed at an American Legion convention, that is now known to have more than 22 different but related forms of a bacteria as the cause; it is now possible to perform agglutination tests on urine, lung tissue, and sputum as a means of proving the diagnosis)

Leishmaniasis
>(a parasitic disease, sometimes called kala-azar disease, most commonly transmitted by sandflies, that causes skin ulcers called Oriental sores; it can also cause serious infections of the mouth, nose, and throat)

Leptospirosis
>(a generalized body infection caused by a spirochetal organism—see **Syphilis**—usually resulting from contact with an infected animal)

Listeriosis
>(a bacterial infection that commonly occurs in the fetus or newborn—it can also occur in adults—that becomes meningitis)

Lyme disease
>(a generalized disease—involving the heart, nerves, joints, and skin—caused by a spirochete-shaped organism [see **Syphilis**] and transmitted by ticks)

Melioidosis
>(a generalized infection common in drug addicts)

Mumps
Pertussis
>(whooping cough)

Q-fever
>(a rickettsial pneumonia; rickettsia are a form of bacteria)

Rat-bite fever
Rocky Mountain spotted fever
>(a severe, generalized infection caused by tick bites)

Salmonellosis
>(primarily a gastrointestinal infection caused by contaminated food or drink; recent outbreaks of this disease have been caused by drinking milk not properly pasteurized or by drinking milk or eating meat from animals who are routinely fed antiobiotics and who then harbor and pass on bacteria that become resistant to drug treatment)

Schistosomiasis
>(swimmer's itch)

Sporotrichosis
>(a *Fungus* disease that affects the skin and lymph glands, sometimes called rose gardener's disease because it is often caused by rosebush thorns)

Streptococcal infections
Tapeworms
Toxic shock
>(antibodies can indicate risk of using tampons)

Toxoplasmosis

Trichinosis
    (primarily from eating raw, infected pork)
Tularemia
    (rabbit-handling fever)
Typhoid fever
    (a salmonellosis infection)
Typhus
Virus conditions, see **Virus Disease**
Yersinia diseases
    (many different conditions caused by a bacteria, the most common being bubonic and pneumonic plague and pseudotuberculosis)

These are but a few of the many disease-specific agglutination-type tests now available; new ones are being introduced almost daily. Your doctor will know if there is a particular test for a disease you may be wondering about.

Agglutination tests are also performed to help diagnose rheumatoid arthritis; to ascertain the specific cause of certain allergic reactions, such as to cow's milk; to diagnose certain anemias caused by the Rh factor; to determine a person's blood type, such as A, B, AB, O, or Rh; and even to ascertain pregnancy.

By noting which type of blood a person's serum agglutinates, the physician can determine that person's blood type and therefore the type of blood that would be safe for transfusion if ever needed. Whether a mother will react to the Rh factor during pregnancy is also determined in the same way. By mixing a woman's urine that contains the hormone human chorionic gonadotropin that increases during pregnancy with the antiserum for that hormone and observing for agglutination, the physician can ascertain if the woman is pregnant (see **Pregnancy**).

Normal values: While agglutination reactions to disease should not be present, an old, forgotten infection can cause a positive test. Usually, though, the titer is quite low, averaging less than 1:64 dilution. Unless this titer suddenly rises (is present in much greater dilutions) within a few days, it is not considered evidence of any active disease. When it comes to blood typing, there are no normal values.

Abnormal values: If the titer of a patient against a specific disease rises within a few days to a week, it can reasonably be concluded that the patient is manufacturing a great many antibodies against that disease and therefore is harboring the organism that causes the disease. Sometimes agglutination tests are performed against a number of different infectious diseases; the one that shows the highest, increasing titer usually indicates the diagnosis. A titer over 1:64 is needed to be of definitive value.

Well over half of all people with rheumatoid arthritis show a positive agglutination test to latex particles (the reason is not known), but then so do some people with systemic lupus erythematosus and chronic infections. A few drugs such as methyldopa (for high blood pressure) and some pain relievers can cause a false-positive test; in contrast, excessive use of certain antibiotics can mask a positive agglutination test, making it appear negative.

Risk factors: Negligible (see general risk factors for blood testing).

Pain/discomfort: Minimal (see general pain/discomfort factors for blood testing).

Cost: Regular agglutination tests, which usually include two blood samples taken two to three weeks apart, average $10 to $30 for both samples. An individual IFA, DFA, or ELISA test averages $25 to $35; paired samples (taken two to three weeks apart) range from $35 to $45 for the pair. Special agglutination tests such as cold or febrile agglutinins can run from $6 to $53. The direct Coombs' can cost from $26 to $50, although a single Rh factor test averages $5. **Typing and cross-matching** of blood for transfusions—performed almost exclusively in hospitals—runs from $53 to $78. Legionnaire's disease testing can cost $100.

Accuracy and significance: Most agglutination tests—and particularly those using IFA, DFA, and ELISA—are considered 90 percent accurate. There are a few exceptions, however. The test for Legionnaires' disease has approximately an 80 percent accuracy, while the test for trichinosis is only about 60 percent accurate. Antibody testing for pertussis (whooping cough) is not very accurate; many cases so diagnosed have later proved to be in error. And, regardless of which disease is being tested for, a positive test result does not always indicate the suspected infection is active; and, in a few instances, a positive test indicating one disease may turn out to come from an entirely different disease. In general, agglutination-related tests are about the best there are to identify infections.

AGGREGOMETER, see *Platelet Count*

A/G RATIO, see *Albumin/Globulin*

AIDS, see *Acquired Immunodeficiency Syndrome*

AIDS-ASSOCIATED RETROVIRUS, see *Acquired Immunodeficiency Syndrome*

AIDS-RELATED COMPLEX, see *Acquired Immunodeficiency Syndrome*

ALA, see *Lead; Porphyrins*

ALANINE AMINOTRANSFERASE, see *Aspartate Aminotransferase*

ALBUMIN/GLOBULIN (A/G Ratio)

Albumin and globulins are the main total plasma proteins in the blood. These proteins aid in maintaining the osmotic pressure of the blood (keeping a balance between the percentage of chemicals and plasma), provide nutritive substance for tissues, and carry essential substances such as hormones, vitamins, drugs, and enzymes throughout the body. There are four different globulins; the largest in number are the gamma globulins, which carry the immune bodies to help fight disease. The average person produces about 15 g of plasma proteins a day. Blood is taken from a vein, and the plasma or serum is tested. The results are stated as a ratio of the amount of albumin to the amount of all the globulins.

The different forms of the primary plasma proteins are also detected through electrophoresis (a technique rather than a test). This method of applying an electrical charge to the proteins and observing their migration on paper gives an indication of the amounts of albumin and the globulins. Although the patterns that result may indicate the presence of disease, they are not considered specific.

Albumin and globulin are also measured in other body fluids; the presence of albumin (protein) in the urine is usually an indicator of kidney disease. However, people with a condition known as orthostatic albuminuria automatically excrete albumin in the urine when they are on their feet for long periods of time. It signifies no known disease.

When performed: If there are problems of food absorption; to distinguish starvation from other diseases; in various liver and kidney diseases; when there is a question of infections, especially when there seems to be no resistance to infection; when cancer is suspected.

Normal values: The total proteins (primarily the sum of the albumin and the globulins) average 7 g per 100 ml. Usually, there is almost twice as much albumin, 4.5 g per 100 ml, as there are globulins, 2.5 g per 100 ml; and when the amount of albumin is divided by the amount of globulins, the normal A/G ratio averages two to one (2:1). Ratios from 1.5:1 to 2.5:1 are within normal limits. No protein should be detected in the urine.

Abnormal values: With diseases that affect the blood proteins, the amount of albumin is usually decreased and the globulins increased, thereby reversing the usual A/G ratio. In liver conditions especially, the amount of albumin decreases because of that organ's inability to manufacture it; gamma globulins increase, since they are made outside the liver. In kidney problems, both the serum albumin and gamma globulins decrease, but the alpha and beta globulins increase. In starvation, because little or no protein is eaten, all the blood proteins are decreased. The same decrease in the proteins is found when food cannot be absorbed because of various diseases.

Alpha antitrypsin (AAT), an antienzyme globulin, is decreased in inherited liver disease in children and lung disease in adults. Another globulin, **Alpha Fetoprotein** (AFP), usually disappears from the blood after birth but is sometimes found in adults with liver and other cancers.

Risk factors: Negligible (see general risk factors for blood testing).

Pain/discomfort: Minimal (see general pain/discomfort factors for blood testing).

Cost: From $8 to $30 for both albumin and globulin. Usually included in a **Comprehensive Multiple Test Screening** panel, which ranges from $7 to $42. When albumin is measured quantitatively in urine, the cost runs from $8 to $30. AAT testing can cost from $25 to $45.

Accuracy and significance: The majority of doctors consider the presence of albumin in the urine to be a reasonably accurate indicator of kidney disease (90 percent). There is one exception. Some physically active people, such as athletes, may show small amounts of albumin in the urine; however, after lying down for several hours, they should have no albumin in the urine. In general, albumin/globulin tests do not specify a particular disease, and they should be viewed as confirmation of other diagnoses. (Also see **Malnutrition**)

ALCOHOL

Testing for the body's ethyl alcohol content—whether in the blood, the breath, or the urine—is most commonly related to the legal question of driving while drunk.

Police and highway officers often measure alcohol concentration in the breath, which reflects blood levels. After alcohol is consumed, it reaches a peak in the blood in about half an hour's time. It takes about three hours to eliminate each ounce of alcohol ingested. Thus, a blood alcohol test is fairly reliable for many hours after the last drink. The blood alcohol test is also an important diagnostic tool when an unconscious person is brought to an emergency facility.

Blood, breath, or urine may be tested. Blood is taken from a vein. Breath is usually collected in a bag or balloon, or it may be exhaled directly into a measuring instrument. In the urine test, the individual must first empty the bladder and then wait a minimum of 20 minutes before the test sample is taken so that the specimen accurately reflects the amount of body alcohol at the time of testing.

When performed: The test is performed not only to determine if alcohol has been consumed but, of greater importance, to determine the degree of alcoholic intoxication so as to apply proper treatment. It can also help determine the cause of coma and is used to discriminate antihistamine or tranquilizer overdosage from alcohol toxicity.

Normal values: Normally, there is no measurable amount of alcohol in the body. When less than 0.05 percent of the blood (50 mg per 100 ml) is composed of alcohol, it is usually not considered intoxication in the legal sense.

Abnormal values: Three ounces of an average (86-proof) liquor will usually produce symptoms of intoxication and cause a blood alcohol level of over 0.05 percent, which in many states is sufficient to cause prosecution as "under the influence." Other states have laws that stipulate more than 0.10 percent as evidence of intoxication; a few states insist on alcohol levels of 0.15 percent before issuing a citation. Ten ounces of liquor will usually produce stupor or coma and will cause blood alcohol levels to measure 0.4 percent. Twelve ounces at one time have caused death. Urine levels are always about 50 percent higher than corresponding blood levels. Breath values parallel blood values. It must be pointed out that measurements of blood/breath alcohol do not indicate the amount of alcohol taken into the body but show the blood's concentration of alcohol. Thus, a large, heavy person would have to drink much more than a small, thin person to show the same percentage. The test therefore takes into account the effect of alcohol on the body regardless of size. The exception to this rule, however, can be shown when someone who is not used to drinking takes in a small amount of alcohol; in such a case, the effect on the body and mind may be much greater with small amounts, such as can occur with teenagers.

Abnormally high test values will result if, just prior to inserting the needle to take blood, the technician wipes the skin with alcohol, or if the individual belches while breathing into a bag or measuring device. The use of alcohol-containing mouthwashes, some inhaled asthmatic medications, and in fact, any medicine or substance containing any alcohol (some medicines are 40 proof) prior to a breath test can cause a false result. Some breath tests are also affected by smoking within 15 minutes before the test is performed.

Risk factors: Negligible (see general risk factors for blood testing).

Pain/discomfort: Minimal (see general pain/discomfort factors for blood testing).

Costs: Blood and urine tests for alcohol average $19 to $74; there is often an additional charge if the findings are to be used for medical-legal purposes. Breath tests are most commonly performed by law enforcement officials and rarely by laboratories.

Breath alcohol analyzers are often found in bars; little or nothing is charged for their use.

Accuracy and significance: If performed properly, the test is considered 85 percent reliable. Any evidence that the specimen has been improperly collected, handled, transported, or evaluated in the laboratory usually disqualifies the test result for legal purposes. Urine tests are not as accurate as blood tests; breath tests, when properly performed, are considered as accurate as blood tests. While a false-positive test result is rare for blood alcohol, a true positive test occurs in only about half of all people afflicted with alcoholism. Evidence has shown that blood taken from a vein may show a smaller amount of alcohol than blood taken from an artery because some alcohol may still be stored in muscle tissue at the time of testing. And a recent government study showed that when identical blood alcohol samples were sent to 284 laboratories, the reported results were so divergent as to be relatively useless; the difference more than 70 percent in some cases. Some courts now require evidence that the device used to test for alcohol was properly calibrated before admitting test results in evidence. Should there be a question as to test results at a later date, and the original blood sample is retested, the new values could be much different depending on how the blood sample was stored.

ALCOHOLISM

The **Alcohol** test (whether from blood, breath, or urine) is a measure of the concentration of alcohol in a person at the time the test is taken. It does not in any way indicate whether the patient is a chronic user of alcohol. There are, however, tests that can reveal whether a person is a heavy drinker, or even an alcoholic, in spite of that person's denial. One such test is the measurement of enzymes, either gamma glutamyl transferase (GGT) or gamma glutamyl transpeptidase (GGTP). Others include the folic acid test (see **Folates**), **Uric Acid** test, measurement of **Zinc** levels in the blood or urine, measurement of **Sweat,** and measurement of certain amino acids in the blood, such as alpha-amino-n-butyric acid and glutamate dehydrogenase (GDH), that indicate liver damage.

Another test for alcoholism is measuring acetaldehyde in the blood. While this metabolic product of ethyl alcohol (from the liver) is a strong indication of excessive alcohol use, it can also come from other exposure (industry, perfumes). Virtually none should be found in the blood (some feel 0.1 mg per liter is still within normal limits); with alcoholism, however, 2 or more mg per liter may be the reported value.

Outside the realm of biochemistry, there is the Self-Administered Alcoholism Screening Test (SAAST). Originally known as the Michigan Alcoholism Screening Test, and subsequently modified and improved upon by the Mayo Clinic, the test consists of 35 questions; the answer to each is designated as "alcoholic" or "nonalcoholic." The questions are quite direct; two examples are: "Have you ever lost friendships because of your drinking?" and "Has your wife, husband, or other family member ever gone to anyone for help about your drinking?" When the test was compared with drunken driving arrest records and enzyme measurements, it was found to be about 95 percent accurate.

When performed: Whenever alcoholism is suspected or when patients are admitted to hospitals in coma or undiagnosed unconscious conditions; to aid in uncovering patients who might become alcoholics; to aid in the treatment of patients who show symptoms of alcoholism but who deny drinking; to follow the progress of a patient's therapy.

Normal values: Normal values range from 30 to 45 units per liter (men usually have higher amounts) for GGT; less than 25 units per liter for GGTP. Amino acids have varying normal values.

Abnormal values: GGT will rise to 500 to 1,000 units per liter, depending on how heavily the person has been drinking and for how long; the GGTP enzyme will usually go above 250 units per liter. Normal amino acids will double in alcoholics. It is possible to have false elevated GGT levels after eating excessive simple carbohydrates or from using acetaminophen drugs. Folic acid will decrease, and uric acid will increase. It takes more than 5 ounces of alcohol a day, on a regular basis, to affect these test values; but the greater the alcohol intake, the higher the test value.

Risk factors: Negligible (see general risk factors for blood testing).

Pain/discomfort: Minimal (see general pain/discomfort factors for blood testing).

Cost: A GGT test averages $18; a GGTP test runs $6 to $30. The bile acid Cholylglycine test, sometimes used to determine the extent of liver damage in alcoholism, averages $24. The GGTP test has recently been included in **Comprehensive Multiple Test Screening** panels, which range from $7 to $42.

Accuracy and significance: The GGT test is considered more accurate than the GGTP, but both tests are only considered to have an accuracy rate between 40 and 80 percent. Other causes of liver disease can result in false-positive tests; some people, on the other hand, can consume a dozen drinks a day and still show negative tests. Questionnaire-type tests are considered more accurate than chemical tests—especially for predicting the possibility of future alcoholism. Patients taking antiepileptic drugs may show a false-positive GGT test.

ALDOLASE

Aldolase is an enzyme that helps convert sugar in the muscles to energy. Like another enzyme, **Lactic Dehydrogenase** (LDH), aldolase is found in increased quantities in the blood when there is severe damage to various body tissues, especially muscles. In addition to its concentration in skeletal muscle tissue, aldolase is found in the liver, heart muscle, and red blood cells. Blood is withdrawn from a vein, and the serum is examined.

When performed: Aldolase measurement is used mainly in muscle disorders, particularly in early diagnosis of spinal muscle atrophy conditions.

Normal values: Values vary with the method used. A range of 0 to 12 units per ml is considered normal.

Abnormal values: Aldolase is increased in the blood primarily with polymyositis (infected muscles), muscular dystrophy, acute hepatitis, infectious mononucleosis, crush injury, malignancies (especially liver and prostate), various anemias, heart attack, pulmonary embolism, delirium tremens, stroke, trichinosis, pneumonia, hemorrhagic pancreatitis, and lead intoxication.

Risk factors: Negligible (see general risk factors for blood testing).

Pain/discomfort: Minimal (see general pain/discomfort factors for blood testing).

Cost: About $11.

Accuracy and significance: A not-too-specific test that shows abnormal values in a variety of conditions. Its main purpose seems to be to help confirm an established diagnosis of tissue damage somewhere in the body. Less than 80 percent accurate.

ALDOSTERONE

Aldosterone is a hormone of the adrenal gland that helps control the electrolyte balance (see **Chloride; Potassium; Sodium**) in the body. (Other adrenal hormone groups are the cortisones and the adrenalins.) By keeping sodium (which holds fluid) in and letting potassium out of the body, aldosterone controls the volume of the blood and therefore, in part, blood pressure. Normally, the amount of aldosterone in the body is regulated by **Renin,** an enzyme produced by the kidney; renin, in turn, reacts to blood sodium changes and blood volume. Renin is sometimes measured alone, usually when blood pressure problems are thought to be caused by only one kidney; more often, it is measured with aldosterone as a means of diagnosing where an aldosterone-forming tumor is located. Blood is taken from a vein, and the plasma is tested. Urine is also measured for aldosterone.

When performed: With high blood pressure; when an adrenal tumor is suspected; when there is a constant problem with sodium and/or potassium control; when there is edema (water retention) that cannot be explained.

Normal values: Plasma levels should not exceed 20 ng per 100 ml. Urine levels should be no more than 20 mg per 24-hour specimen. Normal values from various laboratories may differ markedly.

Abnormal values: Elevated aldosterone values (usually along with decreased potassium and increased sodium) indicate hyperaldosteronism, which can come from an adrenal tumor, kidney disease, or liver disease. Elevated levels may also occur following surgery and during pregnancy. Sometimes a salt-loading test is performed: after several days on a salt-free diet, the patient is given a large amount of sodium; normally, this stops production of aldosterone, and the salt is passed out in the urine. With aldosterone problems, the patient's body retains the sodium and becomes edematous.

Risk factors: Negligible (see general risk factors for blood testing).

Pain/discomfort: Minimal (see general pain/discomfort factors for blood testing).

Cost: From $35 to $75 for each test, whether on blood or urine.

Accuracy and significance: Because abnormal values can signify a number of different diseases, the test is most useful in confirming suspected adrenal gland disorder. It is also increasingly used to study possible causes of high blood pressure; its true significance, however, remains somewhat controversial. It is more valuable as a research tool than in making a specific clinical diagnosis. Less than 80 percent accurate. The use of *Potassium* and *Renin* tests to help confirm aldosterism is not considered sufficiently accurate.

ALKALINE PHOSPHATASE

Alkaline phosphatase is an enzyme normally found in the blood. Different forms of this enzyme are also produced in the intestines, liver, and bone cells. Conditions that stimulate bone cell activity and that deposit excess calcium in the bones create elevated alkaline phosphatase levels in the blood. A single test for alkaline phosphatase is usually insufficient for diagnosis; blood levels must be evaluated several times. Blood is usually taken from an arm vein for serum examination. All urine passed in an 8-hour period (usually overnight) may also be tested. In certain rare diseases, alkaline phosphatase is also observed in white blood cells.

When performed: When cancer is suspected; to differentiate the causes of liver disease; following injury; when parathyroid disease is suspected; to study nutritional problems such as vitamin D deficiency.

Normal values: Values vary with the kind of test measurement used: 2 to 4.5 Bodansky units; 0.8 to 2.3 Bessey-Lowry units; 3.0 to 13.0 King-Armstrong units. Normal values are higher in children because of bone growth activity. Adults may show from 20 to 100 IU per L, with the highest normal values found as age increases; older women may show a normal value up to 125 IU per L. Growing children can have a normal value up to 500 IU per L.

Abnormal values: Higher-than-normal values are found with cancerous and noncancerous bone disease, liver disease, blockage of the bile duct system (gallbladder disease), Gaucher's disease (a type of anemia), healing fractures, rickets, leukemia, thyroid gland infection, and hyperparathyroidism; values may also rise during the latter part of pregnancy. Elevated alkaline phosphatase levels are caused by a number of drugs, including male hormones, tranquilizers such as Thorazine, antibiotics such as erythromycin and oxacillin, some antiarthritic drugs such as gold and Indocin, and oral antidiabetic drugs. Birth control pills will also elevate alkaline phosphatase levels.

Lower-than-normal values are found in patients taking too much vitamin D or too little vitamin C and in conditions of poor nutrition. Patients taking Atromid-S to reduce blood cholesterol levels have been reported to have falsely lowered alkaline phosphatase levels, which could mask the diagnosis of certain liver diseases; it has also been noted that patients who take Atromid-S have a much greater incidence of gallbladder disease.

Risk factors: Negligible (see general risk factors for blood testing).

Pain/discomfort: Minimal (see general pain/discomfort factors for blood testing).

Cost: The routine blood alkaline phosphatase test runs $5 to $30. It is usually included in a **Comprehensive Multiple Test Screening** panel, which ranges from $7 to $42. Urine examination averages $25, and testing white blood cells for alkaline phosphatase is about $20. Isoenzyme measurements run from $30 to $80.

Accuracy and significance: This is a very generalized test that shows abnormal values in the presence of so many different diseases that it is really used only for screening, supplementation, and confirmation. The accuracy rate is less than 80 percent. Unfortunately, this test is usually part of *Comprehensive Multiple Test Screening;* unless there is clinical evidence of a related disease, an abnormal test result should not routinely be considered an indication of disease.

Recent research has shown that abnormally elevated levels of this enzyme (from 7 to 30 times the upper limits of normal) have been found to occur in some very young children who showed no explanation for such abnormal values. The values returned to normal after a few weeks, and the children showed no adverse health problems.

The possibility of such false values should be kept in mind to prevent unnecessary, and possibly dangerous, additional testing to try and uncover a false abnormality. Measurement of isoenzymes (related) of alkaline phosphatase as part of **Amniocentesis** seems to be a fairly accurate way to diagnose cystic fibrosis (see **Sweat**) during pregnancy. The accuracy of this test is best shown by a recent study; over a two-year period, of 661 patients who showed an abnormal value, only nine percent had a diagnosis to explain a positive finding. Thus, for screening purposes, the test's true accuracy is less than 10 percent.

ALKALOIDS, see *Drug Abuse*

ALKALOSIS, see *Carbon Dioxide; pH*

ALKAPTONURIA, see *Aminoaciduria*

ALLERGY

Allergy testing, not too many years ago, was limited to "skin tests" (see **Skin Reaction**). A minute amount of a suspected allergy-causing substance in solution was injected just under the skin, and if a small, red swelling resulted, it was interpreted to mean the patient was allergic to that substance—be it a pollen, a food, hair from an animal, or house dust as but a few examples. Patch testing, where the suspected substance was placed on the skin and covered by a small gauze bandage, was but another technique to achieve the same test result. As technology improved, the **RAST** test came about—considered by some, but not all, doctors who specialize in allergy to be the state of the art in diagnosing the cause of allergic symptoms such as wheezing, itching, running nose, watery eyes, headaches, and stomachaches, to name but a very few. Even the elimination diet, where a patient eats only a few prescribed foods for several days and then introduces one suspicious food at a time to measure its allergic effect, is as much a medical test as skin injections or blood **Immunoglobulin** measurements. People with an allergy are said to have an atopic disease; the word *atopy* indicates a predisposition to a hypersensitive reaction when exposed to an *allergen* (another term for *antigen*; see **Agglutination**) such as a weed pollen, wheat, a drop of dog saliva, or even a very cold molecule of air. An allergen can cause symptoms after being inhaled or eaten or simply after skin contact. Respiratory allergens, such as pollens and fungi, may differ in different parts of the country and the world; allergy testing usually takes such geographical areas into consideration. Skin allergies may differ with the age of the patient and may reveal their cause by their location on the body. Food allergy testing must consider ethnic backgrounds as well as heredity, although many allergists feel that virtually all allergies have a genetic component. Then there are people who are allergic to the sun, to heat, to pressure when applied to certain body surfaces, to drugs, and to myriad chemicals—whether in foods, in the air, or at the workplace. Yet another form of allergy testing is called challenge tests, primarily for diagnosing physical urticaria—the skin reactions to sun, heat, cold, pressure, vibrations, etc. that can look like red blotches. Two examples are the ice cube and cold water tests. Susceptible patients who react to cold will usually develop an itching, redness and swelling of the skin about two minutes after an ice cube is pressed against it for a few minutes. After a patient's hand is placed in cold water for several minutes, the blood histamine levels (see **Cancer**) will increase along with the skin reactions. Other tests for allergy include provocation, or challenge, testing, where the suspected allergen is blown into the nose, throat, and lungs—under controlled conditions, because this can be dangerous (see **Pulmonary Function**); this is somewhat similar to the elimination diet for food allergies. Because of the variety and number of allergy tests, the most common ones are listed under their own headings. In addition, the field of allergy has become aligned with **Immunology**, and together both medical specialties also include autoimmune diseases such as lupus erythematosus (see **Antinuclear Antibodies**). At one time, syphilis was called "the great masquerader" because it could imitate almost every disease known; now that ostensible honor has been allotted to allergy because allergy, and immunology, can affect virtually every body organ and cause virtually every symptom known to man and doctor. And then, with all that is now known about allergy testing, a positive test does not always mean a patient is, in fact, allergic to the substance causing the reaction; false-positive results are quite common. Likewise, a negative result can also be false; failure to show a skin or lung reaction does not automatically rule out an allergy to the test substance. Finally, it is well to keep in mind that a delayed reaction to an allergen, such as when skin testing, could be an indication of a loss or failure of the body's immune system and all that could entail (see **Acquired Immunodeficiency Syndrome; Skin Reaction**).

And there are many allergies for which no specific tests exist at the present time. One example is the allergic response to sulfites—chemicals used in food processing and preservation. Sulfites are found in almost all wines, and they may also be in beer, fruit drinks and many medicines. Many restaurants use these chemicals to make foods— especially salads—stay fresh for days. And they are commonly found in cooked seafoods, commercial and restaurant fried potatoes, vegetables, and even some basic ingredients such as gelatin, beet sugar, and cooking starches. Because they are hidden in foods, especially in restaurant food, where there are no ingredient labels to indicate their presence, they have been reported to cause totally unexpected severe reactions, and even deaths, in individuals who have asthma and eat such foods. Some doctors will test their patients for an allergy to sulfites by actually spraying a form of the chemical into the lungs; this can be quite dangerous, however. It is possible to purchase sulfite-detection kits and dipsticks to test foods and beverages before consuming them. It has been estimated that at least 1 million asthmatics are susceptible to this one food chemical alone.

ALPHA-AMINO-N-BUTYRIC ACID, see *Alcoholism*

ALPHA ANTITRYPSIN, see *Albumin/Globulin*

ALPHA CHOLESTEROL, see *Cholesterol*

ALPHA FETOPROTEIN (Fetal Alpha Globulin)

Alpha fetoprotein (AFP) is the primary serum protein (see **Albumin/Globulin**) of the fetus during pregnancy; it usually disappears totally from the newborn's blood immediately after birth. Should it reappear in later life, it most likely indicates liver cell pathology. Blood is taken from a vein, and the serum is tested. Amniotic fluid (the fluid around the fetus) is also tested.

In recent years, testing a pregnant woman's blood for alpha fetoprotein has been employed as a specific screening test for detecting neural tube defects (spina bifida, anencephaly, and encephalocele). Although the FDA approved AFP testing kits in 1984, there is still a great deal of controversy surrounding their use for this purpose. While many obstetricians feel that measuring and following the levels of AFP during pregnancy can help detect certain birth defects in their very early stages, and can even offer information on the health and viability of the fetus, there have been a great many false-positive and false-negative results. The basic problem is, of course, whether the test result prompts an abortion. Naturally, an abnormal test result should be confirmed by other tests such as **Ultrasound** and **Amniocentesis**. There are many who feel this test should be required or routine once during pregnancy, and some states are considering regular screening programs.

Some doctors even believe that alpha fetoprotein testing should be performed several times on the blood of women during pregnancy. By measuring the changes in the mother-to-be's blood, preferably monthly, it may be possible to predict premature births, low birth weights, and growth retardation in the fetus. Other doctors, however, feel that since the test has only a 60 percent sensitivity or relative accuracy, insufficient knowledge is gained to justify continuous monitoring of this fetal-produced protein.

When performed: When liver disease, especially liver cell cancer, is suspected; when a cancer (most likely from the ovary or testicle) is thought to have spread to the liver; as a means of following the progress of therapy in the treatment of hepatitis; on amniotic fluid, see **Amniocentesis**.

Starting in 1986, California will require that all pregnant women be offered the opportunity to have blood testing for alpha fetoprotein; participation in the testing program, however, will be voluntary.

Normal values: Normally, no alpha fetoprotein is found in the blood except in pregnancy. During pregnancy up to 2.5 mg per 100 ml may be detected in the amniotic fluid, depending on the month of gestation.

Abnormal values: Any amount found in the blood serum of an adult (young children may still have a trace) is abnormal and commonly indicates a liver cell cancer; however, it can on occasion be found in other cancers and thus is not an absolute diagnostic indicator. It sometimes appears during recovery from hepatitis. When alpha fetoprotein is increased in amniotic fluid, it can indicate a problem with the fetus such as spinal cord defects.

Risk factors: Negligible when blood is tested (see general risk factors for blood testing). With examination of amniotic fluid, see general risk factors for catheter and needle insertion. When testing for fetal defects, the risk of false results must always be kept in mind, especially when abortion may be under consideration. Recent reports have shown that simply considering or undergoing the test can cause a great deal of anxiety in pregnant women—to the point of increased smoking and increased drug and alcohol use—thereby possibly causing direct damage to the fetus.

Pain/discomfort: Minimal when blood is tested (see general pain/discomfort factors for blood testing). With examination of amniotic fluid for alpha fetoprotein, see general pain/discomfort factors for catheter and needle insertion.

Cost: From $5 to $40, whether of blood or amniotic fluid.

Accuracy and significance: Considered 90 percent accurate in revealing ovarian and testicular tumors, 80 percent accurate for liver cancer, and about 60 percent accurate for other conditions. When the test is properly performed, any abnormal values found in amniotic fluid are considered very significant. Unfortunately, poor technical procedures lead to false abnormal values.

Note: In a research report issued in 1985, of 15,000 women screened for serum alpha fetoprotein levels during pregnancy, 9,000 had elevated, or abnormal, results. Of those who underwent a second test for the protein, almost half had normal test results (49 percent of those with an abnormal first test chose **Ultrasound** as a means of verifying the alpha fetoprotein levels). This is but one more justification for not automatically accepting a single abnormal test result. The study also points out that such tests should be limited to those with some obvious reason (suspicious history, previous abnormality) for testing rather than making the test a routine screening.

ALPHA HYDROXYBUTYRIC DEHYDROGENASE, see *Hydroxybutyric Dehydrogenase*

ALPHA TOCOPHEROL, see *Tocopherols*

ALPHA-2 MACROGLOBULIN, see *Macroglobulin*

ALPHA WAVE, see *Electroencephalogram*

ALT, see *Aspartate Aminotransferase*

ALTERNATIVE TO AMNIOCENTESIS (ATA), see *Amniocentesis*

ALZHEIMER'S DISEASE, see *Cognitive Capacity Screening*

AMBLYOPIA, see *Visual Acuity*

AMBULATORY BLOOD PRESSURE, see *Blood pressure*

AMBULATORY ELECTROCARDIOGRAPHY MONITORING, see *Electrocardiogram*

AMBULATORY ESOPHAGEAL pH MONITORING (Telemetry), see *Gastroesophageal Reflux*

AMEBIASIS, see *Agglutination*

AMETROPIA, see *Visual Acuity*

AMINOACIDURIA

Abnormal amounts of amino acids appear in the urine whenever there are certain inborn (inherited) errors of metabolism. There are nearly 2,000 known inherited diseases of this type (see, for example, **Phenylketonuria**), but only about two dozen have regular test procedures. There are also a few similar conditions that are acquired after birth. Each condition has some unique way of manifesting itself. For example, cystinuria causes kidney stones; alkaptonuria causes a form of arthritis; Hartnup's disease is primarily a skin condition; maple syrup urine disease (so named because the urine takes on a maple syrup odor) can cause convulsions; homocystinuria can bring about eye problems; tyrosinemia causes liver and kidney disease; and histidinemia victims have speech defects.

In most instances because of the missing enzyme, the kidney cannot handle the faulty metabolism of certain amino acids from proteins that are eaten. There is also a degree of mental retardation associated with many of these difficulties. Urine and blood may be screened for general amino acid abnormalities, but in most instances, tests for specific amino acid excess are performed on the basis of the patient's symptoms.

When performed: Most often on newborn infants, but also on young children (occasionally on adults with appropriate symptoms) who show signs of retardation or other inherited abnormalities. The following states require screening of newborn infants for one or more of the various aminoacidurias: Alaska, Arizona, Colorado, Connecticut, Delaware, Florida, Georgia, Idaho, Iowa, Maine, Maryland, Massachusetts, Montana, Nevada, New Hampshire, New Mexico, New York, Ohio, Oregon, Texas, Wisconsin, Wyoming, and the District of Columbia. In most states, if parents present a written objection, the requirement will be waived.

Normal values: Each of the 29 amino acids and their metabolites has a different normal value. In the blood, the levels are usually high at birth and lessen with age. In the urine, the opposite is the rule.

Abnormal values: Increased amounts in the plasma and urine not only help diagnose the condition but can also indicate specific dietary treatment, which is usually successful.

Risk factors: Negligible (see general risk factors for blood testing).

Pain/discomfort: Minimal (see general pain/discomfort factors for blood testing).

Cost: For generalized screening or qualitative testing, the cost is about $14. For quantitative measurements of amino acids performed on blood or urine, the fees are approximately $200.

Accuracy and significance: The tests are extremely accurate (95 percent) in the detection and measurement of amino acids, but they must be carefully correlated with the patient's family history, symptoms, and signs.

Note: For other legally required newborn screening tests, see: **Galactosemia, Genetic Disorder Screening, Hemoglobin, Phenylketonuria, Red Blood Cell, Thyroid Function.**

AMINOPYRINE BREATH, see *Lactose Tolerance*

AMMONIA

Ammonia is usually produced in the liver, intestines, and kidneys as an end product of protein metabolism. The liver converts ammonia into urea to be excreted by the kidneys. In liver disease, the conversion of ammonia to urea is diminished, producing an increase in blood ammonia levels. Whole blood from a vein is examined. Ammonia may be measured in the urine by taking a sample of all urine passed during a 24-hour period.

When performed: If there is suspicion of liver disease or other conditions that affect liver function. Some doctors also test for glutamine (an amino acid) in **Cerebrospinal Fluid** as a means of noting how much ammonia is affecting the brain.

Normal values: Values vary with different laboratories, but generally 75 mcg per 100 ml of blood is considered normal. The urine usually contains up to 1 g in a 24-hour sample. In international units (IU), the range is from 10 to 35 micromol per L.

Abnormal values: Blood ammonia is increased in liver disease, especially in portal system encephalopathy or abnormal mental states due to poor liver function. It may also be elevated when patients are taking diuretics (thiazides, Diamox) and antibiotics (methicillin) or when there is an increase in certain amino acids (from proteins) in the blood, usually an inherited condition. Decreased levels of ammonia are found in patients taking certain mood-elevating drugs and some antibiotics.

Risk factors: Negligible (see general risk factors for blood testing).

Pain/discomfort: Minimal (see general pain/discomfort factors for blood testing).

Cost: Blood tests for ammonia average $23 to $55; urine tests are about $20.

Accuracy and significance: Abnormal blood ammonia levels are quite specific (90 percent) indicators of liver disease, especially when abnormal mental states are obvious. However, many different drugs produce such variations in ammonia levels that they must be taken into account if the test is to have significance.

AMNIOCENTESIS

Studying the amniotic fluid (the fluid that surrounds the fetus during pregnancy) is becoming commonplace when it is suspected that a child might be born with an inherited defect. In the United States, more than 100,000 children are born each year with some form of developmental disability. The fetus gives off cells while growing, and these cells can be studied directly. The test is usually performed early in pregnancy (after 15 weeks), but it can also be done before delivery to ensure that the fetus is sufficiently mature to survive.

After locating the exact position of the fetus, usually with the **Ultrasound** test, the physician places a long, thin needle through the abdomen into the uterus and withdraws the fluid.

Many different metabolic conditions can be diagnosed prior to birth (Down's syndrome, **Tay-Sachs Disease,** some malformations). The process is called karyotyping **(Chromosome Analysis)**, or comparing the fetal chromosome size, shape, and number to what is known to be normal, thus predicting the genetic status of the unborn infant. Chromosome analysis is also performed on blood samples from young children and adults when there are sex identification problems or a question of an inherited abnormality. The same type of test can be performed on blood cells and other body tissues. (The Tay-Sachs blood-screening test for potential parents can help determine the probability of having children with Tay-Sachs disease.) The test can usually determine the sex of the fetus, but many people do not wish to know this fact before birth (also see **Pregnancy**).

Amniotic fluid is also tested for **Alpha Fetoprotein** and **Bilirubin**.

In 1985, researchers at Michigan State University developed a way to perform chromosomal analysis of the fetus from a sample of the pregnant mother's blood. They claim it is effective when the fetus is only 8 to 12 weeks old. The test is called "alternative to amniocentesis" (ATA) and is claimed to be much safer, as well as far less expensive; it costs about $150.

When performed: The test is especially applicable to pregnant women over 35 years of age, families who have relatives with metabolic problems, families who have children born with Down's syndrome, and families who have past indications of chromosome abnormalities. It is also used when there have been cases of mental retardation in the family; when there is a question of an Rh problem; to offer genetic counseling early enough in pregnancy; to determine the sex and maturity of the unborn child. On rare occasions, it may be performed during the last 3 months of pregnancy to test for blood grouping problems, as a means of evaluating the maturity of the fetus, or if there is suspicion of an infection inside the uterus. At this stage of a pregnancy, the test is considered to be quite dangerous and should be performed only when there are no other means of obtaining vital information. (Also see **Genetic Disorder Screening.**)

Normal values: Chromosomal analysis shows no defect.

Abnormal values: When chromosomal patterns show either excessive or missing genes; when certain genes are translocated or found on the wrong chromosomes; when chromosomes are broken. More than 400 different metabolic diseases may now be diagnosed through chromosome analysis, and additional congenital abnormalities continue to be discovered yearly.

An excess of alpha fetoprotein in amniotic fluid usually indicates a neurological defect; the degree of increase in bilirubin helps predict how serious an Rh baby's condition will be after birth.

Risk factors: Needle injury to the fetus, bleeding, and/or infection occur in less than 1 percent of tests performed. There is a risk of 1 out of every 200 fetuses being aborted by the test.

Pain/discomfort: Minimal (see general pain/discomfort factors for catheter and needle insertion).

Cost: The entire procedure—including the doctor's services, ultrasound to ensure proper placement of the needle, and a complete analysis of chromosomes and pertinent chemicals—averages $700 to $900. Chromosome analysis alone is $500 to $600.

This test is usually performed in a hospital because of the equipment required; hospitalization also allows for careful, continuous observation of the patient following the test.

Accuracy and significance: Generally the test is considered 95 percent accurate in its ability to detect inherited defects in fetuses. Even sex determination is not 100 percent accurate; errors have occurred in 1 out of 20 tests.

AMNIOGRAPHY see *Radiography*

AMOEBA, see *Parasite*

AMPHETAMINES, see *Drug Abuse*

AMSLER GRID, see *Visual Acuity*

AMYLASE

Amylase (composed of several enzymes used in the digestion of starch) is normally found in very small amounts in blood serum. It is produced in the pancreas, the salivary glands, the fallopian tubes, and mostly in the liver. Blood is drawn from an arm vein, and the serum is examined. The urine is also tested.

When performed: When abdominal pain suggests pancreatitis; for mumps, pancreas duct obstruction, acute renal (kidney) insufficiency, and intestinal obstruction.

Normal values: Normal serum levels range from 80 to 150 Somogyi units per 100 ml. Normal urine shows from 1,000 to 5,000 Somogyi units per 24-hour sample.

Abnormal values: Amylase levels are increased primarily with pancreatitis, pancreas duct obstruction, salivary gland or duct problems (mumps), perforated ulcer, intestinal obstruction, and renal insufficiency. Amylase levels may also be elevated by certain drugs, including codeine, a large amount of alcohol, indomethacin (Indocin), meperidine (Demerol), morphine, pentazocine (Talwin), and thiazide diuretics. An elevated amylase level becomes even more specific for pancreatitis if the urine shows an increase in amylase clearance by the kidneys when compared with **Creatinine** clearance. Amylase levels may be lower than normal in hepatitis or liver damage or when there is trauma to or deficient functioning of the pancreas so that it is unable to produce the enzyme.

Risk factors: Negligible (see general risk factors for blood testing).

Pain/discomfort: Minimal (see general pain/discomfort factors for blood testing).

Cost: From $6 to $40 for the testing of blood or urine.

Some health insurance companies and government-sponsored medical programs will not reimburse the doctor or patient for certain parts of the test, usually because they are still of an experimental nature.

Accuracy and significance: Considered from 70 to 80 percent accurate. Although amylase is the primary laboratory test to diagnose pancreatic disease, it is known to show false-positive results in patients with acute alcoholic intoxication. In order to maintain a high degree of accuracy, should there be any doubt about the diagnosis, the different forms of amylase isoenzymes (the S type from the salivary glands and the P type from the pancreas) must be determined.

Note: Within the past few years, less and less reliance has been placed on this test as an aid to diagnosing pancreatitis (see **Pancreas Function**); it is now used primarily to rule out this disease when it shows a normal result in patients who have physical signs of pancreas dysfunction. Most doctors now feel that this test must be done in series—over a period of hours or days—along with **Lipase** testing to have any significance, and even then, it is not considered as reliable as it once was.

AMYL NITRATE INHALATION, see *Finger Wrinkle*

AMYLOIDOSIS, see *Congo Red*

ANA, see *Antinuclear Antibodies*

ANDROGEN RECEPTOR, see *Estrogen Receptor*

ANEMIA, see *Bone Marrow; Hemoglobin; Red Blood Cell*

ANERGY, see *Skin Reaction*

ANGIOGRAPHY, see *Radiography*

ANGIOTENSIN, see *Renin*

ANGIOTENSIN-CONVERTING ENZYME, see *Renin*

ANION GAP, see *Lactic Acid*

ANISOMETROPIA, see *Visual Acuity*

ANTHROPOMETRIC MEASUREMENTS

While weight measurements and their changes, especially in relation to height and body build, have always been a test of general well-being as well as an indirect indicator of disease (the weight loss associated with **Cancer** and the weight gain associated with alterations in **Thyroid Function** are but two examples), more specific weight-related tests have come into being. They are generally referred to as anthropometric measurements and are a means of assessing body composition in terms of percentages of fat and protein. The most common measurement is skinfold thickness. Here, using skinfold calipers (similar to any measuring calipers, such as used by machinists, carpenters, and artists), the thickness of the skin and its underlying fat are measured. The skin is pulled away from any muscle or other tissue beneath it, and its thickness is considered a reasonable indication of overall body fat. The middle of the upper arm is the most usual site for such measurements, and when skinfold thickness is considered along with the circumference of the upper middle arm, it offers valuable clues to **Malnutrition,** malabsorption, protein depletion, anemia, **Depression,** and possible reasons for obesity (see **Xylose Tolerance**). Some doctors, when using a caliper to measure skinfold thickness, may prefer to take their measurements from just under the shoulder blade (subscapula), just above the hipbone (supra-iliac), or the fat pad over the spinal cord where the neck ends and the back begins; others will use the abdomen, chest (usually just in front of the armpit), or even the thigh. One problem that has arisen is that skinfold measurements taken from different parts of the body may not always agree or give consistent findings. Thus, the same test performed by different doctors or technicians may not give the same results. The observations, therefore, must be applied within the context of the particular measurer's standards.

Infrared interactance is yet another way of estimating body composition—primarily the body's fat content. The technique uses a spectrograph over a selected part of the body that acts somewhat as **Computerized Tomography**; it is relatively safe and causes no discomfort.

Other tests to determine the percentage of fat and muscle in the body include **Ultrasound, Computerized Tomography,** and various chemical measurements in the blood **(Calcium, Potassium).** A more recent technique uses bioelectrical impedance measurements and is based on the fact that fatty tissues conduct electricity quite differently from nonfatty tissues, such as muscle. Here, electrodes are placed on the skin—usually on the wrists and ankles—and in a sense, the resistance (impedance) of the body's tissues to a tiny electrical current is said to reveal the percentage of body water, fat, and lean or muscle substance. This test can also reflect body changes due to diet, exercise, or disease states, and it has been applied to dehydration, edema, and other problems related to hydration of body tissues. There are also specific tests to measure the size of fat cells to indicate whether fatty tissue is normal or not as an indication of certain pathologies. With this test, a piece of fatty tissue is surgically removed (see **Biopsy**) and then studied with an image analyzing computer.

Weighing an individual underwater is another way of determining the body's fat in relation to total weight; called hydrostatic weighing, it is considered the most accurate way of ascertaining body composition, but it requires a fairly large laboratory tank sufficient to hold the entire body underwater while attached to a scale and is not very comfortable for the patient.

When performed: To help assess the cause of weight loss that cannot be explained by diet or activity; to assess the nutritional status of an individual, particularly someone elderly, after surgery or prolonged illness and even prior to surgery; when various malnutrition conditions are suspected, including such unusual diseases as maramus and kwashiorkor (inadequate protein intake). And such measurements may be employed in an attempt to uncover the cause of obesity. These tests are also used with athletes as a means of evaluating muscle power and to determine the desirable weight of an individual in relation to activities such as athletics, as a means of evaluating fitness, as a corollary observation in certain illnesses such as diabetes, and as a part of many rehabilitation programs. Such measurements have been shown to help athletes improve their abilities; certain sports seem to require different body fat levels for the most efficient performance.

Normal values: These must be determined using the individual's weight, height, body build, body frame, age, and sex; thus, it is impossible to cite normal values for any individual. There are tables that combine all relevant factors, allowing easy access to a normal range for the person under study; women usually average about 23 percent body fat, while men average about 15 percent. Women athletes, however, may normally have much less body fat as a percentage of their body weight; tennis players average 20 percent, while runners and gymnasts average only 9 percent.

Abnormal values: A determination that the percentage of body fat or protein tissue is either in excess of or less than what would be considered normal for the individual's age, sex, height, and weight, along with the present state of health and nutrition.

Risk factors: Essentially none; for fat cell size measurements, see **Biopsy**.

Pain/discomfort: Essentially none; even the electrical current is rarely noticed. For fat cell size measurements, see **Biopsy**.

Cost: When performed in a doctor's office, there is rarely a charge for skinfold caliper measurements. When performed by a nutritionist or as part of an overall obesity study, there may be a $25 to $50 charge for any of the tests. **Biopsy** charges are in addition to microscopic studies, which run from $10 to $50.

Accuracy and significance: None of the tests is considered very precise, but they are the most accurate (about 70 percent) available; most have been somewhat standardized after being compared to underwater weighing. Despite their lack of precision, they are being used increasingly in cases of obesity, as a guide to nutritional status—particularly in the elderly, in patients of all ages prior to surgery or other drastic forms of therapy such as X-ray or tumor chemotherapy, and as an adjunct way of assessing patients with anemia and other debilitating diseases. Some doctors use these tests as a means of uncovering vitamin and/or mineral deficiencies.

A French study showed that when skinfold fat measurements in the upper part of the body are greater than in the lower part (thigh), it signified a susceptibility to heart disease. A Swedish study showed that when skinfold fat around the abdomen was greater than around the thighs in men, they were predisposed to diabetes.

Note: In 1986, the scheduled Anthropometric Standardization Conference is expected to publish the first standards as to how, and where, to perform skinfold testing.

ANTIBIOTIC SENSITIVITY, see *Culture*

ANTIBODY, see *Agglutination; Complement Fixation; Immunoglobulin; Immunology*

ANTICOAGULANT, see *Prothrombin Time*

ANTICONVULSANT DRUG, see *Drug Monitoring*

ANTIDEOXYRIBONUCLEASE-B TITER, see *Antistreptolysin O Titer*

ANTIDIURETIC HORMONE, see *Vasopressin*

ANTIFREEZE, see *Methanol*

ANTIGLOBULIN, see *Agglutination*

ANTIHEMOPHILIAC FACTOR, see *Fibrinogen*

ANTILYMPHOCYTE ANTIBODIES, see *Acquired Immunodeficiency Syndrome*

ANTINUCLEAR ANTIBODIES (ANA)
Antigens such as bacteria, toxins, tissue cells, or foreign proteins are provocative factors in many illnesses. They induce the body to produce antibodies to fight the antigens. The antibodies attempt to combine with the antigens in order to neutralize them. In certain rare and unique diseases, the body's immune system, whose main function is to resist disease, produces antibodies to parts of the patient's own body. These antibodies are special forms of gamma globulins called **Immunoglobulins** and seem to affect all parts of the body that have nucleoprotein, especially muscles and skin. They are called antinuclear antibodies and are found most commonly in people with systemic lupus erythematosus (SLE); they may also be found in people who have relatives suffering from SLE but who do not themselves have the disease.

Blood is taken from a vein, and the serum is examined under the microscope after a fluorescent dye is added. Antinuclear antibodies will appear to fluoresce if they are present. When the ANA test is positive, the serum is then diluted, first in half, then in a 1:4 dilution, a 1:8 dilution, a 1:16 dilution, and so on. The weaker the dilution that fluoresces, the more positive the test.

The lupus erythematosus (LE) cell test is a form of ANA test that is sometimes more specific for SLE. It is considered "positive" when an antinuclear antibody combines with white blood cells and offers a characteristic LE cell picture (grouping) when viewed under the microscope. Several LE cells must be seen to constitute a positive test. Eighty percent of people with SLE have positive LE cell tests.

Another, more recent test, for SLE is the lupus band test. Here, a **Biopsy** is taken of the skin, usually of the inside forearm—particularly if the skin has been exposed to sunlight—and a specific **Immunoglobulin** zone just beneath the skin is searched for under the microscope after special staining. As with ANA testing, many other, somewhat related conditions such as vasculitis, hepatitis, and some allergic reactions can also cause a false-positive indication of SLE, but when combined with the other tests, the lupus band can be of great help in making this difficult diagnosis. Some doctors use this test to monitor patients who have SLE to note when the disease is in its active or passive stage.

When performed: The ANA test is used primarily when there is suspicion of systemic lupus erythematosus (SLE). It is also performed when a patient has a variety of unexplained symptoms such as mysterious rash, arthritis, or chest pains that cannot easily be diagnosed.

Normal values: Antinuclear antibodies are not usually found in the blood. Their presence, though, does not always mean disease, as when found in close relatives of people with SLE.

Abnormal values: Abnormal levels are found mostly with SLE, which usually produces the highest titers (the presence of ANA in the weakest dilutions of serum); scleroderma (marked thickening of the skin) and rheumatoid arthritis usually cause ANA to be observed but in much lower titers (very little dilution). Some forms of kidney disease and certain infections of the pleura (lining around the lungs) can cause ANA. Many drugs can cause a false-positive test: certain thiazide diuretics, almost all antibiotics (penicillin, Terramycin, isoniazid), some tranquilizers such as Taractin, the oral contraceptive pills, a few drugs used to treat high blood pressure (Apresoline), and procainamide, which is used primarily to treat heartbeat irregularities but is sometimes used as an unproven youth restorer. The presence of ANA may be masked or hidden (false-negative) even with disease if the patient is taking steroid drugs.

Risk factors: Negligible (see general risk factors for blood testing).

Pain/discomfort: Minimal (see general pain/discomfort factors for blood testing).

Cost: From $15 to $60. Occasionally included in **Comprehensive Multiple Test Screening** panels, which range from $7 to $42. The LE cell test averages $30.

Accuracy and significance: Although it is not considered a very specific test (less than 80 percent accurate), it is used to help confirm the diagnosis of systemic lupus erythematosus (SLE). The absence of antinuclear antibodies is probably of greater significance in excluding a diagnosis of SLE. There are many other, much more valuable tests to help diagnose SLE and other unusual skin conditions.

ANTISPERM ANTIBODIES, see *Semen*

ANTISTREPTOLYSIN O (ASO) TITER

Streptococcal infection such as sore throat causes production of a number of antibodies (the body's defense reaction) that can be detected in the blood. One of these is antistreptolysin O. Blood from a vein is withdrawn, and the serum is examined.

Starting in 1984, a new, rapid (less than 5 minutes) test for streptococcal infections became available. Using latex agglutination techniques (see **Agglutination**), it became possible for the doctor to take a throat swab (a sample of the lining of the back of the throat obtained by using dacron on the end of a stick) and determine if the causative bacteria are of the group that could lead to rheumatic fever and kidney disease. This test is considered better than 90 percent accurate and costs the doctor less than $2. The American Heart Association claims that, even with the antibiotics available, more than 10,000 people will still die from rheumatic fever each year because of a failure to recognize this bacteria early enough. And in a survey recently conducted in one state, 17 percent of all throat cultures were positive for the dangerous strain of streptococcus.

Another way of detecting a recent streptococcal infection is by examining the blood for antideoxyribonuclease-B (ADN-B). This search for streptococcal antibodies (see **Agglutination**) is considered more accurate than ASO, but it has only recently been put to use.

When performed: The test is used primarily when rheumatic fever or kidney disease (glomerulonephritis) is suspected as a complication of recent streptococcal infection. A single antibody test is usually insufficient to establish a recent infection. Several serial tests are necessary to show the sudden rise in the antibodies.

Normal values: Normally, antistreptolysin O antibodies are not present or, if present, are found in negligible amounts, usually under 150 Todd units per ml.

Abnormal values: ASO is elevated after a recent streptococcal infection. More than 175 Todd units per ml is indicative of such infection, but of even greater importance is an increasing value over several days' time. High readings have also been found in hepatitis, biliary obstruction, and nephrosis.

Risk factors: Negligible (see general risk factors for blood testing).

Pain/discomfort: Minimal (see general pain/discomfort factors for blood testing).

Cost: From $11 to $35. ADN-B tests run from $17 to $45.

Accuracy and significance: The test helps to confirm a suspected streptococcal infection. It is significant only when two or more tests are performed two to three weeks apart. Because elevated values are also found in several other conditions, ASO accuracy can only be considered to be about 50 percent.

ANTITHROMBIN III

Antithrombin III (ATIII; A-THR3) is one of the body's plasma proteins (a globulin), which slows down or stops the clotting of blood. It is assumed that the drug heparin works as an anticoagulant by activating the body's antithrombin III. In 1965, a deficiency of antithrombin III was discovered in certain young patients who were unusually susceptible to clotting disease and who suffered and even died from unexplained thrombosis in blood vessels (phlebitis) and blood clots that traveled to the lungs (pulmonary emboli). The condition is believed to be inherited, and the disease can now be treated. The test is performed on blood, most often taken from an arm vein.

When performed: Whenever there are repeated episodes of phlebitis (blood clots in a vein), thrombus (clots in an artery), especially in people under the age of 30, and on family members once the condition is diagnosed or suspected; when patients do not react to anticoagulant drugs; prior to surgery.

Normal values: 20 to 45 mg per 100 ml, or from 70 to 140 percent of the value obtained from a normal control serum.

Abnormal values: Less than 20 mg per 100 ml, or less than 70 percent of a control value.

Risk factors: Negligible (see general risk factors for blood testing).

Pain/discomfort: Minimal (see general pain/discomfort factors for blood testing).

Cost: From $35 to $80.

Accuracy and significance: The test is considered 95 percent accurate and very significant, as it can be lifesaving, especially when performed for difficulties of clotting following surgery.

ANTITHYROID ANTIBODY, see Thyroid Function

APEXCARDIOGRAM (ACG)

An apexcardiogram is a variation of the standard **Electrocardiogram** (ECG). In the apexcardiogram, a transducer (an electrical device that detects pressure, vibrations, and temperature and translates that energy into recordable tracings to be viewed) is applied to the chest just above the heart. (The apex of the heart is the point that is usually lowest and farthest to the left—what might graphically be described as the "point" of the heart's shape.)

In essence, the apexcardiograph picks up and records the same heart contraction vibrations that can sometimes be seen on the surface of the chest and that can be felt when a hand is applied to the area. The ACG is considered noninvasive, since it is an external technique and the heart itself is not touched directly. An apexcardiogram is rarely ever performed without an accompanying **Phonocardiogram** (the same instrument is used to perform this test) and an **Electrocardiogram**.

A somewhat analogous form of apexcardiography is called kinetocardiography. This test, which some say is a bit more sensitive, requires a much more complicated apparatus. The kinetocardiograph records from a fixed point above a patient's chest (not directly touching the body), while the apexcardiograph can be directed specifically to the heart's apex.

When performed: To graphically identify the vibrations made by heart sounds, especially when abnormal ones are suspected; to verify heart valve disease; to detect tumors of the heart muscle.

Normal values: As with the ECG, the rises and falls of the lines (waves) produced by the instrument are translated into normalcy, suspicion of, or indication of disease by virtue of the experience of the physician interpreting the waves. Patients who are quite fat or who have large, barrel chests from emphysema may not produce sufficient waves for interpretation.

Abnormal values: The recordings show abnormalities in the way the blood travels through the heart; when there is disease, various notches and interruptions in the normally smooth, consistent recorded lines (waves) are evident. Heart valve problems are particularly detectable by this technique, as are abnormal pressure changes within the heart's chambers.

Risk factors: Negligible (see general risk factors concerning electrical instruments).

Pain/discomfort: Minimal. Requires the patient to lie motionless for prolonged periods of time.

Cost: From $25 to $50; approximately $100 when performed at the same time as a phonocardiogram and standard electrocardiogram.

This test is usually performed in a hospital or research facility because of the equipment that is required.

Accuracy and significance: The test is 95 percent accurate in diagnosing heart pathology when it is performed with a phonocardiogram and an electrocardiogram.

APHAKIA, see *Visual Acuity*

APHASIA, see *Language Function*

APNEA MONITORING, see *Sleep Monitoring*

APOLIPOPROTEINS, see *Lipoproteins*

APPLANATION, see *Tonometry*

ARBOVIRUS, see *Virus Disease*

ARC, see *Acquired Immunodeficiency Syndrome*

ARGENTAFFINOMA, see *Serotonin*

ARGININE-INSULIN, see *Growth Hormone*

ARGININE VASOPRESSIN, see *Cancer*

ARGYLL-ROBERTSON, see *Pupillary Reflex*

ARMY GENERAL CLASSIFICATION, see *Intelligence Quotient*

ARSENIC, see *Mercury*

ART, see *Syphilis*

ARTHRITIS, see *Rheumatoid Factor; Synovial Fluid*

ARTHROCENTESIS, see *Synovial Fluid, Thoracentesis*

ARTHROGRAPHY, see *Radiography*

ARTHROSCOPY, see *Endoscopy*

ARV, see *Acquired Immunodeficiency Syndrome*

ASCORBIC ACID (Vitamin C)

Because of a genetically transmitted defect, the human is one of very few mammals that cannot manufacture its own vitamin C. Although ascorbic acid is not stored in large amounts in the body, it is still essential to the body's defense mechanisms (resistance to all forms of disease) and to the formation of bones and teeth. While scurvy (severe vitamin C deficiency disease) is relatively uncommon, slight deficiencies do exist today. Anemia may occur in infants with vitamin C deficiency. Cancer patients often have low blood ascorbic acid levels even with an adequate diet and vitamin supplements. Blood is collected from a vein, and the plasma is examined. Urinary ascorbic acid may also be examined.

When performed: In patients who present scurvylike symptoms (fatigue, loss of appetite, small hemorrhages under the skin and in the gums, hair problems); in patients with severe burns, infections, or malignancies.

Normal values: Normal values range from 0.6 to 2 mg per 100 ml of plasma, reflecting the 5 g of vitamin C normally found in the body; 20 mg of ascorbic acid is usually excreted daily in the urine.

Abnormal values: Lower-than-normal values are found with scurvy, cancer, severe infections, and alcoholism. Vitamin C deficiency is also found in infants fed only milk and in patients with hiatal hernia.

Risk factors: Negligible (see general risk factors for blood testing).

Pain/discomfort: Minimal (see general pain/discomfort factors for blood testing).

Cost: From $1 to $15 for a test on the blood or urine.

Accuracy and significance: The test is only about 50 percent accurate as it relates to a broad spectrum of medical conditions. Test results showing a deficiency in vitamin C have little significance as a specific medical diagnosis. The relation of vitamin C to cancer remains in the research stage.

ASO, see *Antistreptolysin O Titer*

ASPARTATE AMINOTRANSFERASE (AST)

Aspartate aminotransferase was formerly known as serum glutamic oxalacetic transaminase (SGOT); only the name has been changed, albeit many doctors still use the now out-of-date designation. The same goes for alanine aminotransferase (ALT), the new name for serum glutamic pyruvic transaminase (SGPT). In spite of the name change, they are still the same enzymes that are released into the bloodstream when there is tissue or organ damage, primarily of the heart and liver, but also with muscle damage and as a consequence of **Virus Diseases, Pancreas Function** disorders, surgical procedures, and a host of infectious diseases, including trichinosis and Legionnaires' disease. Kidney, brain, and lung pathology, the use of many drugs, and an excessive intake of alcohol can also cause an increase of these enzymes in the blood. As a general rule, AST is measured more as an indication of heart disease; ALT is considered more of a sign of liver problems. But these tests are so nonspecific that false-positive results can occur if a patient is standing, as opposed to reclining, when blood from a vein is taken for serum measurements. Usually, serial measurements must be made; the AST enzyme increases over a period of 24 to 36 hours after an injury or heart attack and then slowly returns to normal levels.

When performed: Primarily when there is suspected heart damage and to follow the course of the illness after a heart attack. ALT is used as a general screening test when liver disease is suspected, as a surreptitious means of checking a patient for

Alcoholism, when there is an unexplained infection, and as a general screening test on a well person to justify subsequent testing for possible latent disease. Usually, both enzymes, AST and ALT, are tested for at the same time.

Normal values: There is some discrepancy about what levels are normal; at present, any AST value from 10 to 40 units per liter or U/L can be considered within normal limits, although some doctors feel 30 U/L or more indicates disease. Infants and children may have values up to 80 U/L and still be normal. ALT values are usually less; from 5 to 30 U/L are thought to be within normal limits.

Abnormal values: After a heart attack, AST levels may reach well over 100 U/L and remain high for several days. With liver diseases, especially hepatitis, ALT values can exceed 2,000 U/L. Again, the two enzymes are measured at the same time, and with heart disease, AST is higher than ALT; with liver disease, the opposite is more common. Abnormally high values are also suggestive of a host of other, unspecified, conditions. Lower-than-normal values are sometimes found as a side effect of many medicines and with **Pyridoxine** deficiency.

Risk factors: Negligible (see general risk factors for blood testing).

Pain/discomfort: Minimal (see general pain/discomfort factors for blood testing).

Cost: From $4 to $24 for either the AST or ALT; either or both enzyme measurements are usually included in **Comprehensive Multiple Test Screening** panels, which range from $7 to $42.

Accuracy and significance: Although these tests are commonly performed, they reflect so many different diseases and conditions that they have no real significance. They are being applied less and less to help diagnose heart attacks (see **Creatine Phosphokinase** and **Lactic Dehydrogenase**). And there are so many situations that can cause false-positive and false-negative results that the tests are no longer considered sufficiently accurate (less than 60 percent) to help pinpoint a diagnosis.

ASPERGILLOSIS, see *Agglutination; Skin Reaction*

ASPERGILLUS, see *Agglutination*

ASPIRATION BIOPSY, see *Biopsy*

ASPIRIN, see *Salicylates*

ASPIRIN ALLERGY, see *Tartrazine Sensitivity*

AST, see *Aspartate Aminotransferase*

ASTHMA, see *Allergy; Pulmonary Function; RAST; Skin Reaction*

ASTIGMATISM, see *Visual Acuity*

ATA, see *Thyroid Function*

A-THR 3, see *Antithrombin III*

AT III, see *Antithrombin III*

ATOPY, see *Allergy*

ATROPINE, see *Finger Wrinkle*

ATYPICAL LYMPHOCYTE, see *Mononucleosis*

AUDIOMETER, see *Hearing Function*

AUDITORY BRAIN STEM RESPONSE, see *Hearing Function*

AUSTRALIAN ANTIGEN, see *Hepatitis*

AUTISM, see *Serotonin*

AUTOANTIBODY, see *Immunology*

AUTOHEMOLYSIS, see *Glucose 6-Phosphate Dehydrogenase*

AUTOIMMUNE DISEASE, see *Immunology*

AUTOMATED REAGIN, see *Syphilis*

A-Z, see *Pregnancy*

B

BABINSKI, see *Reflex*

BALANCE, see *Cerebellum*

BALLISTOCARDIOGRAM (BCG)

Ballistocardiography screens heart function indirectly by measuring the vibration of the entire body as a consequence of the heartbeat. The patient lies motionless on a special bed or platform connected to instruments that record the slightest movement of the bed. The movement of blood through the body, caused by the heartbeat, sets off a tiny vibration in the body that can be detected when the patient is lying perfectly still. This motion is amplified electrically and recorded as waves on a chart. It is interesting to note that the secondary motion of the body caused by heart movements is about the same in a human as it is in a mouse or a whale.

When performed: While primarily a research test, ballistocardiography is also used to help diagnose heart disease before symptoms appear. It can help measure the result of treatment of heart disease, especially the effect of certain drugs on the heart.

Normal values: Although normal values change with age, certain types of waves indicate the condition of the heart. Unfortunately, there are several different standards of "normal," depending mostly on the experience of the cardiologist performing and interpreting the test.

Abnormal values: Certain categories of abnormal values are obvious to the trained cardiologist; but if three different cardiologists read the same ballistocardiogram, there could be three different interpretations. The test, however, can be helpful in rare instances when a specific diagnosis has been impossible to make.

Risk factors: Negligible (see general risk factors for electrical instruments).

Pain/discomfort: Minimal. Requires the patient to lie still for prolonged periods of time.

Cost: From $25 to $35.

This test is usually performed in a hospital or research facility because of the equipment needed.

Some doctors consider this test outmoded, and it is possible that a health insurance company or government-sponsored medical program will not reimburse the doctor or patient for the cost of the test.

Accuracy and significance: The test has a 60 percent accuracy level. Some doctors feel the ballistocardiogram provides the same information as the electrocardiograph stress test.

BALLOON FLOW–DIRECTED PULMONARY ARTERY CATHETER, see *Blood Pressure*

B AND T CELLS, see *Lymphocyte Typing*

B AND T LYMPHOCYTE, see *Lymphocyte Typing*

BÁRÁNY, see *Caloric*

BARBITURATES

When there is a suspicion of accidental or suicidal ingestion of barbiturates (Seconal, Nembutal, phenobarbital) in an unconscious patient, blood, serum, or plasma (usually from a vein) is examined to ascertain the barbiturate level. Urine can also be examined for barbiturates as a rapid screening test. Body organs such as the liver store barbiturates, and the level can be detected from a **Biopsy**. Occasionally, the stomach contents are analyzed.

When performed: When a patient is unconscious and the cause is unknown; to distinguish the comatose state from that due to other causes such as diabetic coma and alcoholic and/or tranquilizer intoxication; to aid in deciding the type of therapy for the unconscious patient; in medical-legal situations of suspected drug abuse. See **Drug Abuse.**

Normal values: Normally there are no barbiturates in the blood.

Abnormal values: Any barbiturate in the blood greater than 0.01 mg per 100 ml is considered dangerous. It is important to know the kinds and amounts of barbiturates in the blood, because a small amount of a quick-acting barbiturate such as Nembutal or Seconal is far more deadly than a larger amount of a longer-acting barbiturate such as phenobarbital. Certain drugs such as aspirin, aminophylline, and some antibiotics can interfere with the test technique and cause erroneous results.

Risk factors: For blood testing, the risks are negligible (see general risk factors for blood testing). For urine testing when a patient is comatose, see general risk factors for catheter and needle insertion. The risks of passing a tube into the stomach for gastric content analysis are negligible unless the patient is unconscious, at which time there is the possibility of the tube entering the windpipe and the additional danger of vomiting and inhaling portions of the vomitus.

Pain/discomfort: Minimal (see general pain/discomfort factors for blood testing and catheter and needle insertion). Passing a tube into the stomach is uncomfortable but not necessarily painful.

Cost: When urine is tested for rough screening, the charge is approximately $10 to $15. When additional tests are performed on blood, urine, or stomach contents — a chemical analysis for the presence of barbiturates — the cost is $30 to $40. When tests are done to identify the specific type of barbiturate and to estimate the quantity involved, there is an additional charge of $40 to $60.

Accuracy and significance: The tests are quite accurate (90 percent), as long as the presence of all other drugs is known. Determining the specific barbiturate ingested can be lifesaving.

BARIUM, see *Mercury*

BARIUM ENEMA, see *Radiography*

BARIUM SWALLOW, see *Radiography*

BARR BODIES, see *Chromosome Analysis*

BASAL BODY TEMPERATURE, see *Body Temperature*

BASAL METABOLIC RATE (BMR)

The basal metabolic rate is primarily a measure of thyroid function. The patient fasts prior to the test, and the test is performed when the patient is as relaxed as possible, both physically and mentally. The patient breathes into a machine that measures the body's oxygen consumption and the calories expended while at rest.

When performed: The test is used when there is a suspicion of endocrine disease or when metabolic processes must be studied but the patient's iodine intake or exposure precludes the more precise chemical tests (see **Thyroid Function**). Iodine compounds used in some diagnostic tests can stay in the body for five years or more.

Normal values: Normal values range from −15 percent to +15 percent of the amount of oxygen a person of a specific age, height, and weight typically uses at rest.

Abnormal values: The BMR may be elevated (the patient uses more than a normal amount of oxygen) in hyperthyroidism, acromegaly, diabetes insipidus, Cushing's disease, leukemia, pulmonary and cardiovascular disease, acidosis, and anxiety. Tremor, shivering, and generalized movement can accelerate the BMR and give false high values. The BMR is lower than normal with hypothyroidism (cretinism).

Risk factors: Negligible. There is always a slight possibility of infection from the machine's mouthpiece if it is not properly sterilized between patients.

Pain/discomfort: Minimal. In order to perform the test properly, the patient must lie down in a darkened room and remain undisturbed for at least one hour prior to the test. Some patients find this claustrophobic. During the test procedure, all body movements must be restricted. A few patients find holding the mouthpiece tightly inside the mouth for ten to twenty minutes quite uncomfortable.

Cost: From $25 to $50.

Some doctors consider this test outmoded, and it is possible that a health insurance company or government-sponsored medical program will not reimburse the doctor or patient for the cost of the test.

Accuracy and significance: The BMR is seldom performed today, having been replaced with more precise **Thyroid Function** tests. When properly performed, the BMR is considered to have a diagnostic accuracy of 60 percent.

BASE EXCESS OR DEFICIT, see *Bicarbonate*

BASOPHIL HISTAMINE RELEASE, see *RAST*

BAUER-KIRBY, see *Culture*

BAYLEY SCALE, see *Motor Development*

BCG, see *Ballistocardiogram*

BECK DEPRESSION INVENTORY, see *Depression*

BÉKÉSY AUDIOMETRY, see *Hearing Function*

BELLAK, see *Thematic Apperception*

BELL'S PALSY, see "Salivary Gland Scan" in *Nuclear Scanning*

BENCE-JONES PROTEIN

Bence-Jones protein is a nonalbumin protein that is rarely found in the urine. (Albumin is the most common form of protein that is found in the urine; any measurable protein in the urine is abnormal.) Bence-Jones protein is a test primarily for multiple myeloma (a cancer of the plasma cells usually arising in bone marrow). In one out of five patients with multiple myeloma (myelomatosis), detection of Bence-Jones protein (the globulin that comes from the cancerous cells) in the urine is the only way to diagnose the disease. A urine sample is examined by adding an antiserum. Occasionally, the blood or the cerebrospinal fluid is tested.

When performed: When there is a suspicion of multiple myeloma; when there are many unexplained infections; when there is unexplained bleeding into tissues.

Normal values: There may be a very slight trace of Bence-Jones protein in the urine, but it is usually not measurable. There should be no Bence-Jones protein in blood serum or cerebrospinal fluid.

Abnormal values: Bence-Jones protein is primarily associated with multiple myeloma. It may also be found in cases of Waldenström's macroglobulinemia, where lymphocytes (white blood cells) as well as plasma cells are produced in excess numbers. The Bradshaw test, a newer test somewhat similar to Bence-Jones, is positive in 95 percent of cases of multiple myeloma.

Risk factors: None for urine. Negligible for blood (see general risk factors for blood testing). See **Cerebrospinal Fluid** for risk factors associated with spinal tap.

Pain/discomfort: None for urine. Minimal for blood (see general risk factors for blood testing). See **Cerebrospinal Fluid** for pain/discomfort associated with spinal tap.

Cost: For simply measuring the presence or absence of Bence-Jones protein in urine or cerebrospinal fluid the fee is $8 to $20, depending on the method employed. An analysis of the various forms of the protein in blood, urine, or cerebrospinal fluid is $50 to $60. There is usually an additional charge for a spinal tap.

Accuracy and significance: About half of all multiple myeloma patients show Bence-Jones protein in the urine. While the accuracy of Bence-Jones measurements in blood or cerebrospinal fluid is somewhat greater, the test is not considered too specific, as it is also positive in other related diseases such as lymph gland cancers and leukemia. Some 10 percent of patients show no disease even though Bence-Jones protein is present. Considered 50 percent accurate.

BENDER GESTALT, see *Visual Motor Perception*

BENDER-PURDUE REFLEX, see *Reflex*

BENTIROMIDE, see *Pancreas Function*

BENTONITE FLOCCULATION, see *Rheumatoid Factor*

BENZIDINE, see *Occult Blood*

BERIBERI, see *Thiamin*

BERNSTEIN, see *Gastroesophageal Reflux*

β (Beta)-LACTAMASE ACTIVITY, see *Culture*

BETHANECHOL CHALLENGE, see *Gastroesophageal Reflux*

BICARBONATE (HCO₃)

Bicarbonate (sometimes called carbonates) is the most important buffer compound in the blood. A buffer keeps the **pH** (acid-base balance) of the blood at its proper strength. Bicarbonate is a blood electrolyte that works hand in hand with carbonic acid (from which it is derived as part of the metabolism of food) to help regulate blood pH. There is 20 times as much bicarbonate in the blood as carbonic acid; thus, the normal pH is slightly alkaline.

Bicarbonate is easily regulated by the kidney, which excretes it when there is an excess and holds it back when needed; the amount of carbon dioxide in the blood, and the amount breathed out by the lungs, also controls bicarbonate levels. If bicarbonate is lost from the body because of a kidney problem, diarrhea, or other disease, a state of acidosis (too much acid in the blood) exists.

In most instances, the bicarbonate concentration is determined by testing for the total amount of carbon dioxide, but at times bicarbonate itself becomes a valuable measurement. The "standard bicarbonate," or base excess or deficit, may also be measured, but this is rarely done in practice. Blood is taken from a vein, and the serum is tested.

When performed: As a verification of other tests such as the blood gases (carbon dioxide, oxygen, and hydrogen) and the pH; when there is some doubt as to the exact state of the blood pH; to differentiate the type of kidney disease, toxic coma, and certain lung problems.

Normal values: Blood bicarbonate levels normally range from 24 to 26 mEq per liter.

Abnormal values: Bicarbonate is usually increased when there is severe vomiting, when excessive bicarbonatelike products are ingested (antacid preparations for ulcers or burning stomach), when diuretic and steroid drugs are used, and when difficult breathing prevents the release of proper amounts of carbon dioxide. Blood bicarbonate is decreased moderately with rapid breathing (when excessive carbon dioxide is exhaled) and with liver disease; it is decreased markedly with aspirin or other toxic chemical poisoning, with kidney disease, and with diarrhea.

Risk factors: Negligible (see general risk factors for blood testing).

Pain/discomfort: Minimal (see general pain/discomfort factors for blood testing).

Cost: From $5 to $9.

Accuracy and significance: Although sometimes performed alone, the test has real significance when it is performed along with the **pH,** thereby increasing the accuracy (to 90 percent) of a diagnosis of the blood's acidity-alkalinity levels. It is also used to differentiate abnormalities in the acidity-alkalinity relationship of the blood and body fluids and to detect any abnormality due to a metabolic problem or a respiratory disease. When used in conjunction with **Carbon Dioxide** and **Oxygen,** it is considered extremely accurate in differentiating diseases caused by lung or kidney problems. It is also of great significance in helping diagnose a person in coma, especially when drug overdose is suspected.

BILE ACID BREATH, see *Nuclear Scanning*

BILE ACID CHOLYGLYCINE, see *Cholylglycine*

BILE DUCT VISUALIZATION, see *Radiography*

BILIARY SCANNING, see *Nuclear Scanning*

BILIRUBIN

Bilirubin is a gold-colored pigment waste product of the body. It is formed mostly from the hemoglobin in red blood cells when they break down at the end of their usual life span (four months). Every day about 7 to 8 g (a teaspoon and a half) of hemoglobin is released from dying red blood cells to make 250 mg of bilirubin. Bilirubin then becomes part of the bile fluid that goes from the liver to the gallbladder to the intestines; almost all of it is normally eliminated by the bowels.

Excessive production or decreased excretion of bilirubin increases the minute normal amounts in the blood, and its unique color, when increased, causes yellow jaundice in the skin and the whites of the eyes. Before it is acted upon by the liver, bilirubin is attached to albumin protein molecules in the blood; in this state, it is called indirect bilirubin. After it is acted upon by the liver, the portion no longer bound to proteins is called direct bilirubin. The sum of the two equals the total bilirubin.

Blood is taken from a vein, and the serum or plasma is examined. Bilirubin is also measured in the urine (only direct bilirubin is excreted, causing a dark color). Shaking urine in a glass tube will change the normal white color of the foam to a dark yellow or brown if bilirubin is present. Amniotic fluid (the liquid around the fetus during pregnancy) may also be tested for excess bilirubin (it is normally present in tiny amounts and decreases throughout pregnancy).

When performed: The test is performed primarily to distinguish different forms of liver disease, especially liver cell disease from bile duct obstruction such as from gallstones. It can also help determine the cause of certain anemias. When a patient has gray-white or colorless bowel movements, the bilirubin is measured to ascertain the cause.

Normal values: The total serum bilirubin runs from 0.2 to 1.5 mg per 100 ml. The direct bilirubin usually measures from 0.1 to 0.4 mg per 100 ml; the indirect bilirubin runs about the same but may be slightly higher and still be normal. The urine normally contains no bilirubin. Amniotic fluid usually contains a trace of bilirubin.

Abnormal values: Total bilirubin (both direct and indirect) is increased with liver cirrhosis. When something blocks the flow of bile, such as a gallstone or cancer of the pancreas, the total and direct bilirubin is increased, but the indirect bilirubin usually stays within its normal range. Liver disease from Thorazine and other tranquilizers as well as drugs such as male hormones, some antibiotics, and certain arthritic pain products can cause elevated direct bilirubin; usually, the indirect bilirubin stays normal. In contrast, in certain anemias where blood cells break easily, such as erythroblastosis fetalis (the anemia most often caused by Rh problems), the total serum bilirubin and the indirect bilirubin are elevated, but the direct bilirubin stays normal. As red blood cells are destroyed, the bilirubin increases in amniotic fluid, and this is a way of following the course of the disease. Fasting or low-caloric diet causes a marked rise in serum bilirubin in 24 hours.

Risk factors: Negligible when blood is tested (see general risk factors for blood testing). With examination of amniotic fluid, see general risk factors for catheter and needle insertion.

Pain/discomfort: Minimal when blood is tested (see general pain/discomfort factors for blood testing). With examination of amniotic fluid for bilirubin, see general pain/discomfort factors for catheter and needle insertion.

Cost: The total bilirubin test runs $4 to $24. When, in addition, both direct and indirect bilirubin are measured—in blood or urine—there is often another $5 to $15 charge. Although the total bilirubin is usually included in **Comprehensive Multiple Test Screening** panels, which range from $7 to $42, direct bilirubin is included in the panel only when total bilirubin results are abnormal. When amniotic fluid is tested, the fee is $12 to $36.

Accuracy and significance: A bilirubin test is considered 90 percent accurate and is a sensitive measure of liver disease. It has little significance in distinguishing between specific liver diseases. To assure an accurate interpretation of the test, the effects of many different prescription drugs on liver function must always be considered. The test's accuracy is increased when performed in conjunction with **Urobilinogen.**

BING, see *Tuning Fork*

BIOELECTRICAL IMPEDANCE, see *Anthropometric Measurements*

BIOFEEDBACK, see *Electroencephalogram*

BIOMICROSCOPE, see *Fluorescein Eye Stain*

BIOPSY

Biopsy is the removal of a piece of tissue from the body for detailed, usually microscopic, examination. Examination of isolated cells such as blood cells or those obtained for a bone marrow test or Pap smear (see **Cytology**) are forms of a biopsy. Most often, however, a small piece of tissue is excised with a scalpel. (If the lesion is small, as are most skin growths, the entire mass is removed.) The specimen is sliced to extreme thinness (microtomy), stained, and examined through the microscope.

In needle biopsy, a needle is inserted into a body organ, tissue, or suspected lesion, and a minute piece is sucked into the needle tip for microscopic examination. This is usually performed under the fluoroscope so as to be precise about the location of the specimen. In most instances a local anesthetic is used. Needle biopsies of the breast, liver, spleen, pancreas, kidney, and lung are regularly performed. Biopsy of the prostate may be obtained during cystoscopy (use of an instrument that allows a direct view of the urethra and bladder (see **Endoscopy**). In general, the result of a biopsy of a tumor is reported as benign (noncancerous) or malignant (cancerous). A biopsy may also reveal an infection or foreign body as the cause of the lesion. To correctly diagnose diseases of the fingernails and toenails, which are often the result of a fungus, a nail biopsy is necessary.

A needle biopsy is also known as an aspiration biopsy; when a larger opening is necessary, it may be called a punch biopsy. The terms *incisional* and *excisional biopsy* refer to whether only a piece of the lesion to be studied is removed, or whether the entire suspected growth is excised. When an endoscope is used to observe the area in question—such as through the cystoscope—the biopsy may be called an endoscopic biopsy; if the surface area is scraped, as when studying the inside walls of the uterus, the term *surface biopsy* may be used. A percutaneous biopsy is any biopsy obtained by penetrating the skin, most often with a needle.

An improvement on needle biopsy is called fine-needle biopsy; when guided by **Ultrasound,** it is now considered the test of choice to help identify liver tumors. It is considered more accurate than a liver scan (see **Nuclear Scanning**) and poses far less risk.

Biopsy of brain tissue—when the doctor is looking for or trying to identify the type of brain tumor, infection, or other pathology—can be performed by using stereotactic computer-assisted scans and angiography (see **Computerized Tomography** and **Radiography**). The three-dimensional effect allows the doctor to delve deeply into the brain with virtually no damage to adjacent tissues; it is, however, still considered a risky test, and there have been deaths due to the technique, which requires drilling a hole in the skull—albeit only local anesthesia is used.

When performed: Whenever a suspicious lesion is seen (either directly on the skin or in a body cavity), felt (as in the breast), or noted (by X-ray); whenever there is suspected disease in an organ (such as the liver or lung) that cannot be diagnosed.

Normal values: The very existence of a lesion usually contradicts a normal value, but there are various skin growths such as birthmarks that are not disease-related.

Abnormal values: Any biopsy showing pathological cells is considered abnormal. Benign cells can be pathological, or disease-related, even if they are not cancerous.

Risk factors: General risk factors include the remote possibility of hemorrhage and the even more remote possibility of infection: much depends on the part of the body being biopsied. With a skin biopsy, there is the possibility of a scar. Many doctors feel that, when performing a biopsy on a suspected cancer, unless the biopsy is large enough to be outside the suspicious area, the irritation of the cutting or withdrawal of the biopsy needle may accelerate the spread of the cancer.

Pain/discomfort: Much depends on the part of the body being biopsied and whether anesthesia is used. Biopsies taken from inside the body—the bladder, esophagus, stomach, large bowel, liver, lungs, and bone marrow—are usually uncomfortable procedures, even when anesthesia is employed. Discomfort lasting several days is not unusual following such biopsies. If a patient is particularly apprehensive, a general anesthesia is often administered for the procedure. Biopsies from the skin or surface organs involve little discomfort.

Cost: A simple biopsy costs from $35 to $150, including closure of the wound. This does not, however, include such additional costs as: anesthesia if requested or required; **Endoscopy** to explore a suspicious area; hospitalization if the doctor insists, whether it is indicated or not; follow-up care to see that the lesion heals properly; and the pathology report. These additional fees can increase the cost of the biopsy anywhere from $50 to $500. A pathologist usually charges $25 to $100 to prepare, study, and report on a specimen. If electronic microscopy is needed, there is an additional charge, which averages $250.

Accuracy and significance: When a biopsy is properly performed, preserved, handled, stained, and interpreted, its accuracy is near 99 percent. Unfortunately, cancer cells can be missed at times. There are also instances when normal or noncancerous cells appear as abnormal and cause an erroneous diagnosis. This is not common, but it does seem to occur more often when a frozen specimen is studied. Frozen biopsy specimens are utilized when, during an operation for suspected cancer, the surgeon wants an immediate answer as to just how much surgery he will perform (a report from a routine biopsy takes two to three days).

BIOTIN, see *Thiamin*

BIRTH DEFECT SCREENING, see *Genetic Disorder Screening*

BLACKY PICTURES, see *Thematic Apperception*

BLADDER STONE, see *Urinary Tract Calculus*

BLEEDING AND CLOTTING TIME

Although essentially two different tests, bleeding and clotting time are invariably performed together as if they were one. They are crude measures of hemostasis (how quickly bleeding is stopped by normal body responses). More specifically, bleeding time is primarily an indication of the condition of the blood vessels (principally the capillaries) and an indication of platelet function. In addition to clotting factors, the test measures how well and how quickly small arteries and veins will constrict and close off to stop bleeding when injured. Clotting time is a generalized indication of the effectiveness of the many factors within the fluid blood itself (as opposed to the blood vessels) that bring about coagulation (clotting).

The original technique of nicking the earlobe or a fingertip is still used occasionally to measure bleeding time. However, the preferred technique (Ivy bleeding time) is to apply a standard amount of pressure around the upper arm with a blood pressure cuff and then to make two incisions 10 mm (about 7/16″) long and 1 mm (1/32″) deep on the lower arm. Blotting paper is touched to the cut every 30 seconds until the bleeding stops, at which point the time is noted. Most doctors now use a Mielke template device with a spring that controls the length and depth of the incision; this has eliminated some of the factors that can cause false readings.

In tests of clotting time, blood is usually drawn from a vein and placed in several narrow glass tubes. Sometimes the tubes are broken apart; sometimes they are tilted. In either case, the time is noted when the blood visibly clots (the cells go from a liquid to a solid state).

When performed: The test is used when there are unusual bleeding tendencies (either inherited or caused by drugs or other diseases); when liver disease is suspected, and whenever a patient is to have a surgical procedure or extensive dental work. The clotting time alone may be measured as a guide to dosage when a patient receives heparin as part of anticoagulant therapy; it may also be used as a test of platelet function (see **Platelet Count**).

Normal values: Bleeding time usually averages 5 minutes; however, bleeding times of up to 10 minutes are still considered within normal limits by some laboratories. Clotting time usually ranges from 6 to 16 minutes.

Abnormal values: Longer-than-usual bleeding time generally indicates thrombocytopenia (a decrease in the normal amount of blood platelets, which are essential for clotting). It can also mean that the platelets, although normal in number, are not functioning properly. Bleeding and clotting time together are prolonged when there are coagulation defects — either absence of the multiple clot-causing factors normally in blood or interference with one or more of these factors (such as when a patient is given heparin). The clotting time alone is not a specific diagnostic test. It is usually (though not always) increased with hemophilia. Taking large doses of aspirin can cause increased bleeding and clotting times, as can uremia (a form of kidney failure where the by-products of proteins cannot filter through the kidney) and certain kinds of leukemia. Estrogen products such as oral contraceptives and corticosteroid drugs can prolong clotting time (at one time surgeons gave patients estrogens prior to an operation to lessen bleeding), however it has been noted that these drugs can cause thrombophlebitis (vein clots).

Risk factors: Negligible (see general risk factors for blood testing).

Pain/discomfort: Minimal (see general pain/discomfort factors for blood testing). The incisions are so shallow that they rarely cause pain.

Cost: $10 to $35 when both tests are performed. The clotting time test alone is about $8.

Accuracy and significance: The test is 80 percent accurate in detecting bleeding tendencies; however, it is not sufficiently accurate for consistent use on a patient taking anticoagulant drugs. The test is so nonspecific, it is of no major significance in determining a diagnosis (see **Partial Thromboplastin Time**).

BLIND SPOT, see *Visual Field*

BLOOD ACIDITY, see *pH*

BLOOD CELL DIFFERENTIAL

Changes in the amounts of *each type* of **White Blood Cell** (leukocyte) and changes in the size and shape of **Red Blood Cells** (erythrocytes) can be of greater importance than changes in the total white and red blood cell counts. Particularly, ascertaining changes in the proportions of the different kinds of white blood cells helps to define different disease processes. The blood cell differential test also distinguishes abnormalities in red blood cells (such as sickling or insufficient iron; see **Hemoglobin** and **Red Blood Cell Indices**); it can also reveal the parasites of **Malaria,** if present.

The nitroblue tetrazolium test is used to indicate the ability of the neutrophils to destroy bacteria; at least 5 percent of the neutrophils should be able to reduce the color of the dye when it is added to fresh blood. If they cannot, it is considered a suggestion of a white blood cell disorder or a chronic granulomatous (usually lymphocyte) disease.

At times, an eosinophil count alone is ordered by the doctor; this is usually to help confirm suspicions of Hodgkin's disease (a form of lymphoid tumor), when assessing sensitivity to some anticoagulant drugs, and when considering the possibility of acute hypereosinophilic syndrome (a rare, but usually fatal, leukemia-type condition).

At other times, a slide for blood cell examination is made from the buffy coat; this is the thin layer of white blood cells that lies between the large amount of red blood cells and the plasma after centrifuging (see **Hematocrit**). It is supposed to make it easier to detect leukemia cells, lupus cells (see **Antinuclear Antibodies**), and even some parasites. However, it is not considered too accurate.

A drop of blood is taken from the fingertip, earlobe, or heel; or a drop of venous blood taken for other tests may be used. The blood is stained and then examined through a microscope by a hematologist or trained technician. In recent years, optical imagery computers have been developed that can electronically scan a blood sample and perform this test in a minute or two; normally, it will take a technician viewing the stained slide through a microscope from 15 to 60 minutes. Unfortunately, these automated image analyzers are not as accurate as experienced hematologists, especially when it comes to differentiating monocytes. They do seem adequate for routine blood cell differential screening (see **Hemoglobin**).

When performed: When there is an infectious process, an allergy, or a parasitic infestation; with suspicion of any blood disease such as anemia or leukemia.

Normal values: Usually, each of the different kinds of white blood cells is found in the following proportions:

Neutrophils:
    65 percent total, with 58 percent mature neutrophils and 7 percent young neutrophils (neutrophils are the primary cells that ingest and destroy microorganisms and other toxic disease-producing substances).

Lymphocytes:
    27 percent (lymphocytes represent antibody activity in producing immunity to disease).

Monocytes:
 5 percent (while thought of as old lymphocytes, they represent chronic disease processes in the body).
Eosinophils:
 2 percent (eosinophils are related to allergies and parasitic infestations).
Basophils:
 1 percent (the role of the basophil is still not clearly understood).

Abnormal values: An increased proportion of neutrophils usually indicates poisoning, cancer, hemorrhage, or an infectious process (there are a few exceptions; for reasons still unknown, a virus infection, typhoid fever, and malaria do not cause the expected increase in neutrophils). When most of the neutrophils are young, elevated levels usually reflect leukemia. A decreased amount of neutrophils is seen with spleen disorders, lupus erythematosus, vitamin B_{12} and/or folic acid deficiency, and bone marrow damage from drugs or X-rays. Typhoid and malaria are two infections that cause a decrease in neutrophils. Decreased amounts of all white blood cells may be found in a patient taking steroid drugs.

Lymphocytes are increased primarily after radiation exposure and in hepatitis, herpes simplex and herpes zoster (shingles), infectious mononucleosis, syphilis, and leukemia. They are decreased in lupus erythematosus and other conditions where there is reduced immunity to disease. See **Lymphocyte Typing.**

Monocytes are increased with tuberculosis, cancers, anemias, rickettsial diseases (such as Rocky Mountain spotted fever), and typhoid. A decrease in monocytes is rarely seen.

Eosinophils are increased with asthma, hay fever, and similar conditions, and especially with worm and other parasite invasion. The use of diet depressant drugs such as amphetamines, certain tranquilizers, bulk-forming laxatives such as those containing psyllium seeds, and certain antibiotics can also cause a rise in eosinophils. They are decreased with alcohol intoxication.

Basophils may be increased with leukemias and adrenal disease and are sometimes missing with hyperthyroidism and allergies.

Risk factors: Negligible (see general risk factors for blood testing).
Pain/discomfort: Minimal (see general pain/discomfort factors for blood testing).
Cost: When performed as part of a complete blood count, as it most often is, the fee is $5 to $20. The white blood cell differential count performed separately averages $10. The test is commonly part of **Comprehensive Multiple Test Screening** panels, which range from $7 to $42. A buffy-coat smear is $20 to $30.

Accuracy and significance: The test is 85 percent accurate when properly performed. However, it is only significant in the sense that it can point toward diagnostic possibilities. For example, a rise in the percentage of eosinophils will not tell the doctor whether the increase is due to allergy, worms, or some other condition.

BLOOD CLOTTING FACTORS, see *Fibrinogen; Partial Thromboplastin Time*

BLOOD COUNT, see *Red Blood Cell; White Blood Cell*

BLOOD CULTURE, see *Culture*

BLOOD DONOR HEPATITIS, see *Isocitric Dehydrogenase*

BLOOD ELECTROLYTES, see *Bicarbonate; Chloride; Potassium; Sodium*

BLOOD FATS, see *Lipids*

BLOOD GASES, see *Bicarbonate; Carbon Dioxide; Oxygen; pH*

BLOOD GROUPING, see *Typing and Cross-Matching*

BLOOD MATCHING, see *Typing and Cross-Matching*

BLOOD POOL SCAN, see *Nuclear Scanning*

BLOOD PRESSURE

The term *blood pressure* generally refers to the pressure in the arteries as opposed to the veins. To take one's blood pressure is to measure the pressure (tension) of the blood within the artery walls. (Pressures in the capillaries and veins are quite different.) The end result is derived from a number of factors: the force of each heartbeat, the elasticity or resilience of the walls of the artery, the amount of blood flowing through the arteries at any one time, the viscosity (thickness) of the blood, the number of molecules of various substances (such as protein and sodium) in the blood, the amount of certain hormones and enzymes (such as adrenalin from the adrenal gland and renin from the kidney) circulating in the blood, and the functioning of the autonomic or sympathetic nervous system (over which a person has no direct control) in response to changes in posture, stressful situations, and other stimuli. (See **Cold Pressor** and **Finger Wrinkle** tests.)

The blood pressure is altered during every heartbeat, reaching its highest point when the heart muscle is most contracted (forcing blood into the arteries) and its lowest point when the heart muscle relaxes after each heartbeat. The heart muscle contraction is medically called systole, and the highest point of one's blood pressure is known as systolic. The momentary resting phase of the heart is called diastole, and the low point of one's blood pressure is known as diastolic. The difference between these two pressures is called the pulse pressure.

The measurement of blood pressure is recorded by noting how high in millimeters (mm) applied pressure will cause a column of mercury (Hg) to rise on a measuring instrument. A cuff or sleeve is wrapped around an extremity (most commonly the upper arm); air is pumped into the cuff to apply a counterpressure to all the tissues surrounding the artery (skin, muscles, etc.). By reading the level of counterpressure on an air pressure dial gauge or directly observing how high the mercury rises, the physician can note when the artery collapses (similar to applying a tourniquet and then releasing the pressure to allow the artery to fill normally); at that point, the pressure being applied just exceeds the pressure within the artery. Collapse of the artery is most commonly noted by listening for the cessation of the pulse through a stethoscope placed on the inside of the arm in front of the elbow or by feeling for the pulse until the examiner can no longer feel the beat.

When sufficient pressure is applied around the arm to collapse the artery, the pulse will no longer be heard or felt, giving the systolic blood pressure reading. As outside pressure from the cuff is lessened, the pulse can be heard or felt the instant the artery pressure exceeds that of the surrounding cuff (again, the measure of the systolic pressure). The pulse will be heard or felt as long as sufficient pressure is applied from the outside to cause the blood pulsations to rebound off the artery walls. When the outside pressure is low enough so there is no measurable resistance against the artery wall, the pulse will no longer be heard (it will still be felt); this point is noted for the diastolic pressure measurement. Today, there are electronic instruments that translate the pulse sounds into light impulses or noises, which are much easier to record. And some newer blood pressure measuring devices have microphones built into the cuff; the presence and absence of pulse sounds are then electronically translated into digital displays that may be viewed directly. When the microphone is properly placed, these readings are considered as accurate as mercury measurements, which are considered the best.

It is important to measure blood pressure in both arms and both legs; to measure it while the patient is standing, sitting, and lying down; and most of all to measure it when the patient is as relaxed as possible. Most physicians measure blood pressure at the onset of an examination, again about halfway through, and as the last procedure (when the patient is most likely to be at ease). Doctors now ask patients to measure their own blood pressure at home (or have a family member test it) during various times of the day and to note activities at the time in order to arrive at the most usual reading. Blood pressure readings must be abnormal on three different days before a diagnosis of hypertension can be made. Other factors that are known to cause false blood pressure readings include using a cuff that is the wrong size for the particular arm being tested; a cuff that is too narrow will cause a false higher-than-normal reading, while a cuff that is too wide will produce false low readings (five different sizes of cuffs are available to all doctors). Leaks in the tubing system (inside the cuff, there usually is a rubber bladder connected by rubber tubes to the hand pump or electronic pumping device and to the measuring instrument) are more common than realized and, of course, give false results.

Ambulatory blood pressure measurements, usually over a 24-hour period, record a patient's blood pressure repeatedly during the day and night. A small device, about the size of a pocket tape recorder, automatically makes the readings every 15 minutes (the time intervals may vary according to the doctor or the device). The patient also notes regular—and unusual—activities in a diary or through a voice recording device. This form of testing can be valuable when patients are suspected of having "white coat" or doctor-caused hypertension, to help detect an unsuspected provocative cause, and to measure the effect of drugs being used to treat the condition. Usually, a doctor will charge $100 to $200 per day for this prolonged testing.

Venous blood pressure, as opposed to arterial blood pressure, is recorded directly by using a manometer, a thin glass tube with measurement markings connected to a needle. The needle is placed inside a vein in the arm, which is kept at heart level (it may also be placed in a neck vein, with the patient lying down); the actual rise of blood in the tube is noted. Vein pressure can be estimated by observing the veins on the back of the hand when the arm is raised. Normally, the veins collapse when the hand reaches heart level; neck veins usually collapse when the patient is in a sitting position. At times, central venous pressure is measured by observing the jugular veins on both sides of the neck. The patient at first lies flat; then the head of the bed is raised to a 30 to 45 degree angle at which point, if venous pressure is normal, the obvious neck veins should appear to collapse or relatively disappear. If the veins still stand out after the head of the bed has been elevated more than 45 degrees, it could indicate abnormally high pressure between the lungs and the heart or a blockage in the vein.

At times, the pulmonary artery pressure (PAP) is monitored. The pulmonary artery carries blood directly from the heart to the lungs, and the pressure of the blood inside this artery just after it leaves the heart is considered a measure of heart function. To perform this test, a balloon flow-directed pulmonary artery catheter, most commonly called a Swan-Ganz catheter, after the names of its inventors, is introduced into the body and passed through the heart—using the balloon as a wedge to propel the catheter tip through the blood vessels—until it reaches the pulmonary artery. These catheters usually have a second monitor located a short distance from the tip; this monitor lies in the vena cava (the large vein that enters the right side of the heart) or inside the right side of the heart itself and measures central venous pressure. In essence, these tests tell the pressures within both sides of the heart and within each of the heart's chambers on either side. At times, a thermister is placed in the catheter; it detects any temperature changes in the blood. Although this catheter test is being used with increasing frequency—primarily to monitor the administration of intravenous fluids so that the patient will not become overloaded with water, which can cause edema—it is considered an extremely dangerous test. Many doctors feel it is being overused when the benefits vs. the risks are considered, especially when employed as a test of heart function. Studies have shown that, in most instances, the test results offer no real benefit to the patient.

When performed: Arterial blood pressure is routinely measured during a physical examination to detect early stages of hypertension (high blood pressure), a condition that exists in 1 out of every 10 Americans. It is also followed closely in patients who are overweight; patients who have thyroid and other hormone diseases, kidney diseases, or lung diseases; and during pregnancy (see Rollover). During surgical procedures, the blood pressure is monitored constantly as a guide to the patient's condition, especially to check for blood loss.

Venous blood pressure is measured primarily in heart disease to determine which side of the heart is in difficulty. It is also measured when blood transfusions are given to make sure the patient does not receive too much blood (which can cause congestion of the lungs) as well as when intravenous fluids are administered to patients in diabetic coma.

Normal values: The most generalized figures given for arterial blood pressure are 120/80, which means the systolic pressure is 120 mm Hg and the diastolic pressure is 80 mm Hg when a person is at rest and relaxed. But blood pressure seems to rise naturally as people get older. Even with age, however, the diastolic pressure should not rise as much as the systolic. A consistent blood pressure of greater than 140/85, regardless of age, should be thought of as a warning sign. Venous blood pressure normally ranges from 40 to 80 mm Hg. The pulse pressure averages 40 mm Hg.

Abnormal values: In general, a systolic blood pressure reading over 150 mm Hg and/or a diastolic blood pressure reading over 90 mm Hg is considered evidence of hypertension. Three out of four people with high blood pressure readings (excluding those obtained erroneously) have essential hypertension (although it is believed to result from some direct body dysfunction, the cause will probably never be known); one out of four cases of hypertension has a secondary cause that can be diagnosed, such as kidney disease, connective tissue disease, nervous system involvement, lung disease, or hormonal problems. Certain drugs, such as those used for asthma, can cause high blood pressure readings.

High blood pressure is more a cause of heart disease than a result of heart problems. When blood pressure is elevated in the arms but normal or low in the legs, or when blood pressure in the right arm is greater than in the left, it usually indicates coarctation (constriction) of the aorta. Hypotension, or low blood pressure, most commonly occurs when a person moves from a sitting to a standing position (postural or orthostatic hypotension). It may also be caused by diuretic and other antihypertensive drugs, by many tranquilizers, by certain Parkinson-type diseases, and of course, by shock or severe bleeding.

A major cause of erroneous arterial blood pressure readings is faulty measurement technique. Putting the cuff on wrong, not inflating the cuff properly, and failing to hear the proper pulse sounds (either because of inattentiveness or because of other distracting noises) are the three most common reasons for erroneous, usually elevated, blood pressure readings. Performing a single test, on one arm, at the onset of an examination can also lead to inaccurate high blood pressure readings. Failure to take into account any apprehensiveness on the part of a patient will invariably give false results.

Venous blood pressure rises primarily with heart conditions such as right-sided heart failure or heart valve damage to the point that blood cannot easily enter the heart chambers. A rapid fall in venous pressure usually indicates internal bleeding such as from an ulcer.

A pulse pressure greater than 40, even without high blood pressure, can mean heart or thyroid trouble, or it could reflect anxiety. When the pulse pressure is less than 30, it may be a sign of a heart valve problem.

Risk factors: There is no physical risk in measuring blood pressure with the standard blood pressure apparatus when properly used. Should the device be improperly calibrated, should the technique be incorrect—such as with a wrong-size cuff, improper positioning of the cuff, or defects in the equipment—or should the patient's attitude and environment not be taken into account, a false reading can occur. The risk this entails—either wrongful, unnecessary, dangerous treatment or the failure to obtain necessary treatment—can be far more perilous than any hazard posed by the equipment itself.

Some other risk factors exist if the doctor is hurried or preoccupied, exhibits a facial expression of worry or concern or fails to inquire about the use of drugs, or even if the patient smoked within an hour prior to the measurements; even a full bladder can cause a false elevated reading. And then, if that part of the arm being tested (where the cuff is located) is not at the same level as the heart, or is not resting on something solid, a false reading can result. For the measurement of pressure by a needle inserted in a blood vessel, see general risk factors for blood testing and catheter or needle insertion.

When it comes to the use of the Swan-Ganz catheter for blood pressure measurements, there have been reports that nearly 4 out of every 10 patients who underwent catheterization died after the procedure, and the morbidity (illness attributed to the catheter's use) is even higher. Recently, acute thrombophlebitis (an infected clot) blocking circulation in the arm used for 24-hour blood pressure monitoring has been reported. This could be a fatal complication.

Pain/discomfort: Normally, pressure from the measuring cuff is minimal, but over-inflation of the cuff can be uncomfortable. When needles are used to measure blood pressure, see general pain/discomfort factors for blood testing and catheter or needle insertion.

Cost: Usually, there is no charge for blood pressure measurements. When blood pressure is measured with needles or catheters, most often in a hospital, the average charge is $40 to $150. Pulmonary artery pressure measurements can cost from $500 to $1,000, depending on the doctor's fee, how many days the catheter is left in place, and how many measurments are made; then there is the hospital cost in addition to the doctor's fees.

Accuracy and significance: Properly performed blood pressure readings are 95 percent accurate. When the newer electronic blood pressure measuring devices that detect pulse sounds are used—as they are at health fairs, in drug stores, etc.—it should be remembered that loud noises at the time of testing can produce abnormal results. Blood pressure measurements are very significant in following the course of many different diseases and during pregnancy and surgery.

The latest studies on the accuracy of blood pressure measurements have shown that the test is far more accurate when it is performed at home than when it is performed in a doctor's office; in addition, it usually measures 20 to 30 mm Hg lower than when it is performed by a doctor.

The Swan-Ganz catheter-use tests are not considered very accurate. Many technical errors occur, and errors in reading the measurements are not uncommon.

The most recent evaluation of blood pressure measurements made in doctors' offices, when compared with measurements made by patients wearing blood pressure monitors for 24 hours, showed that at least one out of every three patients were wrongly diagnosed as having high blood pressure and were being treated unnecessarily.

BLOOD TYPE, see *Agglutination*

BLOOD UREA NITROGEN, see *Urea Nitrogen*

BLOOD VISCOSITY, see *Macroglobulin; Osmolality*

BLOOD VOLUME, see *Hematocrit*

BMR, see *Basal Metabolic Rate*

BODY SCANNING, see *Computerized Tomography*

BODY TEMPERATURE

Most people associate the measurement of body temperature with an infection—from a simple cold or pneumonia to abscesses and appendicitis. In actuality, a rise in body temperature (fever) reflects increased metabolic activity; in the case of an infection, the elevated temperature indicates increased **White Blood Cell** production and action as they attempt to destroy invading microorganisms—whether they are bacteria, fungi, parasites, or some viruses—along with immune body production usually specific to the cause of the disease. At times, the presence of fever may be the only indication of a hidden illness. Tuberculosis may be present within the body in lesions too small to be detected by any other tests; food poisoning whose symptoms are only a mild annoyance may be accompanied by an elevated temperature; other infections of the gastrointestinal tract such as colitis or diverticulitis may have a fever as their initial warning sign.

At other times, various tumors (cancerous or not) produce a rise in body temperature. Leukemias and cancers of the liver and lung seem to do this most often. Conditions related to **Immunology,** such as systemic lupus erythematosis, as well as other diseases that cause abnormal values in **Antinuclear Antibodies** tests, may also bring about fever. Various forms of arthritis can cause a rise in body temperature before pain is felt in the joints. And disruptions in the hormone system, especially those causing water retention or excretion problems, may alter body temperature.

It is also possible for the body's temperature to drop below normal—this condition is called hypothermia. While a slight drop may routinely occur in elderly people or in those who reside in cold climates, a drop in body temperature can also be present in patients with circulation problems or diabetes and in those who abuse alcohol, barbiturates, and some tranquilizers. In certain instances, hypothermia can be as dangerous as a high fever.

Body temperature also rises slightly during the menstrual cycle. The basal body temperature test indicates the time of ovulation (when the ovum, or egg, is released from the ovary ready for fertilization or pregnancy). The body temperature is taken each morning on arising (usually by mouth) and recorded. It generally remains slightly below normal (normal is 98.6° F, or 37° C) until ovulation occurs, when it rises to normal or slightly above and stays elevated until menstruation. Thus, if a woman is having difficulty becoming pregnant, the couple is told to wait for the temperature to rise before having intercourse. The test can, of course, also be used as a contraceptive guide to show when conception would be impossible. The basal temperature test is used in conjunction with the Pap test (see **Cytology**) to study the menstrual cycle phase.

The measurement of temperature inside the penis has been used as a test for **impotence.** When penile temperature is 3 degrees or more lower than normal body temperature, it could indicate a problem of blood circulation to and inside the penis. The test is sometimes used as a means of evaluating psychological from physical impotence; with psychological problems, the temperature difference is rarely greater than 1 to 1½ degrees.

The most recent epidemiological studies have revealed that from 3 million to 5 million couples are affected by infertility every year. A new test, called ovulation predictor, is said to predict ovulation from 12 to 24 hours in advance. A test kit, to allow testing for six days, costs about $30; three-day refill kits cost $15. The latest test for ovulation timing is called OvuSTICK; here, a dipstick is placed in the urine, and a color change indicates the onset of ovulation. This test allows a few days' advance notice, eliminating some of the anxiety suffered by men when the timing of intercourse was on such short notice. (Also see **Tackmeter**.)

Many prescription drugs can cause a rise in body temperature. (Most doctors initially call this FUO, fever of unknown origin.) The drugs include the amphetamines, numerous anticholinergics (used to relax gastrointestinal spasm), a few blood pressure medications, procainamide, and surprisingly, several aspirinlike products used to reduce pain. An elevated temperature after vaccination and other immunizations is also not unusual. Body temperature is commonly measured by inserting a thermometer in the mouth under the tongue, in the rectum, or under the armpit (axillary). Some new devices measure skin surface temperature and convert it to body temperature.

Temperature may also be measured in the urine. There are times when a patient has a persistent high fever, yet no body pathology is detected. Measuring the temperature of the urine immediately after it is passed will indicate which patients have a false high temperature—that is, which patients are employing devices to deliberately raise the temperature of the thermometer.

When performed: In almost all instances of illness, especially infection, as an indication of the severity of the disease and to measure the success or failure of treatment. The basal body temperature is measured when patients have fertility problems; when chemical contraception is obviated; and when gynecological problems are suspected. The urinary temperature test is used when patients are suspected of faking fever.

Normal values: Normal body temperature is usually between 98° and 99° F, or around 37° C; there is usually a 1° rise in temperature at the time of ovulation. Normal skin surface temperature is about 86° F.

Abnormal values: Any elevation of body temperature greater than 100° F, failure of the body temperature to rise about 1° in the midmenstrual cycle, and a difference of more than 1° between body and urine temperature are all considered abnormal.

Risk factors: Breakage of the thermometer; the risk is, of course, relative to the thermometer's location. Should breakage occur, the amount of mercury released is not considered very dangerous. If thermometers are not properly sterilized prior to each use, there is the risk of transmitting infection.

Pain/discomfort: Minimal.

Cost: Rarely any additional charge for temperature measurements taken in the doctor's office. Most people own their own thermometers. A mercury glass thermometer costs $1 to $3; an electronic instant-reading thermometer is $10 to $20. Disposable thermometers average 10 cents apiece.

Accuracy and significance: Virtually all types of thermometers are 98 percent accurate. When using body temperature readings for ovulation time or birth control, special ovulation thermometers, with larger spaces between the pertinent degree divisions, are much easier to read.

BOECK'S SARCOID, see Kveim

BONE MARROW

Red and white blood cells and platelets are produced in the bone marrow. When a disease process affects the bone marrow, there is either an increase or a reduction of these essential blood elements. Also, depending on the nature of the disease, **Iron** may be increased in, or lost from, the bone marrow. A tiny amount of bone marrow can be aspirated (withdrawn) for examination with a syringe and special needle. The most common sites for bone marrow aspiration are the crest of the hipbone and the sternum (breastbone). Bone marrow may also be cultured for infection (see **Culture**).

One particular type of anemia, called aplastic anemia, needs confirmation by bone marrow studies. It is most commonly caused by exposure to a toxic agent; this could be an industrial chemical or insecticide, radiation, or even a therapeutic drug such as an antibiotic. It can also come following exposure to **Hepatitis,** and some believe it can be genetic in origin. While it is quite rare, it is a very serious, not easily cured, disease (see **Hemoglobin, Lymphocyte Typing,** and **Red Blood Cell**).

When performed: When leukemia, certain anemias, blood diseases such as hemolysis (self-destruction of red blood cells) or polycythemia (too many red blood cells), drug toxicity, or tumor growths such as lymphoma, myelofibrosis, and multiple myeloma are suspected; to follow the effectiveness of therapy in these diseases.

Normal values: A normal bone marrow specimen contains 15 different kinds of cells in varying stages of growth and in varying amounts. Normally, a small amount of iron is found in the marrow (detected using a special stain). Examination and determination of the normalcy of the different kinds of cells and the amount of iron must be made by a hematologist.

Abnormal values: Evidence of red cell destruction, presence of sickle or other diseased cells, absence of normal cells, and excess of diseased cells are all considered abnormal. Iron absence is found with iron deficiency anemia (usually due to blood loss); an increase in iron is seen with pernicious and hemolytic anemia and anemia caused by infection.

Risk factors: Negligible (see general risk factors for catheter or needle insertion).

Pain/discomfort: Even with a local anesthetic, there is often moderate to severe pain when the bone marrow aspiration needle penetrates the bone surface (see general pain/discomfort factors for catheter or needle insertion).

Cost: There is usually a charge of $25 to $75 to obtain a bone marrow specimen. If the specimen is analyzed by a hematologist, there is an additional fee of $35 to $100. When this test is performed in a hospital, most often for the doctor's convenience, the cost averages $350, excluding room charges.

Accuracy and significance: A bone marrow study is considered 95 percent accurate, better than a **Blood Cell Differential** study, especially to determine the leukemias and to ascertain the specific cause of anemia. Bone marrow studies are particularly significant in measuring adverse effects of toxic substances, including many of the drugs used to treat cancer.

BONE MINERAL DENSITY ANALYSIS

The density, or mass, of bone is determined by many factors, including one's diet, ethnic background, age, and sex. And it has been shown that even weight-bearing activities can stimulate new bone to form and prevent the loss of bone substance. Astronauts can lose 4 percent of their heel bone mass after two weeks in space, where they bear no weight, and even bedridden patients can lose 1 percent of their bone density a week—from their spinal column as well as from other bones. Normally, new bone is formed throughout life—even after the menopause in women—but at the same time, bone resorption (loss of mass) also takes place; bone loss or replacement with new bone is quite normal, but an excess of bone resorption can also be caused by various diseases or metabolic conditions. The most common one is called osteoporosis, so named because it leaves the bones porous, with what should be hard bone substance being replaced by empty vacuoles or air cavities. This, in turn, causes the bones to be brittle and break more easily. Other, somewhat similar diseases include osteomalacia (bone softening, usually due to a vitamin D and calcium lack) and osteodystrophy (defective bone, usually from a kidney and/or a parathyroid gland disease; it is most common in children).

Although doctors disagree as to the incidence of osteoporosis in women, especially after the menopause, it is estimated that from 10 to 25 percent of all women past 40 will suffer from this condition—and that usually means a bone fracture, most commonly of the spine. Studies do show that more than 1 million women have such fractures every year. And since it is now believed that it is possible to prevent or minimize osteoporosis, a test that will accurately reveal susceptibility to brittle bones could be extremely valuable. At the present time, there are several different tests that measure the density of bone, and while each has it supporters, there is no one absolutely accurate test. **Computerized Tomography** (CT) is one such test, but it is one of the most expensive ways to measure bone density, and it does involve exposure to a large amount of radiation. A modification of CT scanning, called densitometer CT scanning, has recently been introduced; this adaptation lessens the exposure to radiation and is said to be more accurate. Densitometer CT scanning can show the type of bone that first deteriorates in osteoporosis (in the body, there is trabecular, or spongy, bone and cortical, or hard, bone) and can therefore also be used to measure the progress of treatment for that disease. But as with CT, only the bones of the arms and legs can be adequately studied; the spine, where osteoporosis afflicts most women, is in too thick a portion of the body for this particular test. Regular X-rays are considered useless for measuring bone mineral density; almost half of a bone's density must be gone before a standard X-ray picture of an arm or hand will reveal a related abnormality. A newer, radiographically related test is called photon absorptiometry; here, the outer layer of the bones of the forearm is "scanned" (see **Nuclear Scanning**) by projecting beams of radioactive material through the bone and, with a computer, noting just how much of that radioactivity was absorbed. There are two types of photon absorptiometry: single-beam, or single-energy (SPA), and dual-beam, or dual-energy (DPA); SPA is usually used on the forearm, while DPA can measure bone density of the spine and the femur (the large bone of the thigh). Yet another test, called photodensitometry, combines photon absorptiometry and X-ray pictures; it is considered an indirect measure of bone density.

There are other, indirect methods of assessing calcium utilization in the body as a means of detecting the existence of, or susceptibility to, osteoporosis. Measuring **Calcium** in the blood or urine may offer clues to bone density. The Sulkowitch test, where calcium is measured in the urine over a period of several days—after a normal diet and then after first eating an excess of calcium, either in food or as supplements, and then after going without any calcium in the diet—has long been a simple screening test of calcium metabolism. Tests for **Phosphorus** and **Alkaline Phosphatase** can contribute to bone density estimates. **Parathyroid** hormone measurements are sometimes used to help differentiate the cause of brittle bones. Even **Estrogen** testing can offer bone density information; a decrease in the amount of this hormone in the blood seems to parallel a loss of bone substance. A bone **Biopsy** is yet another means of assessing bone density.

The most recent test is a measurement of bone gla-protein to indicate whether bone production equals or is less than bone loss. This protein, called osteocalcin, is part of bone manufacture.

When performed: To follow changes in bone minerals as a means of preventing osteoporosis or to follow the treatment of same. To help diagnose other bone diseases and calcium metabolism problems, when searching for the cause of certain gland or hormone deficiencies, to differentiate between cancer and other bone conditions, and in patients with some kidney diseases. To monitor therapy for bone disease.

Normal values: Bone mineral density varies with age and sex, and test results are compared with known standards; much depends on the experience and interpretation of the doctor "reading" the graph or computerized scan. The value is usually expressed in grams of mineral per square centimeter of bone when compared to what density would be expected in a "normal" individual of the same sex and age.

Abnormal values: When the patient being tested shows less than a normal amount of bone density. Abnormal values may also come from a condition called familial benign hypercalcemia, and although the emphasis is on testing women, men are also tested for similar bone disorders—especially when there are related symptoms. Young patients who have anorexia nervosa (severe weight loss because of an unwillingness to eat) also show decreased bone mineral density.

Risk factors: For blood tests, negligible (see general risk factors for blood testing). For urine tests, none. All other tests do involve exposure to radiation (see **Radiography**) to some degree, with photon absorptiometry causing the least amount of exposure. Bone density measurements of the spine naturally require greater radiation exposure than do tests of the arm.

Pain/discomfort: There is usually no pain or discomfort, other than the necessity of sitting or lying still for several moments at a time. For blood tests, see general pain/discomfort factors for blood testing.

Cost: Radiographic absorptiometry is considered the least expensive test; it runs

$65 plus the cost of the X-rays (two are taken at different exposures as a check on accuracy). SPA can cost from $35 to $200; DPA runs from $100 to $300. CTs range from $100 to $500, depending on which bones are studied. The Sulkowitch test may cost from $1 to $10, depending on whether it is performed by the doctor in the office or by the patient at home; some doctors do not charge for the solution to perform the test. Other blood tests can run from $5 to $500, depending on how many different ones are performed. A bone biopsy will cost from $100 to $300.

In 1985, some health insurance companies would not reimburse the doctor or patient for densitometer CT scanning, single- and dual-energy absorptiometry, and photodensiometry, claiming the efficacy of, and medical necessity for, these procedures has not been established.

Accuracy and significance: While none of the tests is very precise, they may indicate bone mineral density loss; they may also offer early warning signs of osteoporosis in time to prevent extensive bone damage. The doctor who interprets the test must always take into consideration the individual's size and weight; too much fatty tissue can cause misleading results. The real significance of these tests, at present, comes from following changes in an individual's bone density over a period of time — either to initiate treatment or to assess the value of therapy. It is believed that DPA and densitometer CT scanning are relatively the most accurate tests, followed by radiographic absorptiometry and then SPA. But none of the tests is infallible when it comes to predicting which patients are most subject to osteoporosis fractures. At the present time, the consensus is that most of these tests are about 50 percent accurate. And many doctors feel that the clinics now claiming to diagnose osteoporosis, or to identify women at risk for that disease, are misleading because of the lack of accuracy — at this time — of their testing.

BONE SCAN, see *Nuclear Scanning*

BORTNER, see *Jenkins Activity Survey*

BOTULISM

Botulism is considered the deadliest form of food poisoning. It comes from the causative bacteria's toxin (a substance given off by the bacteria rather than the bacteria itself), and although it may not cause any symptoms for up to 36 hours after ingestion — there have been cases where symptoms did not occur for eight days — it can be fatal within a day or two after symptoms appear. The bacteria are common in soil and can easily contaminate all sorts of foods; they must, however, be kept away from air to propagate. Proper food processing will eliminate the danger of the disease; careless home canning and meat smoking are the primary causes (boiling canned food for at least 20 minutes and never using cans that are swollen or jars that are not properly sealed are the best preventive measures). The first symptoms of botulism are usually visual: double vision and the inability to focus on near and far objects. There may be an inability to hold up the eyelids. A dry throat and difficulty in talking or swallowing usually follow. Ultimately, there is muscle weakness to the point of respiratory paralysis (breathing stops).

There are several forms of botulism. Infant botulism can occur within the first six months of life, and no specific cause is known (it is not believed to come from ingesting the toxin, although feeding honey has been implicated, and some feel it might come from dirt-contaminated floors). Wound botulism can come from contamination of an infected injury or even after a surgical incision. It has also been reported in drug abusers who inject drugs into themselves. And there have been cases of botulism where no food or wound can be incriminated.

The disease may imitate myasthenia gravis (see **Edrophonium**), poliomyelitis, the consequence of a tick bite, and even a stroke, to mention but a few of the problems in diagnosis. In 1985, the Public Health Service's Centers for Disease Control reported on cases of botulism that came from improperly handled fresh food (as opposed to home-canned food). Foods such as meat loaf, pot pies, baked potatoes, and fried onions that are allowed to stand at room temperature for several hours—or even a day or two—and then eaten without proper reheating have, in the past, been the source of this disease. All food to be eaten at a later time should be refrigerated and then thoroughly reheated before serving.

The most common ways of testing for botulism are by culturing (see **Culture**) the blood, the feces (see **Feces Examination**), and if at all possible, the foods eaten within the past several days. It is also possible to test for the botulism toxin in a patient's blood, feces, or a wound. First, a mouse is injected with material from a patient suspected of having the disease; if botulism was the cause, the mouse usually shows signs of paralysis and then dies within 24 hours. At the same time, another mouse is given botulism antitoxin and also injected with the same material; it should show no signs of the disease. It is also possible to test vomitus, stomach washings, and even spinal fluid for the toxin. While some state health department laboratories can perform these tests, in most instances, it is necessary to send specimens to the Centers for Disease Control in Atlanta, Georgia, for fast evaluation (toxin testing takes only one day; culture, at least three days).

When performed: On a patient who suddenly becomes ill with neurological symptoms and signs, especially with associated vision problems. Even though this disease is a form of food poisoning, there may or may not be nausea and vomiting, and there rarely is diarrhea. The most important aspect in diagnosing botulism is thinking of its possibility; evidence of home canning or of bad-tasting food from misshapen containers warrants immediate botulism testing, even before serious nerve or muscle abnormalities become evident. Infant botulism should be considered in a baby who suddenly becomes limp all over, especially after a period of constipation.

Normal values: No evidence of the bacteria or the toxin.

Abnormal values: Any evidence of the bacteria or the toxin. The bacteria and toxin can be found for a month after the disease onset.

Risk factors: For blood, negligible (see general risk factors for blood testing); for spinal fluid, see **Cerebrospinal Fluid;** for other specimens, virtually none.

Pain/discomfort: Minimal (see general pain/discomfort factors for blood testing); see also **Cerebrospinal Fluid** and **Feces Examination.**

Cost: In most instances, the cost of the test is borne by a government agency; detecting this disease is a public health measure. When private facilities do attempt testing for botulism, the cost can range from $30 to $100.

Accuracy and significance: The tests are 98 percent accurate when they show a positive result. Because this disease can be fatal within a very short period after symptoms appear, the significance of performing such tests where there is even the slightest thought of botulism is obvious.

Note: Some doctors feel that infant botulism may be one cause of sudden infant death syndrome (SIDS), at times called "crib death." (Also see **Sleep Monitoring**.)

BOVINE CERVICAL MUCUS, see *Semen*

BOWEL BLEEDING, see *Occult Blood*

BRADSHAW, see *Bence-Jones Protein*

BRAIN SCAN, see *Nuclear Scanning*

BRAIN STEM EVOKED RESPONSE, see *Hearing Function*

BRAIN STEM RESPONSE, see *Hearing Function*

BRAIN WAVE, see *Electroencephalogram*

BREAST CANCER, see *Biopsy; Cytology; Radiography; Thermography; Ultrasound*

BREAST STIMULATION STRESS, see *Nonstress Fetal Assessment*

BREATH ALCOHOL, see *Alcohol*

BREATH ANALYSIS, see *Lactose Tolerance*

BREATH CARBON MONOXIDE, see *Hemoglobin*

BREATH HYDROGEN, see *Lactose Tolerance*

BREATHING, see *Pulmonary Function; Smell Function*

BRODIE-TRENDELENBERG, see *Tourniquet Test for Varicose Veins*

BROMIDES

Before the introduction of tranquilizers, bromides were commonly prescribed as a sedative and a sleeping medicine. Today, some over-the-counter medications for insomnia may still contain bromides; as patients are known to take more medication than the directions advise, it is still possible to suffer from bromism or bromide poisoning. Bromide drugs, though rarely prescribed today, are used in some instances to treat epilepsy when all other drugs fail. A sensitivity to bromide drugs or an excess of bromides in the blood can produce all sorts of mental manifestations that imitate schizophrenia. Bromide intoxication can cause hallucinations, a condition of total apathy, and loss of appetite. Blood is taken from a vein, and the serum is examined. The urine can also be examined for bromides.

When performed: The test is one of many usually performed on an unconscious patient when there is no known cause for coma. It is also performed when excess intake of bromides is suspected and on patients who are confused or appear to be psychotic, especially when such behavior is new.

Normal values: Normally, there is no measurable amount of bromide in the blood serum and none in the urine.

Abnormal values: When a toxic amount of bromide has been ingested, more than 150 mg of bromide per 100 ml of serum is usually detected.

Risk factors: Negligible (see general risk factors for blood testing).

Pain/discomfort: Minimal (see general pain/discomfort factors for blood testing).

Cost: Blood testing for bromides is $5 to $30; urine testing is $30 to $35.

Accuracy and significance: If bromides are present, the test is 95 percent accurate in detecting them. It is of major significance in diagnosing an unconscious patient and of value in helping differentiate between psychotic behavior and drug-induced mental illness.

BROMSULPHALEIN (BSP)

Bromsulphalein is a trade name for sulfobromophthalein, and the Bromsulphalein retention test is used primarily to evaluate liver function when jaundice is *not* present. BSP is a dye that is injected into a vein after the patient has fasted for at least 12 hours (water is permitted). A normal working liver will immediately take up almost all the injected dye from the blood and secrete it into the bile. After 45 minutes, a blood sample is taken (from a different vein), and the amount of dye still remaining in the serum is measured. The dye is irritating and must be injected very carefully so that it does not seep around the vein under the skin, where it can cause tissue damage. It can also cause severe allergic shock in susceptible people. BSP is being replaced by a new dye, indocyanine green (ICG), which seems to cause less irritation or allergy.

When performed: The test is used when there is a suspicion of liver disease or some related condition of the gallbladder or bile ducts. It is primarily a screening test, since it does not reveal any specific diagnosis, and is used mostly when other, more precise liver function tests cannot be employed. The test is sometimes performed to follow the progress of a known liver condition during treatment.

Normal values: After the 45-minute period following injection of the dye, the blood normally retains less than 5 percent of that dye. With advancing age, up to 10 percent of the dye normally may still be found in the blood. A normal value, however, does not positively exclude liver disease.

Abnormal values: When there is liver disease, the blood may still have 80 percent of BSP after 45 minutes. Excess BSP retention in the blood can also be caused by gallbladder inflammation, intestinal hemorrhage, obesity, and drugs such as barbiturates, oral contraceptives and other estrogens, medication to help lower cholesterol levels, and phenolphthalein (in Ex-Lax and some other laxatives). If albumin (a normal serum protein) is lower than normal, an artificially low BSP will result.

Risk factors: In addition to the general risk factors for blood testing, catheter and needle insertion, and contrast substance use, it must be pointed out that reports indicate that allergic reactions even to injections of the less irritating substance, indocyanine green (ICG), cause death in 1 out of every 50,000 tests.

Pain/discomfort: In addition to the general pain/discomfort factors for blood testing and catheter and needle insertion, there can be pronounced discomfort if the dye seeps from the vein into adjacent tissues.

Cost: For pretesting for allergic reactions, injecting dye, and withdrawing blood for sampling, the fee is $10 to $30. An analysis of the blood to determine the amount of dye remaining in the serum averages $20.

Accuracy and significance: The BSP or ICG test is considered 50 percent accurate and significant as a means of diagnosing liver disease and as an aid in evaluating treatment for liver problems. Due to adverse reactions to the dye, the test is no longer widely used.

BRONCHIAL INHALATION CHALLENGE, see *Pulmonary Function*

BRONCHOALVEOLAR LAVAGE, see *Endoscopy*

BRONCHOGRAPHY, see *Radiography*

BRONCHOSCOPY, see *Endoscopy*

BRUCELLOSIS, see *Agglutination; Skin Reaction*

BSP, see *Bromsulphalein*

B$_{12}$, see *Schilling*

BUBO, see *Frei*

BUCCAL SMEAR, see *Chromosome Analysis*

BUFFER, see *Bicarbonate*

BUFFY COAT SMEAR, see *Blood Cell Differential*

BUN, see *Urea Nitrogen*

C

C, see *Complement*

CADMIUM

Although cadmium has been recognized as a body poison for some years, only recently have there been sufficiently accurate tests to diagnose toxicity from the metal. An accumulation of cadmium in the kidneys is believed to cause high blood pressure. It is also suspected as a cause of learning disabilities, loss of bone substance, liver damage, and anemia. Cadmium poisoning is the cause of Itai-Itai disease or osteomalacia, a softening of the bones that leads to bending, associated with kidney impairment. Cadmium is found in most foods and is particularly evident in oils and fats made from plants, a majority of alcoholic beverages, fish, and poultry. Usually, these foods also have a sufficient **Zinc** content (it seems that the more zinc these foods contain, the less likely it is that the cadmium will cause toxic effects). At one time, incidentally, cadmium was used as a lotion to treat dandruff. Symptoms of cadmium poisoning include: excessive salivation, nausea and vomiting, back and leg pain, and difficulty in breathing. These are pronounced among those industrial workers who inhale particles of the metal—people engaged in making batteries and dental supplies and those in the printing trade seem especially susceptible to cadmium's effects. Most people accumulate cadmium with age. Furthermore, it seems that cigarette smoking contributes to a buildup of cadmium. Both blood and urine can be examined for cadmium; **Hair Analysis** is also being evaluated for use in cadmium detection, especially in industrial and community surveys.

When performed: Primarily to detect and monitor increasing cadmium accumulation in those engaged in certain industries and in areas around industries that use cadmium-containing products—for example, where paint and other metal coatings are applied. Also, as part of a toxicological survey when heavy metal poisoning is suspected; where evident bone disease is difficult to diagnose; in chronic lung disease of an undetermined nature; and in children with learning problems, especially in an area where such problems seem more frequent than would be expected.

Normal values: If there has been no exposure to cadmium, the blood should reveal less than 10 ng per ml and the urine less than 10 mcg per liter. If there has been exposure, perhaps in industry or through pesticides, the blood often contains up to 40 ng per ml and the urine up to 600 mcg per liter, with no evidence of toxicity.

Abnormal values: A blood value greater than 50 ng per ml or urine containing more than 600 mcg per liter.

Risk factors: Negligible (see general risk factors for blood testing).

Pain/discomfort: Minimal (see general pain/discomfort factors for blood testing).

Cost: Precision testing for cadmium in the blood averages $40 and in the urine about $60. It is not usually included in generalized chemical screening groups for heavy metal testing; however, it may be included in hair analysis for toxic metals.

Accuracy and significance: Although the values obtained by testing are 95 percent accurate, it is questionable as to the amount of cadmium the body must accumulate before toxic symptoms appear or before there is actual body damage.

CAFFEINE

The active ingredient in coffee, tea, some cocoa, and many cola drinks is caffeine. Some consider caffeine the most commonly used mood-altering drug. While it is difficult to know the amount of caffeine in each of these beverages, because of the many variations in the original product (coffee bean, tea leaves, etc.) and the many different ways the beverages are brewed, it seems safe to say drip coffee averages the highest caffeine content (145 mg in a 6-ounce cup), followed by percolated coffee (100 mg), filter-brewed coffee (80 mg), and instant coffee (60 mg). Tea, when brewed for five minutes loose or in bags, averages from 30 to 60 mg per cup, depending on the brand. Cocoa contains anywhere from 5 to 50 mg per cup, while a cola drink can be as high as 100 mg per 12-ounce can. Numerous nonprescription drugs offered for headaches and colds and as aids in staying awake contain from 50 to 100 mg in each pill.

Caffeine produces a sense of feeling "good," "high," "alert," and "active," depending on the amount taken and how accustomed the body is to the drug. Unfortunately, caffeine can also cause anxiety, aggressive behavior, and insomnia and has been known to bring on schizophrenic reactions. Caffeine has even caused convulsions and death when self-administered by enema. It is now possible to measure the caffeine level in the blood and urine and to distinguish this drug from similar drugs, such as the xanthine drugs used to treat asthma. Caffeine is also measured, after ingesting a fixed amount, to determine how quickly the drug reaches active levels in the blood and how long it takes to be metabolized or leave the body.

When performed: In comatose patients; to evaluate the relation, if any, of caffeine to headaches, heart rhythm irregularities, eye problems, and other difficult-to-diagnose symptoms. Caffeine has been used, successfully at times, to commit suicide. To detect drug abuse, especially when caffeine is substituted for amphetamines and similar drugs (athletes sometimes use caffeine as a performance enhancer).

Normal values: If a patient does not use any products containing caffeine, there should be no measurable caffeine in the blood or urine.

Abnormal values: Blood levels greater than 10 mcg per ml, particularly when associated with the onset of symptoms. Urine should show about half that amount within two hours after ingestion. (The drug should be almost completely excreted within 48 hours.)

Risk factors: Negligible (see general risk factors for blood testing).
Pain/discomfort: Minimal (see general pain/discomfort factors for blood testing).
Cost: From $20 to $30 for each test, whether on blood or urine.
Accuracy and significance: Measurement of caffeine levels is 95 percent accurate, but the significance in each individual varies. Past experience with the drug must always be considered. If elevated blood levels are associated with symptoms, it is reasonable to assume a relationship.

CALCIFEROL, see *Vitamin D*

CALCITONIN

Calcitonin is a hormone produced by the thyroid gland. Its principal task seems to be to help the body get rid of excess **Calcium.** It acts in opposition to the parathyroid gland hormone, in that it slows down the release of calcium from the bones to the serum. Blood is taken from a vein, and the serum is tested. Calcitonin from salmon is even more potent in humans than human calcitonin and is used to treat certain bone disease.

When performed: When X-rays or other **Bone Mineral Density Analysis** tests show the bones to be losing minerals; when thyroid cancer or certain adrenal tumors are suspected; to verify high levels of calcium in the blood.

Normal values: From 5 to 300 pg per ml (usually less than 400 pg per ml) is considered normal.

Abnormal values: Calcitonin levels are increased with certain thyroid cancers, stomach cancers, anemia, and kidney disease.

Risk factors: Negligible (see general risk factors for blood testing).
Pain/discomfort: Minimal (see general pain/discomfort factors for blood testing).
Cost: From $35 to $65.
Accuracy and significance: The test is only about 85 percent accurate, as it has been

known to show normal values in some patients with the type of cancer that produces elevated values. Its significance is in differentiating among various forms of thyroid cancer. Calcitonin measurements are now being studied to follow the course of osteoporosis.

CALCIUM

There are approximately two pounds of calcium in the body at all times, almost all in the bones and teeth. About 0.03 ounce of calcium is taken in each day in a normal diet. This is the bare minimum required to fulfill the body's regular needs, because 80 percent of ingested calcium is excreted (in urine and sweat and through the bowels). Calcium is needed to maintain many body processes, such as muscle contraction and nerve transmission, to keep cells from being destroyed, and to ensure that blood will clot.

The body's calcium need and use are controlled by the hormone from the parathyroid glands (four separate, tiny glands buried within the thyroid gland but distinctly different from it) and almost as much by the amount of phosphorus and vitamin D in the body (see **Alkaline Phosphatase** and **Phosphorus**). When there is an excess of parathyroid hormone, calcium increases in the blood and phosphorus decreases; with insufficient parathyroid hormone, the opposite occurs. The thyroid gland exerts a serum-lowering effect on calcium through the production of a unique hormone called **Calcitonin.**

Three different forms of calcium are in the blood: the ionized, or active, form, which comprises approximately half the total amount; 45 percent in a form attached to the serum protein albumin; and a form attached to phosphates, which comprises about 5 percent of the total. The usual test for calcium measures all three forms and is called the total calcium (there are special tests to measure only the ionized portion). Blood calcium is measured in the serum from venous blood. It is also measured in the urine (Sulkowitch test), in the feces, and in the spinal fluid.

When performed: The test is used primarily when there are suspected abnormalities of the parathyroid gland; when there are mysterious symptoms such as memory problems, unusual sleepiness, or nerve and muscle problems; and in contrast, when there is excessive muscle irritability. When a patient has difficulty swallowing, tongue problems, or certain forms of deafness, measuring calcium levels in the blood may aid in discovering the cause. Other gland dysfunctions, such as a lack of adrenal hormones or too much thyroid hormone, may be diagnosed by testing for calcium. The test is also used when there is suspicion of vitamin D poisoning or unexplained bleeding and to differentiate various bone diseases, including the unique bone problems of women after the menopause, called osteoporosis (also see **Bone Mineral Density Analysis**), and when cancer is suspected.

Tests are now available for measuring **Parathyroid** hormone directly.

Normal values: Normal values in serum range from 8.5 to 10.5 mg per 100 ml (4.25 to 5.25 mEq per liter); in urine, no more than 150 mg in a 24-hour sample; in feces, about 800 mg a day (depending on diet); and in spinal fluid, 4 to 5 mg per 100 ml. Normal values may be higher in children and teenagers.

Abnormal values: Serum calcium is increased in hyperparathyroidism, certain bone tumors, and rarefaction or demineralization of bone (osteoporosis); adrenal disease; hyperthyroidism; when too much vitamin D or milk is taken; when too much antacid medication (usually for ulcers) is consumed; when diuretics are taken; and in rare lung diseases. Serum calcium is decreased when the parathyroid glands are inactive or if those glands have been accidentally removed during thyroid surgery; when there is insufficient vitamin D or when vitamin D cannot be absorbed; with kidney disease and certain bone diseases such as rickets; and in nutritional problems when insufficient calcium is eaten or absorbed. When serum calcium levels are lower than normal, total serum proteins (especially albumin) must be evaluated; decreased albumin will give a decreased calcium value (see **Albumin/Globulin**). Cancer is the most common cause of increased serum calcium levels.

Calcium levels in the urine fairly well reflect serum calcium levels, but they are increased when patients are taking certain diuretic drugs (which cause decreased levels in serum). Calcium is increased in feces when there are problems with intestinal absorption. Calcium levels are increased in the spinal fluid with tuberculous meningitis.

Risk factors: Negligible (see general risk factors for blood testing).

Pain/discomfort: Minimal (see general pain/discomfort factors for blood testing).

Cost: Routine calcium measurements in blood or urine are $5 to $25. The test is usually included in **Comprehensive Multiple Test Screening** panels, which range from $7 to $42. The fee to determine the ionized form of calcium, which usually includes the total calcium, is from $20 to $100.

Accuracy and significance: If correctly performed, the test is about 90 percent accurate in verifying the existence of numerous conditions. (A common error is using improperly cleaned glassware that contains traces of calcium.) As abnormal calcium levels are common to a variety of diseases and nutritional problems, the test's significance is particularly dependent on such factors as the doctor's observations, **Bone Mineral Density Analysis,** and corroborative hormone tests. In the past few years, the importance of measuring ionized calcium has increased; many doctors feel the usual total calcium values alone, although accurate in themselves, are relatively useless when diagnosing calcium-related diseases such as osteoporosis.

CALCULUS, see *Urinary Tract Calculus*

CALORIC

The caloric test is so named because it uses differences in temperature as the basis for diagnosing ear nerve damage that can cause dizziness.

Dizziness or vertigo can also accompany hearing loss, vision problems, brain disease, or alcoholism. Patients describe feelings of turning, twirling (or things around them twirling), and faintness. Vertigo is most often a result of disease to the vestibular part of the nerve that allows hearing; the vestibular part controls balance. In the caloric test, one teaspoon of ice water is instilled in the ear canal with a rubber syringe (similar to the technique used when washing wax out of the ear). This should cause nystagmus (the eyes move quickly away from the ice water and then slowly back). If nystagmus does not occur, two more teaspoons of ice water are used. Should the eyes still fail to move, four and then eight teaspoons of ice water are used.

At times, hot water is used as well as ice water. The hot water should cause an opposite eye movement pattern from the ice water. Performing the test with both hot and cold temperatures will give more accurate results. As a confirmation for vertigo, the Romberg test is used. The patient stands with feet together and eyes closed; with vertigo, the patient will tend to fall to one side.

The Bárány test is another way of evaluating whether the cause of dizziness is from the inner ear. Here, the patient sits in a special chair that can be rotated in a complete circle of one turn every 2 seconds; after from 20 to 30 seconds, the chair's motion is abruptly stopped. Although the body is no longer moving, the fluid in the inner ear canals continues to move and may reveal several signs to aid in the diagnosis; one sign is called nystagmus (involuntary movements of the eyeball in any direction). Another test for nystagmus is called past-pointing; here, a patient, with the arms outstretched and the eyes closed, places one fingertip of each hand on the tips of the doctor's matching fingers. The patient then raises his fingers and tries to relocate them on the doctor's fingertips. Those with inner ear problems cannot do this. This test is also done in conjunction with the caloric test as a confirmatory measure.

Electronystagmography provides a graphic recording of the eye movements, as opposed to visual observation. Here, the patient's eye movements can also be recorded behind closed eyes (with a band around the head over the eyes) with the patient's head and body in different positions as a means of determining if, in fact, body position affects the inner ear. Using electronystagmography, the optokinetic test projects a pattern of black stripes on a white background before the patient's **Visual Field** as a means of helping locate the exact site of the pathology. If the trouble is thought to be in the brain, as opposed to the ear or its nerve, a saccadic velocity test may be performed (saccades is the ability to move the eyes rapidly from one point to another—such as when reading). People with nystagmus, from ear disease or certain neurological conditions, cannot make these rapid eye movements; instead, their rate of eye shifting shows up as quite slow. This test is also said to reveal drug abuse (being under the influence of various intoxicants and mind-altering drugs) in drivers and some police departments are now applying the test in the field (using a disposable head band).

When performed: Primarily when there is dizziness or fainting, especially after ear injury or in ear disease; whenever impaired hearing exists; with patients taking certain antibiotic drugs and with anemias; when psychological problems are suspected; with a comatose patient to determine the extent, if any, of brain damage.

Normal values: Nystagmus should occur after one teaspoon of water is instilled in the ear canal.

Abnormal values: If nystagmus does not appear until after two or more teaspoons of ice water are placed in the ear, the ear nerve may be diseased, but the possibility of cure exists. If eight teaspoons of ice water in the ear do not produce nystagmus, it may be assumed that the nerve is permanently damaged.

Vertigo can be caused by any disease or injury that affects the vestibular nerve as well as damage inflicted by many antibiotic drugs (usually when given in large doses for long periods of time). Atherosclerosis of the blood supply to the ear, cholesteotomas (growths), and certain poisons can also cause vertigo.

Risk factors: Negligible. Too much water pressure can injure a previously damaged eardrum, but this rarely occurs.

Pain/discomfort: Minimal, although some patients find cold water in the ear mildly uncomfortable.

Cost: Approximately $10 to $15. Nystagmography runs from $100 to $300. There is usually no charge for the Bárány test.

Accuracy and significance: Considered 80 percent accurate in differentiating between treatable and permanently nontreatable ear disease.

CANCER

At the present time, there is no absolute, or even consistently reliable, test for early cancer detection; nor is there a reasonably accurate test to screen for hidden cancers. If any one test comes close, it is the **Carcinoembryonic Antigen** (CEA), once considered specific for colon and rectal cancers (some doctors think it justifiable for lung cancers, but that is now considered inadequate by the National Institutes of Health). The **Acid Phosphatase** test for prostatic acid phosphatase (PAP) is considered useful in diagnosing early prostate cancer. Some doctors use the **Alpha Fetoprotein** test to substantiate liver cancers; others use a version of the ferritin (see **Iron**) test, which measures isoferritins, to confirm suspicions of liver cancer as well as other cancers. A particular ferritin substance is occasionally found on the T cells and B cells (see **Lymphocyte Typing**) of breast cancer patients; T and B cells are also examined for lymph cell cancers. **Hydroxyproline** tests are employed when bone cancer is suspected, and a few doctors use hydroxyproline measurements for breast cancer evaluation. **Alkaline Phosphatase** values are considered to be of diagnostic aid in bone and liver cancers (or when cancer cells from other parts of the body migrate to the bone or liver, a process known as metastasis); even the enzyme tests used to evaluate **Alcoholism** are considered of value in discovering metastasis to the liver. The alpha-antitrypsin test (see **Albumin/Globulin**) is a generalized, though nonspecific, indication of cancer, as is the **Haptoglobin** test, another form of globulin. **Lactic Dehydrogenase** (LDH), while nonspecific, can offer a clue that cancer may be present somewhere within the body, most likely in the breast, lung, or bowel. **Catecholamines** can signal the possible presence of an adrenal gland tumor or some abnormal nervous system growth.

Some hormone tests can point to cancer. **Calcitonin** values may help diagnose thyroid cancer; human chorionic gonadotropin (see **Pregnancy** and **Testis Function**) and lactogenic hormone (see **Prolactin**) abnormalities are known to result from various tumors; **Gastrin** values are extremely abnormal when certain stomach tumors exist; and antithyroglobulin levels are sometimes used to aid in the diagnosis of thyroid cancer (see **Thyroid Function**). The **Estrogen Receptor** test helps determine which cancers will respond to hormone therapy instead of surgery. **Serotonin,** which some doctors believe is a hormone, is used experimentally as a diagnostic aid for certain cancers. **Glucagon** and **Insulin** tests are performed when there is a suspicion of a pancreas tumor. **Cortisol** measurements can direct attention to the possibility of an adrenal gland tumor, especially when coordinated with a test for **Catecholamines.**

Immunoglobulin tests can offer early warning signs for certain cancers, particularly multiple myeloma (see **Bence-Jones Protein**).

Cancer markers: Many of the tests mentioned are also known as cancer markers or tumor markers; while some are associated with a particular tumor, others may be indicative of more than one form of cancer. A cancer marker can be an antigen, collagen breakdown product (collagen is the matrix, or supporting tissue, of skin and other body tissues and organs), enzyme, or protein; it is usually produced by, or in association with, a cancer and is thought to signal a cancer's presence. Although not absolute in their diagnostic abilities, many of these tests are nevertheless being used more and more as a means of screening for unsuspected growths in various parts of the body. In addition to those tests already cited, some doctors measure ACTH (see **Cortisol**) when looking for lung and intestinal cancers; 5-nucleotide phosphodiesterase in suspected breast and liver cancers; **Placental Lactogen** when considering genitourinary and testicular cancers; erythropoietin, a kidney-produced hormone that stimulates **Red Blood Cell** production, when kidney or liver tumors are under study; **Fibrin Degradation Products** for suspected liver tumors; and even blood group antigens (see **Typing and Cross-matching**) have been tried for various growths thought to be cancer, especially in the bladder. The red cell adherence test uses the principle that tumor cells will attach themselves to certain blood group antigens. Some patients with systemic mastocytosis (an invasion of mast or connective tissue cells into the skin) and those who develop a tumor called an argentaffinoma (see **Serotonin**) produce an excess of histamine in their urine; this, too, can be a cancer marker, although people who eat large amounts of spinach, eggplant, and certain cheeses and drink red wines will also show large amounts of urinary histamine without having cancer. And even monoclonal antibodies (see **Agglutination**) are becoming tumor markers. At Oxford University, they have developed one, called Ca 1, that is said to attach itself to the antigen of several different cancers, especially those found in the fluids that surround a tumor such as in the intestines. The failure of this monoclonal antibody to reveal cancer antigens is, at present, thought to indicate the absence of a cancer. Arginine vasopressin (see **Vasopressin**) has been found in patients who have lung and pancreas cancers, while vasoactive intestinal polypeptide (a hormone made by cells in the intestine) has also been found in pancreatic and lung cancers; it has been found as well in patients who have pheochromocytoma (an adrenal tumor that causes high blood pressure).

Other indirect tests for cancer, tests whose positive results could just as well indicate a noncancerous condition, include: Pap smears (see **Cytology**), **Occult Blood, Sputum, Dilitation and Curettage,** and what might well be the three most useful cancer screening tests of all—the digital rectal examination, breast self-examination, and testicle self-examination. Even self-surveying of one's skin and body for unusual markings, blemishes, and swellings can be a valuable cancer screening test—if you seek professional advice regarding any observed changes.

At the present time, however, most doctors believe a combination of tests affords a better opportunity for a diagnosis than the use of only one or two tests. There are also other forms of medical testing such as **Radiography, Nuclear Scanning, Ultra-**

sound, **Computerized Tomography,** and even variations on the **Agglutination** test that may help detect hidden cancer.

In 1985, the director of the National Cancer Institute revealed that viruses probably cause more cancers than previously thought (see **Virus Disease**). One example is where the virus invades T cells (see **Lymphocyte Typing**); these are the cells that are part of the body's immune system (see **Immunology**). Another example is liver cancer; it is now believed that this disease is preceded by viral hepatitis. Unlike virus-caused colds and similar conditions, it is postulated that very intimate contact is needed (such as sex or blood transfusions) to transmit a virus-caused cancer.

CANCER MARKERS, see *Cancer*

CANCER RESPONSIVENESS TO HORMONES, see *Estrogen Receptor*

CANDIDA EXTRACT, see *Skin Reaction*

CANDIDIASIS, see *Agglutination; Fungus*

Ca 1 ANTIBODY, see *Cancer*

CAPILLARY FRAGILITY (Rumpel-Leede)

In a number of diseases of blood vessels — such as thrombocytopenia (decreased thrombocytes or platelets needed for clotting), disorders of platelet function, scurvy, and purpura — the small blood vessels near the skin surface become very fragile. In the capillary fragility test, a blood pressure cuff is placed on the forearm and inflated until it is approximately midway between the diastolic and systolic pressure — usually from 80 to 100 mm of mercury (see **Blood Pressure**). This pressure is maintained for five to ten minutes. The cuff is removed, and the arm is inspected for the number of petechiae (small hemorrhages) that have appeared under the skin in a premarked area. The test is sometimes used to help detect eye pathology in diabetics; there is, however, no general agreement on its value for this purpose because of a great many false positives.

The petechiometer is a new device now available to measure capillary fragility. A small suction cup is applied to the forearm, and pressure, measured and controlled by a gauge, performs the same function as it does with the blood pressure cuff.

When performed: As one of many tests to determine hemostatic function (blood clotting and blood vessel structure).

Normal values: Normally, the cuff pressure will not produce petechiae. For some unknown reason, women with red hair are sometimes more sensitive and have a slightly positive reaction without any disease condition.

Abnormal values: The appearance of multiple petechiae indicates weakness of the tiny blood vessels and/or a platelet defect.

Risk factors: Negligible, as this is a noninvasive test.

Pain/discomfort: Minimal; some patients find the tightness of the blood pressure cuff uncomfortable.

Cost: Usually, no additional charge over and above the doctor's fee for an office visit. When performed in a hospital, the charge runs from $15 to $20.

Some doctors consider this test outmoded, and it is possible that a health insurance company or government-sponsored medical program will not reimburse the doctor or patient for the cost of the test.

Accuracy and significance: Although the test indicates susceptibility to spontaneous bleeding under the skin, it is of no major significance, as it cannot differentiate among defects in the capillaries or platelet disease. Although it is considered only about 50 percent accurate, there are some doctors who regularly use this test as a confirmation of diabetic retinopathy when *Fundoscopy* is equivocal.

CAPNOGRAPHY, see *Carbon Dioxide*

CARBAMATES, see *Cholinesterase*

CARBOHYDRATE ANTIGEN 19–9, see *Carcinoembryonic Antigen*

CARBONATES, see *Bicarbonate*

CARBON DIOXIDE (CO_2)

Carbon dioxide and water are end products of oxygen metabolic processes. Carbon dioxide's primary route of elimination is through the lungs (during respiration, the blood gives off CO_2 and picks up oxygen); a small amount of CO_2 is changed into bicarbonates and is excreted in the urine. The depth and rapidity of a person's breathing help to control the blood CO_2 levels.

There are several different ways to measure carbon dioxide in the blood. The oldest and probably the most common test (although it is considered the least precise) measures the *carbon dioxide combining power*. A more accurate evaluation is obtained by measuring the *carbon dioxide content* (called capnography); when performed with the **pH** test, it will also demonstrate the exact amounts of free bicarbonate and carbonic acid in the blood. The preferred method of evaluation is testing for *carbon dioxide tension*, or PCO_2 (sometimes called partial pressure or carbonic acid concentration).

Regardless of how CO_2 is determined, the primary purpose of the test is to measure ventilation, or how well air moves in and out of the lungs. A secondary purpose is to determine what is affecting the acid-base balance, or pH (acidity or alkalinity), of the blood, which is an extremely important and very sensitive reflection of potentially disastrous bodily disorders. Blood is taken from either an artery or a vein in a special syringe to avoid any contact with air, and the serum is tested.

When performed: Whenever there are respiratory problems; whenever there is suspicion of acidosis (excessively low blood pH) or alkalosis (excessively high pH), both of which are usually brought about by metabolic or respiratory disorders; when a patient has suffered severe injuries, is in coma, or is severely disoriented; when there are severe muscle cramps, severe vomiting, or diarrhea.

Normal values: Carbon dioxide tension (PCO_2) normally ranges from 35 to 45 mm Hg in arterial blood (slightly lower in women) and 38 to 50 mm Hg in venous blood; CO_2 content, from 19 to 25 mM per liter in arterial blood and 22 to 30 mM per liter in venous blood; and CO_2 combining power, from 24 to 32 mEq per liter in arterial blood and 38 to 50 mEq per liter in venous blood.

Abnormal values: Increased carbon dioxide is found primarily in respiratory acidosis from lung conditions that prevent CO_2 from being exhaled (such as asthma, emphysema, and severe chest injuries) and during anesthesia when the patient rebreathes his own air. It is usually elevated with metabolic alkalosis caused by taking diuretic drugs, steroid hormones, or antacid preparations; with vomiting, intestinal obstruction, and starvation; and with hyperactive adrenal glands. Decreased carbon dioxide is found with metabolic acidosis caused by drug poisoning (especially from aspirin and from ammonium chloride that is sold for use as a diuretic without a prescription) and with diarrhea, liver disease, kidney disease, and diabetes that is out of control. It is also lower than normal when respiratory alkalosis exists (most commonly caused by hyperventilation, or deliberate rapid breathing).

Risk factors: Negligible (see general risk factors for blood testing).

Pain/discomfort: Minimal (see general pain/discomfort factors for blood testing).

Cost: In most instances, carbon dioxide is determined along with oxygen and pH. When the three tests are performed together, they are usually performed in a hospital, as patients requiring such tests are almost always seriously ill. The cost for testing for all blood gases as a group averages $40 to $60. Carbon dioxide alone can be measured, either as carbon dioxide content or as **Bicarbonate;** the charge for bicarbonate is $9 to $24. The carbon dioxide test alone is occasionally included in **Comprehensive Multiple Test Screening** panels, which are $7 to $42.

Accuracy and significance: The measurement of carbon dioxide tension, along with oxygen tension and pH, is considered 90 percent accurate to evaluate the function of the lung, which is to permit oxygen to reach and saturate the blood. Measurements of the blood gases are the most significant **Pulmonary Function** tests in diagnosing the body's ability to carry adequate oxygen to the tissues and to dispose of carbon dioxide as a waste product of metabolism.

CARBON MONOXIDE (CO)

Carbon monoxide is a colorless, odorless, tasteless gas that is a deadly poison in the tiniest amount. It can come from heaters, furnaces (especially those that are defective), engines that burn gasoline (even power lawn mowers), charcoal barbecue fires, and cigarette smoking. Industrial plants, refineries, and any other sites where incomplete burning takes place can be a source of CO. Obviously, any enclosed place such as a garage—including one at home—or a motor vehicle tunnel can accumulate dangerous amounts of the gas. CO causes illness by replacing normal oxygen-carrying **Hemoglobin** in the blood with carboxyhemoglobin, which cannot carry life-supporting oxygen to the brain and all other body organs. Inhaling minute amounts of this gas can cause symptoms that mimic many different illnesses (dizziness, shortness of breath, fainting, giddiness, headache, impaired judgment, memory loss, muscle paralysis, ringing in the ears, unconsciousness, and vomiting, to name but a few). Exposure to CO can make existing heart disease much worse, and it can decrease the amount of **Estrogens** in women and testosterone (see **Testis Function**) in men, causing **Impotence**. In a study of runners in urban areas, it was shown that traffic-produced CO caused a fourfold increase in their carboxyhemoglobin blood levels.

There are several ways to test for CO; most commonly, it is measured in the blood, but breath testing is considered just as accurate. Many doctors feel it is equally important to test for CO in the patient's environment, using monitors, at the workplace, at home—especially in the garage or where water and room heaters are stored—and inside the patient's motor vehicle. Smokers are frequently tested during pregnancy; a pregnant woman who smokes can cause a marked loss of oxygen to the fetus.

When performed: Usually, when the doctor happens to think of CO exposure as a possible cause for the patient's illness. Some doctors do CO testing when they are considering anemia, especially if the patient reports episodes of deep-red skin color. When headaches are recurring, especially when accompanied by dizziness or fainting. As a means of discouraging smoking.

Normal values: Although there should never be any CO in the blood, just about everyone will show from 1 to 3 percent blood carboxyhemoglobin (or CO directly with breath testing). Those who smoke (cigarettes, cigars, pipes, plants) can show CO levels up to 20 percent; although this may be usual for such individuals, it is not normal. Those who work in and around motor vehicles, especially in enclosed areas, may show blood levels from 10 to 15 percent.

Abnormal values: Although any amount of CO is abnormal, it usually takes 10 percent or more to cause symptoms; some tests, however, have shown that even 3 percent can produce mental impairment. When blood levels reach 20 percent or more, the consequences can be very dangerous; when 50 percent is approached, it almost always causes unconsciousness; and 60 percent is fatal. A 10 percent level of carboxyhemoglobin in the blood requires only 30 parts per million of CO in the air.

Risk factors: Negligible (see general risk factors for blood testing).

Pain/discomfort: Minimal (see general pain/discomfort factors for blood testing).

Cost: Blood testing averages $30; breath testing can cost anywhere from $1 to $15, depending on the technique and instrument used. Home monitors cost from $1 to $5 each, although there are pocket digital monitors that sell for hundreds of dollars.

Accuracy and significance: While blood testing is considered 95 percent accurate, breath testing is sufficient for most purposes. Environment testing, especially when related to symptoms, is most significant when it detects a CO source.

CARBOXYHEMOGLOBIN, see *Carbon Monoxide; Hemoglobin*

CARCINOEMBRYONIC ANTIGEN (CEA)

Originally, the carcinoembryonic antigen (CEA) test was used to detect **cancer** of the colon, but the antigen has since been found to appear with other cancers, as well (pancreas, lung, breast, and prostate). Blood is drawn from a vein, and the serum is examined. Other body fluids (joint fluid, peritoneal fluid, amniotic fluid) may also be tested. A newer antigen, carbohydrate antigen 19–9 (CA 19–9) used along with CEA has been reported to detect a recurrence of gastrointestinal cancer sooner than when CEA is used alone. It is also claimed CA 19–9 is more sensitive in detecting pancreas cancer (see **Pancreas Function**).

When performed: The test is performed primarily to follow the course and treatment of patients with known cancers. It is also used to determine the extent of cancer, since CEA can return to normal values following successful surgery. When a cancer patient has a checkup, the level of carcinoembryonic antigen may rise months before new symptoms appear, alerting the doctor to the need for immediate further therapy. The test may also be performed to diagnose certain causes of jaundice.

Normal values: Levels below 2 ng per ml are not considered indicative of pathology. Carcinoembryonic antigen is found in very small amounts in many pregnant women, in infants, and in other normal individuals.

Abnormal values: A CEA greater than 5 to 10 ng per ml is found in a majority of patients with known cancer. Increased values are also found in patients with alcoholic cirrhosis, colitis, ulcers, and emphysema, and in heavy smokers. A subspecies of CEA called CEA-S is specific for gastrointestinal cancers without being elevated for other conditions.

Risk factors: Negligible (see general risk factors for blood testing and catheter and needle insertion).

Pain/discomfort: Minimal (see general pain/discomfort factors for blood testing and catheter and needle insertion).

Cost: From $25 to $80.

Accuracy and significance: The CEA test has a high sensitivity rating—it is usually elevated in a cancer patient, particularly one with cancer of the colon—however, it has a low specificity. Less than half the patients with early cancer show a positive test. The test is most useful in following the progress of cancer patients who have had treatment, as it helps evaluate which type of treatment is the most effective. The CEA should not be considered a routine screening test for cancer. It is thought to be 70 percent accurate.

CARDIAC CATHETERIZATION, see *Nuclear Scanning; Radiography*

CARDIAC CINERADIOGRAPHY, see *Radiography*

CARDIAC GLYCOSIDE, see *Digitalis Toxicity*

CARDIAC OUTPUT (CO), see *"Angiography," in Radiography*

CARDIAC PACING, see *Electrocardiogram*

CARDIAC SCAN, see *Nuclear Scanning*

CARDIOGRAM, see *Electrocardiogram*

CARDIOTOCOGRAPHY, see *Fetal Monitoring*

CAROTENE, see *Retinol*

CAROTID ARTERY PULSE, see *Pulse Analysis*

CAROTID SINUS MASSAGE

The carotid sinus, although not a true sinus such as the air cavities in the head, is really a dilatation of the carotid artery on both sides of the neck where that artery divides in two; one branch carries blood inside the skull to the brain, eye, and other adjacent tissues, while the other branch carries blood to the organs, glands, and tissues in the front of the face. There are two carotid "bodies" (as the sinuses are frequently called), one on each side of the neck at about the level of the upper part of the thyroid gland. Each tiny carotid body, inside each carotid sinus, is a small bundle of extremely sensitive nerves that react to minute changes in the blood (pH, pressure, oxygen content, carbon dioxide content) and even to pressure applied from the outside on the skin of the neck over the areas where the carotid bodies lie. An irritation of the carotid body can cause changes in blood pressure, a change in the heart rate (pulse), and alterations of the rhythm of the heart. Standing, from a sitting or lying position, can also cause the carotid body to send out nerve impulses that will alter one's pulse and blood pressure. Sudden head movements, especially rotation, and the wearing of tight collars have been known to irritate the carotid body to the point of causing syncope (fainting). In the days when men routinely wore stiff, tight collars, it was not unusual for a man to faint while standing in front of a urinal; the "habit" of looking up toward the ceiling while urinating could cause sufficient pressure on the carotid body to lower the blood pressure and lessen the pulse so that insufficient oxygen was carried to the brain for several seconds—just enough time to produce fainting.

Because of carotid sinus/body sensitivity, deliberate massaging of the areas has been used as a test to evaluate patients who have frequent fainting spells. With a physician performing the test, or at least present during the testing, the patient's blood pressure and **Electrocardiogram** (ECG) are observed while pressure—of a massaging nature—is applied to each carotid sinus area. Usually, the test is first performed while the patient is lying down, and depending on the response or lack of same, the test may be repeated in the sitting or standing position. At times, certain drugs may be administered during the test, either as a means of confirming the observations or as a way of reversing some of the effects caused by the test. For some as yet unexplained reason, the carotid body on the right side of the neck is usually more sensitive than the body on the left side, but sensitivity on either side can cause a test reaction. Some doctors perform this test before they prescribe certain drugs, such as digitoxin or the "beta blockers," for their patients; these drugs seem to make the carotid bodies more sensitive than usual.

When performed: To help uncover the cause of fainting. To aid in uncovering the cause of irregular heart rhythms. To assess a patient's reaction to certain drugs.

Normal values: When pressure is applied to the carotid sinus, most people have a 10-point drop in blood pressure and a slowing of the heart by about five beats per minute. Patients who have high blood pressure or some forms of heart disease usually experience a greater lowering of their blood pressure and a more pronounced slowing of their heart rate. Blood pressure and heart rate usually return to normal within a few minutes after massage is stopped.

Abnormal values: A large decrease in blood pressure (more than 30 points) and a severe slowing of the pulse (more than 20 beats a minute) accompanied by a fainting-type episode (it may be called a blackout, light-headedness, a weak spell, or even a dizzy spell). The feeling should reproduce the symptom being investigated. In a few instances, the dizziness may occur without any real changes in blood pressure or pulse.

Risk factors: This can be a dangerous test, especially if the patient has some blockage of one or both carotid arteries; strokes and even death have happened while the test was being performed. Expert professional help and corrective drugs must be at hand during the test.

Pain/discomfort: Those who have a normal reaction to carotid sinus massage usually feel no discomfort; those who experience a fainting sensation generally have no other discomfort.

Cost: Much depends on the staff assigned to perform the test. Some doctors insist it be performed in a hospital with an anesthetist standing by in the event of an emergency. Since an ECG must be performed along with blood pressure monitoring, the cost of these procedures must be included. In general, when performed in a hospital, the test runs from $100 to $500, plus the cost of hospitalization. When performed in a physician's office, the cost averages $200.

Accuracy and significance: In patients who have been through a great many different tests to diagnose the cause of fainting, the test can be very significant. If the test produces the same symptoms the patient has been suffering, it is 90 percent accurate in uncovering the underlying cause of the illness—one that is often not even considered by many doctors. Dangerous as the test can be, it can also be lifesaving if it helps detect patients who are unusually sensitive to certain heart drugs.

CAT (X-RAY), see *Computerized Tomography*

CATECHOLAMINES

Catecholamines are produced by the medulla, or central part of the adrenal gland, as opposed to the outer area, or cortex, where cortisone-type hormones originate (see **Cortisol**). Epinephrine (adrenalin) and norepinephrine (noradrenalin) are the two principal catecholamine hormones. They are called pressor amines because of their ability to constrict blood vessel walls, thus elevating the blood pressure. Norepinephrine is also necessary to transmit nerve impulses in the brain.

The two catecholamines can be tested in the blood, but they are most commonly measured in the urine, along with their metabolic end products, vanillymandelic acid (VMA), homovanillic acid (HVA), and metanephrines. Recently, it has been found that decreased amounts of norepinephrine in the brain cause patients to experience symptoms of depression; excessive amounts seem to be associated with manic symptoms.

Decreased amounts of norepinephrine in the urine, accompanied by decreased amounts of 3-methoxy-4-hydroxyphenyl glycol (MHPG), another related catecholamine, are considered good evidence for a diagnosis of psychologically caused depression, particularly when exhibited as manic-depression. Increased values point to depression engendered by a physical rather than a psychological condition. There is tentative evidence that decreased MHPG with increased norepinephrine, VMA, and HVA signifies schizophrenia.

At times, clonidine (a drug used to lower blood pressure) is given to patients, and then their blood is tested for norepinephrine three hours later as a means of detecting the cause of unexplained high blood pressure. It is called the clonidine suppression test.

There is now a filter-paper urine test for catecholamines that parents can perform at home on 6-month-old babies; the urine-wetted paper is mailed to the testing laboratory as a means of screening for a neuroblastoma (a tumor of nervous cells that occurs mostly in very young children).

When performed: When pheochromocytoma (a tumor of the adrenal gland that causes high blood pressure) is suspected; to assess adrenal function; in certain cases of depression when a specific cause cannot be found; when neuroblastoma is suspected.

Normal values: Urine levels should not exceed 100 mcg per 100 ml in a 24-hour sample. A single urine sample should not exceed 15 mcg per 100 ml. Plasma epinephrine averages 20 ng per 100 ml; norepinephrine, 60 ng per 100 ml. Urine VMA should not exceed 8 mg per 100 ml in a 24-hour sample.

Abnormal values: When total urine catecholamines exceed 200 mcg per 100 ml and/or VMA is greater than 25 mg per 100 ml, disease is present, most likely pheochromocytoma. However, several other nerve tumors can cause increased values (in which case, HVA is also increased), as can myasthenia gravis and muscular dystrophy. Certain drugs such as those used to treat depression, aspirin, some antibiotics, and coffee, tea, chocolates, fruits, and vanilla extract can cause false high values. Stress or exercise can increase catecholamines. Increased norepinephrine has been found in autism.

Risk factors: Negligible (see general risk for blood testing).

Pain/discomfort: Minimal (see general pain/discomfort factors for blood testing).

Cost: Urine evaluations of all the catecholamines average $23 to $33. Blood evaluations are $35 to $50. When catecholamines are individually identified, the cost is $65 to $75. A determination of VMA and HVA in the urine is $13 to $45.

Accuracy and significance: Catecholamine measurements are 90 percent accurate in the diagnosis of pheochromocytoma, but at this time they have little significance in other conditions. The test's accuracy is affected by a variety of foods and drugs and can also show a misleading value related to the amount of physical activity prior to testing.

CAT SCAN, see *Computerized Tomography*

CAT-SCRATCH DISEASE, see *Skin Reaction*

CEA, see *Carcinoembryonic Antigen*

CellSoft-CASA, see *Semen*

CELLULOSE TAPE, see *Feces Examination*

CENTRAL VENOUS PRESSURE, see *Blood Pressure*

CENTRAL VISUAL FIELD, see *Visual Field*

CEPHALIN FLOCCULATION (Cephalin-Cholesterol Flocculation)

Cephalin flocculation is used to measure liver cell function. Cephalin is a plasma lipid. It will not normally flocculate, or clump, if there are balanced levels of serum albumin and gamma globulins. When the **Albumin/Globulin** ratio is upset, the woolly looking precipitation (flocculation) of cephalin is increased. Blood from a vein is tested. A **Thymol Turbidity** test is usually performed as a parallel check on cephalin flocculation.

When performed: As a general screening test when liver disease is suspected; to follow the progress of patients with known liver disease.

Normal values: From negative to no more than a 1-plus (very slight) flocculation is considered normal.

Abnormal values: Readings of 2-plus to 4-plus (visibly increased clumping) suggest liver disease from within the liver itself, as opposed to a bile tract obstruction.

Risk factors: Negligible (see general risk factors for blood testing).
Pain/discomfort: Minimal (see general pain/discomfort factors for blood testing).
Cost: From $5 to $10.

Some doctors consider this test outmoded, and it is possible that a health insurance company or government-sponsored medical program will not reimburse the doctor or patient for the cost of the test.

Accuracy and significance: Although the test indicates liver damage 50 percent of the time and may help differentiate between direct liver damage and bile duct blockage, its significance is minimal, as it makes no distinction among the different causes of liver disease. The test is no longer widely used, especially where more sophisticated liver evaluations are available.

CEREBELLUM

The cerebellum is the part of the brain that helps control balance and coordination. Loss of coordinated movements can result from cerebellum disease as well as from certain nerve conditions that cause inability to feel pressure and other sensations. The cerebellum tests help to determine if the problem is in the brain itself, as opposed to the spinal cord and its nerve extensions.

The easiest coordination test is to have the patient stand up with feet together and close his eyes; with cerebellum disease the patient tends to fall. Attempting to walk heel to toe with eyes closed is an extension of the same test. In another simple coordination test the patient may be asked to touch the tip of his nose with his finger (with the arm first extended out); the test is repeated with the eyes closed. Trying to touch the fingers in rapid succession with the thumb is another cerebellum test, as is trying to point to objects with the big toe while lying down.

When performed: In cases of ataxia (loss of muscle coordination or irregular muscle actions); when brain disease is suspected; following head injuries; to differentiate alcoholism, drug, or hysterical reactions from physical disease.

Normal values: Normally, patients perform the simple tasks of coordination without difficulty.

Abnormal values: Patients with impaired coordination are unable to perform the simple movements described. Usually, only one side of the body is affected with cerebellum disease; both sides of the body are generally involved with conditions that arise from below the brain level.

Risk factors: Negligible. Attendants should be on hand to prevent injury as a result of a fall.

Pain/discomfort: None.

Cost: No charge; it is usually part of the routine physical examination.

Accuracy and significance: When all the cerebellum tests are performed in sequence, the test is 95 percent accurate in diagnosing loss of coordination as a specific brain condition.

CEREBRAL ANGIOGRAPHY, see *Radiography*

CEREBROSPINAL FLUID

Testing the spinal fluid—more accurately described as the cerebrospinal fluid, since it surrounds the brain as well as the spinal cord—is a valuable diagnostic aid in many nervous system diseases (infections and brain and spinal cord damage associated with injury or cancer). Many tests may be performed on the spinal fluid; the usual examination consists of measuring the pressure of the fluid within the spinal canal, observing the transparency and color of the fluid, and counting the white blood cells. The most common chemical tests performed on spinal fluid to establish or prove a diagnosis are chloride, sugar, proteins, and quantitative VDRL (Venereal Disease Research Laboratories) reactions to follow the treatment for syphilis. A small needle is placed in the back, between the lumbar (lower back) vertebrae, and the fluid is withdrawn (hence, the terms *lumbar puncture, spinal puncture,* or *spinal tap*). While the test is most commonly performed with the patient sitting up and bent slightly forward, there are times when the patient lies on his side with an assistant bending the head toward raised knees. The test should not be performed when increased intracranial pressure is suspected.

When performed: Following head or back injury or when such injury is suspected but not proved; when symptoms suggest brain tumor or stroke; when there is a severe infection (virus, meningitis, poliomyelitis, encephalitis) that seems to be affecting the brain or muscles; when there are suspected birth injuries.

Normal values: The spinal fluid has a normal pressure equal to 70 to 200 mm of water (in the sitting position; it is slightly lower when lying down). The fluid should be transparent and without color. There should be no white blood cells in the spinal fluid; however, a cell count of up to 10 is still considered normal by many physicians. Normally, the fluid contains 5 to 15 mg per 100 ml of protein, 45 to 80 mg per 100 ml of sugar, and 110 to 125 mEq per liter of chloride.

Abnormal values: The spinal fluid pressure may be lower than normal when there is a spinal cord tumor or shock, or even after fainting. In diabetic coma, the pressure is decreased. The pressure is increased following brain and spinal cord injury and in infection.

The color may have a reddish tinge if there is bleeding into the spinal canal following injury or stroke. With infection or with old blood from previous damage, the color may change to yellow or gray.

The cell count rises with infection, tumor, and most conditions that directly affect the brain, spinal cord, and their coverings.

Chemical tests for sugar and chloride are used to differentiate poliomyelitis from meningitis. Protein is elevated in almost all diseases that are reflected in the spinal fluid.

Risk factors: A lumbar puncture (spinal tap) might occasion a hemorrhage in the area of needle penetration, especially if the needle is improperly placed or the patient moves. Other risks are included in general risk factors for catheter or needle insertion. Approximately 1 out of every 1,000 patients who undergoes cerebrospinal fluid testing suffers nerve paralysis; in most instances, the paralysis is reversible. A test for cerebrospinal fluid when there is increased intracranial pressure (brain tumor, etc.) can be fatal.

Pain/discomfort: Minimal. Most patients tolerate needle insertion without anesthesia. Some patients feel that assuming the fetal position, lying on one's side, is the most uncomfortable aspect of the test. There is the possibility of a headache a few hours after the test is completed. Medical opinion on the subject varies; some doctors require bed rest for several hours after the test to help prevent headaches, while others believe that headache seems to occur most often in patients who are told to expect a headache.

Cost: From $40 to $50 for lumbar puncture; additional costs for the chemistries, cultures, and blood cell examinations range from $5 to $80 for each individual examination.

Accuracy and significance: When properly performed, the test is 95 percent accurate in helping to diagnose brain and spinal cord disease. It is especially significant in determining the specific cause of meningitis and/or encephalitis. Although the test is frequently used to help diagnose dementia (see **Cognitive Capacity Screening**), it is not considered of real value. And, although testing cerebrospinal fluid was once fairly routine when neurosyphilis was being considered or treated, it is no longer recommended in patients who have had this disease for more than a year.

CEREBROSPINAL FLUID SCAN, see *Nuclear Scanning*

CERULOPLASMIN, see *Copper*

CERVICAL VISCOSITY, see *Tackmeter*

CERVICOGRAPHY, see *Cytology*

CERVIX, see *Schiller*

CHEMICAL SCREENING, see *Comprehensive Multiple Test Screening*

CHEMILUMINESCENCE, see *Agglutination*

CHILDREN'S APPERCEPTION (CAT), see *Thematic Apperception*

CHLAMYDIA IDENTIFICATION

Chlamydial infections have become so common that knowledgeable doctors are requesting laboratories to perform specific searches to isolate these unique bacteria. Public health officials report that the diseases caused by chlamydial infections are not only extremely dangerous but have reached epidemic proportions in the United States. Unfortunately, unless the doctor is aware of the bacterium and the damage it causes, its diagnosis is missed and the diseases are left untreated. Among the illnesses caused by chlamydia are: trachoma blindness, pneumonia and eye infections in newborn infants, ectopic pregnancy (the fetus develops outside the uterus), lymphogranuloma venereum (see **Frei** test), generalized pelvic inflammatory disease (a major cause of infertility), spontaneous abortion, psittacosis pneumonia (also called "parrot fever," in the belief that it is spread by pet birds), fatal infections in new mothers immediately after childbirth, and most commonly, nongonococcal urethritis (NGU), or nonspecific urethritis as it was named before the cause was discovered (an infection of the urethra—from which urine is discharged—that is thought to be three times as common as **Gonorrhea**). There are two species of chlamydia; one responds to certain antibiotic drugs, while the other does not. Although it is possible to test for antibodies signifying chlamydial conditions through various **Agglutination** and **Complement**

Fixation techniques that use blood taken from a vein, the most common method is by **Culture**. Samples are taken from any part of the body with abnormal secretions (urethra, vagina, eye, sputum, even the back of the throat), treated to eliminate any potentially contaminating organisms, and then, because these unusual bacteria need body energy to multiply, grown on special cells. A specific diagnosis can take two to three days.

When performed: When a patient's symptoms imply a sexually transmitted disease that is not easily diagnosed, and especially if that patient is in the later months of pregnancy; when flulike or pneumonia symptoms persist; with eye infections that are not easily diagnosed; following sudden infant death syndrome; when rectal inflammation or itching persists; when undiagnosed vaginitis persists. Many public health officials recommend routine chlamydia cultures for all pregnant women.

Normal values: No growth of the organism on the culture; no evident titer when blood is tested for antibodies.

Abnormal values: Evidence of chlamydial organisms after culturing; antibody titers greater than 1 to 64.

Risk factor: Negligible (see general risk factors for blood testing and for catheter or needle insertion).

Pain/discomfort: Minimal (see general pain/discomfort factors for blood testing and for catheter or needle insertion).

Cost: From $30 to $50 for each culture (sometimes several areas of the body are tested at the same time); from $10 to $25 for antibody testing, depending on the technique used.

Accuracy and significance: Culture growths, when properly performed, are considered about 90 percent accurate. Antibody observation studies are only about 50 percent accurate.

Note: Newer tests for chlamydia now take from 30 minutes to 4 hours (compared to the several days for a culture); they use ELISA or monoclonal antibody techniques (see **Agglutination**) and are considered more than 90 percent accurate in patients with related symptoms. They cost from $5 to $10. Because of the increasing infection rate (up to 20 percent of all women screened at family planning clinics), it has also been recommended that the test be performed regularly on women who are sexually active, especially with multiple partners.

CHLORIDE

Chloride, a salt of hydrochloric acid, is mostly taken into the body as part of salt (sodium chloride). It is usually tested along with **Bicarbonate, Potassium,** and **Sodium,** since they all act reciprocally to balance the body's acid-base system and control water metabolism. The major concentration of chloride is in the tissues around cells and in stomach secretions (a very dilute hydrochloric acid). The kidney usually excretes about as much chloride as is taken in. Blood is collected from a vein, and the serum is examined. Urine, spinal fluid, and **Sweat** may also be examined for chloride content.

When performed: When dizziness, weakness, or unconsciousness cannot easily be diagnosed; when adrenal disease is suspected.

Normal values: Normal values in the serum range from 100 to 110 mEq per liter (350 to 385 mg per 100 ml); in the urine, from 100 to 250 mEq per 24-hour sample; in the spinal fluid, from 120 to 130 mEq per liter.

Abnormal values: Serum chloride levels are occasionally elevated with kidney disease (but can be normal), dehydration, and aspirin toxicity. They are decreased with vomiting, diarrhea, excessive sweating, diuresis (with or without drugs), heart disease, and diabetic acidosis. Spinal fluid levels are usually decreased with meningitis; urine levels are decreased with hypoactive adrenal disease.

A special test called Robinson-Power-Kepler is used occasionally to help diagnose Addison's disease (inadequate adrenal function). After drinking a great deal of water, patients with the disease excrete higher-than-normal amounts of chloride in the urine but lower-than-normal amounts of water.

Risk factors: Negligible (see general risk factors for blood testing).

Pain/discomfort: Minimal (see general pain/discomfort factors for blood testing).

Cost: From $5 to $30. This test is usually included in **Comprehensive Multiple Test Screening** panels, which run from $7 to $42.

Accuracy and significance: Although the test is 90 percent accurate in measuring body chlorides, it is of little significance when used alone, because there are so many different conditions that alter chloride levels. It is considered useless as a spinal fluid test.

CHLORINATED PESTICIDE SCREENING, see *Toxic Chemical Exposure*

CHLORINATED PHENOLS SCREENING, see *Toxic Chemical Exposure*

CHOLANGIOGRAPHY, see *Radiography*

CHOLECYSTOGRAPHY, see *Radiography*

CHOLECYSTOKININ STIMULATION, see *Pancreas Function*

CHOLESTEROL

Cholesterol is an essential body product that is manufactured by many organs such as the liver, the skin, and the intestines. It is not a fat, as is erroneously believed, but is a solid alcohol called a steroid; steroid compounds also include hormones, vitamins, and drugs. It has been estimated that the average person ingests about 600 mg of cholesterol each day. Cholesterol is found in most foods of animal origin; plant foods are usually free of the substance. Cholesterol is indispensable for brain and nervous system growth and development (nerves cannot transmit impulses without it), as well as for the body's manufacture of sex hormones.

Cholesterol measurements are not very specific for diagnosing disease, and for many years, the test was virtually abandoned; recently, it has had a resurgence as a possible predictor of heart problems. Its actual predictive value has not yet been proved, however, and it is not totally accepted as a reliable heart risk measurement by most scientists and many cardiologists. Cardiac surgeons, who usually treat the most severe heart and artery disease, report that 80 percent of their patients have normal blood cholesterol levels.

Attention should be called to a particular observation being reported in medical journals with increasing frequency; that is, the adverse effects associated with the attempt to lower one's cholesterol level—by means of either diet or drugs. Epidemiological studies repeatedly show that patients who have low blood cholesterol levels have a much higher incidence of cancer. And as cholesterol levels are lowered, the incidence of gallbladder problems—especially those requiring surgery—also increases. Yet another observation related to people with low cholesterol values has been in the area of behavior and the test is being tried as a personality indicator. Studies in Finland and the United States show a statistically significant relationship between low cholesterol levels and violent behavior, aggressiveness, and other forms of antisocial personality traits, especially suicide. When homicidal offenders were tested for low cholesterol levels, the results were considered to be a good indicator of dangerousness.

In the 1985 report of the heart disease prevention trial that used the drug cholestyramine as a means of lowering blood cholesterol levels, not only did the drug not statistically lessen heart problems or deaths from heart disease (when common and proper statistical methods are applied), but the group taking the drug also showed 200 percent more deaths from accidents and/or violence (100 percent more homicides and 100 percent more suicides) than those who took a placebo as a control group. Incidentally, in that same study, those who took the drug to lower cholesterol also had a 700 percent increase in cancers over those who took a placebo.

Another, more recent study using two other drugs to lower cholesterol levels (probucol and clofibrate) seems not only to confirm the failure of cholesterol-lowering drugs to prevent heart disease and heart attacks, but also to substantiate the evident adverse effects of such drugs. Those who took the drugs had four times as many heart-caused deaths as those who took no drugs. And those taking the drugs had four times as many "accidents" as those who took no drugs; in the cholestyramine study, there were more than twice as many deaths from automobile and motorcycle accidents in those taking the drug—a possible reflection of aberrant personality caused by the drugs.

The usual laboratory test measures total cholesterol, or all the cholesterol that is attached to various fats and proteins floating in the blood. However, when it comes to studying heart disease prediction, the specific protein-fat complexes (see **Lipoproteins**) to which the cholesterol is attached are more important. An excess of certain cholesterols—called alpha, or high-density lipoprotein (HDL), cholesterols—is associated with a *decrease* in heart disease. Low-density or very low density lipoproteins (LDL, VLDL) appear to be "bad" cholesterols, and epidemiologically, they seem to be the ones associated with heart disease.

The most recent application of cholesterol measurements is the ratio of total cholesterol to HDL cholesterol; the less HDL in proportion to total cholesterol, the alleged greater risk of heart disease. While some doctors feel that this ratio, as well as the proportion of HDL to LDL, is more significant than other **Lipoprotein** values, a 1985 British study cast doubt on the validity of any association; one more example of the lack of a true scientific basis for all so-called risk factors.

Blood cholesterol levels will rise almost instantaneously when an individual is frightened, under anxiety, or in pain, and even when an individual is exposed to an uncomfortably loud noise. For example, many income tax accountants have a great increase in their cholesterol levels during the weeks before April 15; the elevated levels return to normal by May 1. Blood is taken from a vein, and the serum is examined.

When performed: When there is suspicion of thyroid disease; with liver disease when there is a question of drug damage or hepatitis; with people who have xanthomatosis (yellowish plaques around the eyes, on the eyelids, over the elbows, and on the palms), although more than half of all people with xanthomatosis have normal cholesterol values; to measure the body's reaction to adrenal hormones; to measure an individual's response to stressful situations; as an experimental aid in the prediction of heart disease.

Normal values: Normal serum cholesterol levels range from 150 to 280 mg per 100 ml. These figures are not absolute. Higher values are normally found in older people; and with patients over 50 years of age, most laboratories consider 350 mg the upper limit of normal. Normal values also vary with the technique used (automated testing is considered less accurate and produces higher values).

In the last few years, there has been a disagreement among physicians as to the "normal" value of cholesterol. While the "normal values" cited here reflect the typical United States population, there are doctors who feel that these values should be considered abnormal and that much lower values should be applied as normal. At this time, the lower values reflect more of an opinion than a scientific fact.

Abnormal values: Serum cholesterol is increased with familial hypercholesteremia (an inherited trait); with hypothyroidism (cretinism), hepatitis, herpes, and kidney disease (nephrosis); and when the flow of bile from the gallbladder is obstructed. Elevated cholesterol levels also result from pregnancy (after the second month); from fear of the test results at the time the test is performed; and from taking male hormones, certain tranquilizers, cortisone products, vitamins A and D, some diuretic drugs, and epinephrine (adrenalin) products such as those used by asthmatics. Eating a great deal of cholesterol within a few hours of the test may have a slight effect on test results in some people, but it is not constant. Most physicians believe that cholesterol values are not influenced to any significant degree. Abnormal values can come from postural changes, however; values may be completely different when blood is taken when the patient is lying down, as opposed to after the patient has been standing for several minutes.

Lower-than-normal cholesterol values are usually found with hyperthyroidism (Graves' disease), cirrhosis of the liver, certain anemias, and severe infections. Taking female hormones, thyroid hormones, aspirin, vitamin C or B_3 (niacin), certain antibiotics, and drugs used to treat diabetes will lower cholesterol values.

Decreased cholesterol esters indicate liver disease (hepatitis or active cirrhosis).

Risk factors: Negligible (see general risk factors for blood testing).

Pain/discomfort: Minimal (see general pain/discomfort factors for blood testing).

Cost: From $4 to $24. When cholesterol esters are evaluated, the cost is approximately $20. HDL cholesterol evaluations are $20 to $40. Complete analysis of cholesterol, including LDL and VLDL, is $50 to $75. Cholesterol and HDL are usually included in **Comprehensive Multiple Test Screening** panels, which run from $7 to $42.

Accuracy and significance: Cholesterol measurements are neither very accurate (less than 80 percent) nor considered significant for any one particular disease. So many variables can affect blood cholesterol that, should the blood be tested hourly throughout the day, or even once daily over a month's time, it would not be unusual to find a wide variation in blood cholesterol values. Whenever an HDL cholesterol test is performed, the serum must be packed in dry ice immediately until the analysis is undertaken; otherwise, false values will be reported. Starting in 1986, The National Heart, Lung and Blood Institute will attempt to standardize cholesterol testing for the first time. Recent surveys have shown that different laboratories will report a difference of 50 mg per 100 ml on the identical blood specimen—considered a serious error when this test is used as a heart disease predictor.

As but one example of how cholesterol values fluctuate, consider yourself lying in bed late at night when you are awakened by a noise that makes you think of an intruder. You know how long it takes for your heart to start pounding—give or take 5 seconds. That is how long it took for your brain to signal your adrenal glands to give out adrenalin that causes the heart rate to accelerate—amongst other signs of nervousness. Adrenalin can markedly raise cholesterol levels that fast. Keep that in mind when your blood is being taken for a cholesterol test, when you consider the test's accuracy.

CHOLINESTERASE

There are two different forms of cholinesterase: one may be referred to as true cholinesterase, or acetylcholinesterase, and the other as pseudo-cholinesterase. Both enzymes are necessary for proper functioning of the parasympathetic nervous system, which controls the body's involuntary processes that transmit nerve impulses to the heart, gastrointestinal tract, tear ducts, etc. When these processes are reduced or interfered with—either by disease or by inhalation, ingestion, or skin contact with organic phosphate insecticide such as malathion—the patient has increased parasympathetic nervous system activity. Symptoms include increased stomach acidity, increased intestinal motility, erratic pulse and heart rate, difficulty in breathing, increased sweating, salivation, and watering of the eyes.

In almost all instances, pinpoint-sized pupils are an early sign of interference with the parasympathetic nervous system. Severe reactions include headache, muscle twitching, convulsions, and diarrhea. Some physicians believe ingestion of monosodium glutamate can also cause these reactions. True cholinesterase is measured from red blood cells; pseudo-cholinesterase is measured from serum. Both are obtained from blood taken from a patient's vein.

A special test to measure the presence of cholinesterase is the succinylcholine reaction. Succinylcholine is administered, and if cholinesterase is missing, the patient will experience severe difficulty in breathing and muscle inactivity. The test is sometimes given by an anesthetist just prior to surgery to make sure that cholinesterase is present. Succinylcholine may also be used to aid in relaxation during surgery.

At times, dibucaine (a very toxic local anesthetic) is given to patients to see how much cholinesterase activity the drug will suppress; normal individuals, with adequate amounts of cholinesterase, show the greatest amount of restricted activity, with the actual amount called the dibucaine number. This test is usually performed when the other tests are ambiguous, and especially if a breathing problem is anticipated.

A recent application of acetylcholinesterase has been in testing for this substance as part of **Amniocentesis;** an increased amount is said to be an indication of a neural-tube defect in the fetus (see **Alpha Fetoprotein**).

When performed: When a variety of symptoms that result from excessive parasympathetic nervous system activity are observed (as described above), especially after possible exposure to an insecticide; in certain skin, liver, and kidney diseases.

Normal values: Cholinesterase values in serum average at least 0.5 pH units per hour. In red blood cells, true cholinesterase levels should be at least 0.7 pH units per hour. Some laboratories report cholinesterase values in their own units; these may range from 40 to 80 units as a total value.

Abnormal values: Decreased values indicate interference with the enzyme, usually as a result of organic phosphate poisoning. (Some physicians believe that the lower the value, the greater the intensity of the phosphate poisoning.) Cholinesterase may also be decreased during pregnancy and with cancer, liver disease, and certain skin conditions. Rarely, the levels are increased in kidney disease and hyperthyroidism.

Risk factors: Negligible (see general risk factors for blood testing).

Pain/discomfort: Minimal (see general pain/discomfort factors for blood testing).

Cost: Direct measurements of cholinesterase in serum or in red blood cells are $11 to $30. When pseudo-cholinesterase is included, there is often an additional charge of $15. The dibucane test averages $70.

Accuracy and significance: The test is 95 percent accurate for organic phosphate insecticide toxicity. It is especially significant when administered prior to surgery during which certain muscle relaxants are to be used.

Note: This test is now being used to identify the presence of carbamates, a herbicide that can cause skin and kidney disease. (See **Toxic Chemical Exposure**.)

CHOLYLGLYCINE (Bile Acid Cholylglycine)

Cholylglycine is a component of bile acids that are made by the liver, stored in the gallbladder, and excreted into the small intestines whenever fats are eaten. The bile emulsifies the fats so they can be absorbed by the bowel. Once these bile acids have performed their function, they travel back to the liver, where they are stored or re-manufactured as needed. If liver disease exists, however, cholylglycine remains in the blood in larger-than-normal amounts; what makes this liver test somewhat different from others is that is shows abnormal values very early—even before actual liver disease becomes evident physically. And it helps to differentiate between the causes of liver disease, as the early effect from alcohol is not reflected in this test. Blood is taken from a vein for study.

When performed: When liver disease or beginning liver involvement is suspected. To help ascertain the cause and extent of liver disease.

Normal values: Less than 70 mg per 100 ml.

Abnormal values: More than 70 mg per 100 ml.
Risk factors: Negligible (see general risk factors for blood testing).
Pain/discomfort: Minimal (see general pain/discomfort factors for blood testing).
Cost: Approximately $10; approximately $25 if all bile acids are measured.

Accuracy and significance: Some doctors believe this might be the best test to detect early signs of liver damage. (The sooner such illness is diagnosed, the easier it is to treat successfully.) It is also thought that the increase in abnormal values could be a valid indicator of the extent of the liver damage; values of up to 10,000 mg per ml are not unusual, and the extremely large range of abnormal values allows a very sensitive way of measuring the degree of the disease. Considered to be 90 percent accurate.

CHORIONIC GONADOTROPIN, see *Pregnancy; Testis Function*

CHORIONIC VILLI SAMPLING (CVS)

This is a new test to help uncover chromosomal and other genetic defects in the fetus; while the end result is similar to that obtained by **Amniocentesis,** which usually cannot be performed until 15 weeks into pregnancy, chorionic villi sampling can be performed after only 8 weeks of pregnancy—allowing the results to be made known to the parents months earlier. Moreover, the results are available in 24 hours, compared to several weeks after amniocentesis (see **Chromosome Analysis** and **Genetic Disorder Screening**). Although this method of prenatal testing has been used in Europe and China for nearly two decades, it has only been researched in the United States since 1983. Unlike amniocentesis, which most often takes place in a hospital setting and can be quite time-consuming, CVS can be performed in the doctor's office or on a hospital outpatient basis and takes from 5 to 30 minutes. With the woman in the usual pelvic examination position, a small catheter is inserted into the uterus (similar to the insertion of an intrauterine device for contraception) using **Ultrasound** as a means of guiding the catheter to the exact position. When the chorionic villi (tiny protrusions from the outermost layer of the sac surrounding the fetus and placenta) are reached, a small sample **(Biopsy)** is removed for study. These villi contain cells identical to those from the fetus and may therefore allow an early diagnosis of various genetic and biochemical defects if they exist (e.g., **Tay-Sachs Disease,** Cooley's anemia, Down's syndrome, and sickle-cell anemia). Much of the success of this test depends upon the skills of the physician obtaining the sample and the ultrasonographer guiding the physician's catheter. At the present time, the test is not usually performed on women with bleeding or spotting problems, those who may have fibroids (muscular growths in the uterus) or cervical polyps, or those who have a sexually transmitted disease (it is not unusual to require testing for **Gonorrhea** before CVS is performed). One advantage of CVS is that if the results are not clear, the patient can still undergo amniocentesis.

It is also possible to obtain a villus sample using aspiration (suction) instead of surgical removal, and the chorionic tissue can also be reached using a needle (again, directed by ultrasound) through the abdomen. If ultrasound is contraindicated, **Endoscopy** can be used to guide the biopsy forceps.

When performed: To screen, prenatally, for genetic diseases, especially in women over 35 years of age, those with the slightest suspicion of metabolic or genetic problem births in the past, and those who are disturbed over the possibility of having an abnormal child.

Normal values: No evidence of any genetic defect or metabolic abnormality.

Abnormal values: Abnormal chromosomal patterns; missing, defective, or mislocated genes; or a suspicion of abnormal development.

Risk factors: There is no universal agreement about the risks of this test; some feel it carries a greater risk of spontaneous abortion than does amniocentesis, but others claim the risk is much less. With CVS, there is usually no need to penetrate the abdomen and uterine wall with a needle, nor any need to touch the fetus. The primary complication, after CVS, is uterine bleeding; nearly 20 percent of women show spotting or bleeding for up to 48 hours. Bleeding for more than 72 hours is considered abnormal enough for hospitalization. Sexual intercourse within a week after CVS can be the cause of an infection.

Pain/discomfort: Pain is reported to be rare, and the discomfort has been compared to that with a routine pelvic examination. Much possible discomfort depends on the position of the woman's uterus; if it is "tipped," it makes the procedure more difficult.

Cost: From $100 to $200, plus the cost of chromosome analysis. As of 1985, some health insurance plans will not reimburse the doctor or patient for this test, claiming the safety, efficacy, and appropriate indications have not been established.

Accuracy and significance: The most significant aspect of this test is its ability to reveal fetal defects early in pregnancy. While the ultimate decision as to what action to take depends on the test results, it has been reported that those women who do decide to undergo abortion feel far fewer psychological consequences when the abortion takes place so early during pregnancy. Because the test allows a greater sample of fetal tissue, it can be more accurate than amniocentesis for certain conditions. To date, no "normal" test result has been followed by an abnormal birth, and in general, the cell study has been at least 95 percent accurate. There have been reports, however, that a positive test could reflect an abnormality in the chorionic villi or membrane rather than in the fetus. And this test cannot detect all the defects that can be revealed through amniocentesis.

CHRISTMAS TREE, see *White Blood Cell*

CHROMATIN, see *Chromosome Analysis*

CHROMIUM, see *Mercury*

CHROMOSOME ANALYSIS (Cytogenetics, Chromatin, Karyotyping)
All normal body cells have 46 chromosomes, including a set of sex chromosomes, called chromatin cells. In the chromatin test, the inside of the cheek is scraped for a minute specimen (called a buccal smear), and the cells are stained and examined under the microscope; these cells will reveal the presence or absence of a particular active sexual identity cell called the Barr body. The normal female cell has one Barr body and no Y-chromatin. The normal male cell shows no Barr body and one Y-chromatin. (The **Amniocentesis** test is a more detailed study of the chromosome makeup of the unborn infant.) Chromosome analysis also includes the evaluation of their number,

structure, and the location of specific genes to determine the existence of other genetic problems such as Down's syndrome. In addition to buccal smears, tissue from the skin, lung, ovary, and testicle can be tested, as well as bone marrow. White blood cells (from blood taken from a vein) seem to be the preferred material for study.

Sometimes the term *Southern blot* is used when referring to chromosome analysis; this is simply a term that describes the technique of investigating gene locations and descriptions; it is also used to chart the "pedigree" of a family to help predict where gene mutations might be revealed. While the Southern blot reveals deoxyribonucleic acid (DNA) segments (see **Genetic Disorder Screening**), the Northern blot test discloses ribonucleic acid (RNA), made mostly from DNA, which also aids in assessing genetic information (e.g., sickle-cell anemia; see **Hemoglobin**) prior to pregnancy.

When performed: Whenever there is some doubt about the gender of the individual; whenever abnormal sexual development seems evident—either mentally or physically (undescended testicles; abnormal hair distribution; abnormal fat distribution; growth problems; infertility; failure to menstruate; and gynecomastia, or large breasts in a male); whenever a woman has repeated episodes of spontaneous abortion; whenever there is evidence of physical or mental development disability in siblings or in relatives of the prospective parents.

Normal values: There should be no Barr body in the male and one Barr body in the female. Each cell should contain exactly 46 chromosomes.

Abnormal values: Abnormal values include finding only 45 chromosomes with no Barr body and finding 47 or more chromosomes with one or more Barr bodies. Most of these conditions produce physical sexual developmental abnormalities that usually become obvious with growth.

Other abnormalities may be predicted when the genes are incorrectly located on the chromosomes or a specific chromosome is physically defective (when chromosome number 21 is abnormal, it is indicative of Down's syndrome).

Risk factors: Negligible (see general risk factors for blood testing and catheter and needle insertion).

Pain/discomfort: Minimal (see general pain/discomfort factors for blood testing and catheter and needle insertion).

Cost: Routine chromosome analysis is $600 to $700. If more specific studies are necessary—as they are when mental retardation is a consideration—there is often an additional $300 to $400 fee. A buccal smear limited to Barr body detection is about $25.

Accuracy and significance: Total chromosome analysis is considered about 95 percent accurate. Accuracy increases when more specific studies are performed. The significance of the tests is relative and depends on the action taken following diagnosis.

CIA, see *Macroglobulin*

CIE, see *Counterimmunoelectrophoresis*

CINEANGIOGRAPHY, see *Radiography*

CINERADIOGRAPHY, see *Radiography*

CIRCULATING IMMUNE COMPLEX, see *Immunology*

CIRCULATION TIME

The circulation time test determines just how fast the blood travels through the body. Usually, a substance with a distinctive taste (saccharin, magnesium sulfate, or Epsom salts) is injected into an arm vein, and the exact time from the injection to the moment the patient "tastes" the substance (indicating its arrival at the tongue) is noted. The test may also be performed with dyes or with radioactive substances that are detected by nuclear scanners. The circulation time is affected by the amount of blood in the arteries and veins, especially by the speed with which the blood passes through the heart and lungs. A newer version of circulation time testing involves the use of DMSO (dimethyl sulfoxide), the same drug unofficially, at times, applied to the skin to treat aches and pains. The DMSO is dabbed on the inside of the forearm; the time from the application to the skin to the moment the patient tastes and/or smells the garliclike chemical is a noninvasive way to measure circulation time.

When performed: Primarily as an index of heart failure and its degree; sometimes as a measure of the circulation through the lungs, when the heart is known to be normal.

Normal values: In the "taste" test, it should take from 8 to 16 seconds for the drug to go from the arm vein to the heart, through the lungs, back to the heart, and then into the arteries, particularly the arteries of the tongue, when the patient will taste the drug. Dye and radioactive tests take less time.

Abnormal values: Failure to "taste" the drug within 20 seconds is usually indicative of heart failure.

Risk factors: Negligible (see general risk factors for blood testing).

Pain/discomfort: Minimal (see general pain/discomfort factors for blood testing).

Cost: The test can be performed in the doctor's office or in a hospital, and the charge ranges from $10 to $20 for each test material.

Some doctors consider this test outmoded, and it is possible that a health insurance company or government-sponsored medical program will not reimburse the doctor or patient for the cost of the test.

Accuracy and significance: Although the test is no longer in vogue, there are doctors who find it still serves as a measure of the degree of heart failure and thus provides an index of improvement. Considered to be 50 percent accurate.

CISTERNOGRAPHY, see *Nuclear Scanning*

CK, see *Creatine Phosphokinase*

CLAP, see *Gonorrhea*

CLONIDINE SUPPRESSION, see *Catecholamines*

CLOSTRIDIAL TOXIN, see *Feces Examination*

CLOTTING FACTORS, see *Fibrinogen; Partial Thromboplastin Time*

CLOTTING TIME, see *Bleeding and Clotting Time*

CMV, see *Cytomegalovirus*

COAGULATION FACTOR(S), see *Fibrinogen; Partial Thromboplastin Time*

COAGULATION TIME, see *Bleeding and Clotting Time*

COAGULOMETER

Because the drug heparin is being used more and more, not only for the treatment of clotting disease but also for the prevention of blood clots, a new, simple test has been devised to measure the activity of this anticoagulant drug. Unlike the **Partial Thromboplastin Time** test, which requires venous blood, the coagulometer test can be performed with a blood sample from the fingertip and is similar to the **Bleeding and Clotting Time** tests. The blood is placed in the coagulometer tube, which is immersed in a solution at body temperature.

Because the coagulometer is a relatively new device, the test results are often compared with the partial thromboplastin time at regular intervals. The coagulometer test is especially valuable in controlling the dosage of heparin.

When performed: Before patients undergo surgery, especially surgery that will require a prolonged inactive convalescence (such as hip operations); when patients are being treated with low-dose heparin injections for thromboembolism.

Normal values: Blood in the special coagulometer tube usually clots within 1 to 2 minutes.

Abnormal values: If blood in the coagulometer tube clots sooner than 1 minute, this is considered a sign that the patient is prone to develop thrombosis. If the blood takes longer than 2.5 minutes to clot, this indicates that the patient has had too much heparin or has a tendency to bleed easily.

Risk factors: Negligible (see general risk factors for blood testing).

Pain/discomfort: Minimal (see general pain/discomfort factors for blood testing).

Cost: From $5 to $10.

Accuracy and significance: The test is about 80 percent accurate in detecting patients who might be prone to thrombosis or have a tendency to bleed, but it is not considered sufficiently accurate to measure the effects of all anticoagulant drugs. (See **Prothrombin Time.**)

COBALAMINE, see *Schilling*

COCAINE, see *Drug Abuse*

COCCIDIOIDOMYCOSIS, see *Complement Fixation; Skin Reaction*

CODEINE, see *Drug Abuse*

COFFEE, see *Caffeine*

COGNITIVE CAPACITY SCREENING

The cognitive capacity screening test aids in making one of the most difficult of all diagnoses: whether ostensible mental illness is organic (caused by brain damage or metabolic problems) or functional (caused by an inability or unwillingness to behave properly). Conventional mental status examinations (simple talking with a patient) may miss mental problems caused by physical disease, chronic brain syndrome, or dementia.

At the present time, primary degenerative dementia or Alzheimer's disease is receiving the most attention. Sometimes called presenile or senile dementia, Alzheimer's disease is, in essence, a diminishing—even to a total loss—of one's usual intellectual abilities to the point of impaired judgment (memory loss, especially of recent events, language difficulties, inability to travel to a known destination, inability to concentrate, and a denial that such things are happening). The most obvious sign of the disease, to others, is the individual's inability to function normally in social situations or, if relevant, in his employment.

In the cognitive capacity screening test, the patient is asked 30 questions. (For example: "Listen to these numbers—8, 1, 4, 3. Now count from 1 to 10 out loud and then repeat 8, 1, 4, 3." "Take 7 away from 100 and what do you have? Now take 7 away from that answer and keep taking 7 away from each answer.")

This test is becoming more and more important because of the increasing nursing-home population. Some institutions (as well as some public and private mental hospitals) tend to medicate their patients with tranquilizers and antidepressant drugs before determining if the patient's behavior has an organic or psychological basis. Such drugs will make true dementia cases seem much worse than they really are.

Two of a great many new tests to aid in detecting dementia include the Set test and the mini-object test. In the former, a patient is asked to name as many colors as possible (10 is considered normal), then as many animals as possible, followed by as many fruits and as many towns (at least 10 each should be identified). In the mini-object test, the patient is asked to identify various plastic objects that make up the child's game sometimes called jackstraws. These are usually miniature shovels, ladders, rifles, etc.; after identification, the patient is asked to explain their purpose. With dementia, patients fail to identify several objects and have no idea of their use. (Also see **Facial Recognition**.) There are many more similar tests for detecting mental decline; they go by various names such as the Mini-Mental State (MMS), digit span, controlled oral word association, etc., and some doctors devise their own techniques and then append their own name to their test to help determine cognitive capacity.

When performed: To ascertain a patient's ability to think, reason, and remember; to distinguish between organic dementia and functional delirium; to help diagnose brain pathology.

Normal values: Answering 20 or more questions correctly usually indicates no organic mental disease.

Abnormal values: Fewer than 20 correct answers should cause further investigation into the possibility of brain disease. Answering more than 20 questions correctly and still acting in a bizarre fashion usually indicates a psychotic reaction. Loss of memory for recent events with clear recall of incidents long past is another indication of many forms of dementia, especially Alzheimer's disease (senile dementia).

Risk factors: None.

Pain/discomfort: None

Cost: Administration of the test is approximately $25. If the test is performed by a psychologist outside the doctor's office, there is usually an additional $20 charge for the test administrator's written report.

Accuracy and significance: While the test must be performed by someone well-trained to recognize the influence of drugs and/or malingering, it is still considered only about 50 percent accurate. All other related tests are about as accurate and all are extremely dependent on the examiner interpretations; in most instances, a combination of tests is used before coming to a conclusion.

COLD AGGLUTINATION, see *Agglutination*

COLD BRONCHIAL PROVOCATION, see *Pulmonary Function*

COLD CALORIC, see *Caloric*

COLD FACE, see *Reflex*

COLD IMMERSION, see *Cold Pressor*

COLD PRESSOR

Pressor refers to stimulation of the nerves that control the walls of the arteries. When the autonomic nervous system is excited (see **Finger Wrinkle**), it causes the artery's walls to shrink, which, in turn, produces a rise in blood pressure. One way to stimulate these nerves is to place the hand in ice water (1° above freezing) for one minute. Not only will blood pressure increase temporarily, but the pulse rate will also increase and the heart will use more oxygen. This is a normal response. Once the hand is removed from the cold water, blood pressure and pulse quickly return to their previous levels. If the patient has artery disease, usually in an extremity, the blood pressure's return to normal is delayed for a long time. If a patient has some degree of coronary artery disease (i.e., in the arteries that feed the heart muscle), the cold pressor stimulation may elicit evidence of the disease by causing chest pain, or it might produce corroboration from an **Electrocardiogram, Radiography,** or **Nuclear Scanning**. In addition, the test may precipitate heart arrhythmias (disorders in the heartbeat such as palpitations). The cold pressor test can, in fact, substitute for the exercise stress electrocardiogram; it is easier than walking on a treadmill or cycling, especially while X-rays or nuclear scanning studies are being done at the same time.

When performed: To note the reaction of a patient's blood pressure to cold as a measure of the body's response to stimuli affecting the autonomic nervous system; to help diagnose particular diseases of the arteries such as Raynaud's phenomenon (spasm of the blood vessels, especially in the extremities, causing numbness); to help ascertain the presence of heart disease; at times, the test is performed in association with an **Echocardiogram** to help uncover problems of the heart valves.

Normal values: After the hand is removed from the cold water, the blood pressure should return to its previous level within five minutes; the pulse should return to its usual rate within three minutes. The test should not provoke pain, shortness of breath, dizziness, or any graphic change on the electrocardiograph or X-ray if these tests are being performed concurrently.

Abnormal values: When the blood pressure and/or pulse take longer than 30 minutes to return to previous levels after removing the hand from the cold water. Any physical or technical evidence of impairment of the heart's circulation, rhythm, or valves.

Risk factors: The test can precipitate serious heart problems, but it happens very rarely. The test should always be performed in the presence of a doctor prepared to cope with any emergency.

Pain/discomfort: Minimal. Some people find it uncomfortable, but not painful, to keep their hand in ice water for a full minute. If heart disease is present, it is possible for the test to bring on severe chest pains, but doctors usually consider this and do not perform the test on those who might have such a reaction.

Cost: When performed in a doctor's office, there is usually no charge added to the cost of the office visit. When performed along with other heart diagnosis tests, a charge of $50 can be added to the fees for the radiography, nuclear scanning or electrocardiogram.

Accuracy and significance: A number of doctors prefer this test to the stress electrocardiogram, which uses physical exercise, finding it more accurate and less dangerous. A few diseases of the blood vessels, some bleeding conditions, and an occasional tumor may cause an abnormal cold pressor response and must be considered by the doctor; workers who use chain saws, jackhammers, and grinders also may show an abnormal response (their constant exposure to vibrations seems to make their skin unusually sensitive). About 75 percent accurate.

In a 1985 study performed at the Mayo Clinic, 142 individuals were followed for 45 years to determine the significance of the cold pressor test as a means of detecting those who might later develop high blood pressure. The subjects were first tested to see how they would react to the ice water when they were children, again around 20 years later, and again after another 20 or more years. Of those who had abnormal values, more than 70 percent later developed hypertension, while less than 20 percent of those who had normal values ultimately had some elevation in blood pressure. It was felt that this simple test is a potentially useful predictor of patients who are more than usually susceptible to high blood pressure and that this early detection might help those people avoid serious consequences.

COLD SORE, see *Herpes*

COLD SPOT, see *Nuclear Scanning*

"COLD SPOT" IMAGING, see *Nuclear Scanning*

COLD WATER, see *Allergy*

COLONOSCOPY, see *Endoscopy*

COLON X-RAY, see *Radiography*

COLOR BLINDNESS

About 1 in every 25 men (and 1 in every 250 women) cannot perceive the difference between red and green. This condition is almost always inherited. Very rarely, people cannot tell the difference between blue and yellow. The color blindness test usually consists of a special color plate made up of various colored dots that form numbers or figures. For example, a triangle or number 7 in red, orange, and yellow dots may be surrounded by many blue, green, and violet dots. The plate is shown to the patient, who is asked to describe the numbers or shapes.

Several different tests of color blindness (Ishihara, Hardy-Rand Rittler [HRR]) are used, since people sometimes memorize a particular test in order to pass. Various colored lamps may also be used to detect those who either pretend to be color blind or who try to hide the condition.

When performed: On people whose occupation requires color discrimination (pilots, truck drivers, etc.).

Normal values: No matter how many different colored dots make up a color plate, a normal individual can distinguish the number or figures imprinted within a design of other colors.

Abnormal values: Someone who is color blind will be unable to discriminate a specific number or object among the many colored dots. Color blindness may be a consequence of alcoholism, with blue-yellow defects being the most common.

Risk factors: None.

Pain/discomfort: None.

Cost: Most often the test is part of a complete vision examination. When performed separately, one of several versions may be used, and the charge is $10.

Accuracy and significance: The test is 95 percent accurate; there are sufficiently different forms to counteract any attempt to mislead the doctor.

COLPOSCOPY, see *Endoscopy*

COMPATIBLE TRANSFUSION, see *Typing and Cross-Matching*

COMPLEMENT

Serum complements are proteins in the blood that are part of the antigen-antibody system, which both fights and sometimes causes autoimmune disease (see **Agglutination; Antinuclear Antibodies**). At least 15 different forms of complement are known at the present time; they are usually tested for as total complement, but they can be measured individually. Some forms of complement help neutralize viruses and destroy bacteria; others produce allergic reactions. To give a few examples: complement-1, referred to as C-1, is usually reduced in patients with chronic urticaria (hives; red, raised blotches; and itching); a C-2 deficiency points to autoimmune disease (systemic lupus erythematosus, or SLE); decreased C-3 values suggest kidney or liver disease; C-4 is used to follow the progress of SLE; decreased C-5 values indicate an inability to fight off infection; the remaining specific complement values are studied in relation to specific disease susceptibility.

The complement decay rate test, also called the complement-1 esterase inhibitor test, is specific for diagnosing hereditary angioneurotic edema (a condition in which the skin, mucous membranes, and body organs, especially the lungs, suddenly swell up and become red). Blood is taken from a vein, and the complement is measured from serum.

When performed: To differentiate familial angioneurotic edema from the noninherited allergic form of the disease (a far less serious condition); whenever autoimmune disease such as lupus erythematosus or scleroderma is suspected; in undiagnosed arthritis and kidney disease; when there is an overwhelming infection without a known cause.

Normal values: Total complement ranges from 50 to 100 CH_{50} units per ml. Normal values may vary with the method used. Normal values for individual components of complement (such as C-1, C-2, C-3) vary too widely with each laboratory to list any standard; the reported value is really a relative increase or decrease in the total complement and each component.

Abnormal values: Increased amounts of total complement are found with infections, jaundice, gout, after heart attacks, and sometimes with rheumatoid arthritis. Increased C-3 is found with cancer. Decreased amounts of complement (which are of greater significance) are found in a great many conditions, including chronic kidney disease, severe liver disease, lupus erythematosus, serum sickness (a severe allergic reaction), and myasthenia gravis.

Risk factors: Negligible (see general risk factors for blood testing).

Pain/discomfort: Minimal (see general pain/discomfort factors for blood testing).

Cost: Total complement testing is $50 to $100. Individual complement evaluations are $14 to $54. The complement decay rate test averages $75.

Accuracy and significance: Basically, complement testing is still in the research and experimental stage, but it is used to evaluate mysterious medical conditions, especially those relating to immunity. Because such a variety of conditions affects the components of complement, the tests are minimally significant except when employed to confirm suspected rare diseases; no accuracy rate has been determined.

COMPLEMENT FIXATION

The complement fixation test, which aids in the diagnosis of many diseases, relies on forms of serum antibody proteins (called **Complement**) being present in the blood to identify the specific disease under consideration. Antibodies are formed when the body is exposed to infections; if the antigens (specific causes) of the disease are mixed with a patient's serum, along with specially prepared sheep red blood cells, the antibodies and the antigens will combine, and the blood cells will remain whole. If, on the other hand, the patient's serum does not contain complement antibodies to the disease, the sheep red blood cells will dissolve (a process called hemolysis).

Blood is taken from a vein, and the serum is tested. The serum is diluted to the lowest concentration (highest dilution) that will give a positive reaction (no hemolysis) and is reported as that dilution, called titer. The test is related to the **Agglutination** reaction test, except that agglutination depends on the clumping together of the red blood cells as opposed to their staying whole and separate or their destruction. (At times, the same disease will give a positive reaction to both the complement fixation test and the agglutination test.)

The precipitin reaction is another form of complement fixation test. It is particularly valuable in diagnosing suspected fungus diseases, especially aspergillosis of the lung (an infection that usually accompanies and aggravates asthma).

When performed: The test is used most often when there is suspicion of a virus-caused disease that cannot be accurately diagnosed. A few bacterial and fungus diseases also show a positive complement fixation test. Some specific diseases that can yield a positive high-dilution complement fixation include:

Blastomycosis
    (a fungus-caused lung disease)
Chlamydia
    (see also **Chlamydia Identification**)
Coccidioidomycosis
    (a fungus-caused disease that begins in the lung, sometimes called valley fever)
Dengue fever
    (breakbone fever)
Encephalitis
    (also to differentiate the kind)
Gastroenteritis
Gonorrhea
Hemorrhagic fever
Hydatid disease
    (echinococcosis)
Influenza
    (also to distinguish types A, B, and C)
Lassa fever
    (a new African disease)
Legionnaire's disease
    (a pneumonialike infection)
Meningitis
    (primarily virus-caused)
Pneumonia
    (primarily virus-caused)
Poliomyelitis
Psittacosis
    (a pneumonia-type disease from bird droppings)
Syphilis
Tick fever
Trachoma
Tuberculosis
Venereal diseases
    (now referred to as sexually transmitted diseases, or STDs)
Virus Disease

Normal values: Because of possible past unknown or unremembered infections, an unchanging low-titer positive reaction (a reaction in a very strong or slightly diluted solution) to many diseases is not considered unusual.

Abnormal values: A high titer (a reaction in a very weak or highly diluted solution) to a suspected disease, especially a titer that rises even higher (becomes positive in a more highly diluted solution of serum) after a week or two, indicates the presence of disease. Although the test is used mostly to diagnose suspected disease, it can also be positive in cases of thyroid infection, gout, and severe allergic conditions. Some of the 15 different forms of complement may be reduced with a variety of diseases, usually of the inherited type, but also with various forms of arthritis, certain anemias, malaria, and systemic lupus erythematosus.

Risk factors: Negligible (see general risk factors for blood testing).

Pain/discomfort: Minimal (see general pain/discomfort factors for blood testing).

Cost: From $10 to $70, depending on which disease is being evaluated. Frequently, the test is repeated after two or three weeks to confirm the diagnosis.

Accuracy and significance: A positive test, indicating the presence of specific disease antibodies, is considered 90 percent accurate (there are rare instances when a patient with the disease shows no antibodies; there are also times when a patient with a positive reaction does not have the disease under consideration).

COMPLETE BLOOD COUNT, see *Blood Cell Differential; Red Blood Cell Indices; White Blood Cell*

COMPREHENSIVE MULTIPLE TEST SCREENING

One of many terms used to describe a group of tests (anywhere from 12 to 40 different ones) performed at the same time. A doctor may use the term *SMA,* for Sequential Multiple Analyzer, one of the earliest machines that could perform several different tests concurrently. The original machines could complete 12 tests on 60 patients in one hour; today's machines perform 7,200 tests on 240 patients in the same time. Other terms used for comprehensive multiple test screening are *chemistry panel, chemical screening, chemical scan,* and *profile.* When screening is ordered, it may include any or all of the following tests, depending on the laboratory and its equipment:

Albumin
Albumin/Globulin ratio plus total protein
Alkaline Phosphatase
Antinuclear Antibodies
AST and ALT (formerly called SGOT and SGPT; see **Aspartate Aminotransferase**)
Bilirubin, direct and total
Blood Cell Differential
Calcium
Carbon Dioxide
Chloride
Cholesterol plus high density **Lipoproteins,** or **HDL**
C-Reactive Protein
Creatine Phosphokinase
Creatinine
Gamma glutamyl transpeptidase, or GGPT (see **Alcoholism**)
Globulin
Glucose

HBsAg (see **Hepatitis**)
Hematocrit
Hemoglobin
Iron plus iron binding capacity and transferrin
Lactic Dehydrogenase
Magnesium
Phosphorus or phosphates
Potassium
Red Blood Cell count
Red Blood Cell Indices
Sodium
T_4 and/or T_3 uptake (see **Thyroid Function**)
Triglycerides and total lipids (see **Lipids**)
Urea Nitrogen
Uric Acid
White Blood Cell count

Each of the above tests is described in detail elsewhere in the book. In most instances, chemical screening is more in the nature of a survey of a patient's health status than directed toward a specific diagnosis. Because of the automated equipment, when several tests are performed at the same time, the total cost for the group is far less than when each is performed separately. In 1985, some laboratories performed 24 different tests for $7.95 (the charge to the doctor); in general, anywhere from 12 to 42 different tests can be performed at one time at a cost of from $7 to $42, depending mostly on the competition in any one locality. Unfortunately, the accuracy of tests performed as a panel is not considered as good as when the tests are performed separately. And there are studies that show that when comprehensive multiple test screening is performed on apparently healthy people, at least one out of every seven tests will show a false-positive (erroneously abnormal) result and that one out of every three people will have one or more false-positive values.

COMPUTERIZED ELECTROENCEPHALOGRAM MAPPING, see
Electroencephalogram

COMPUTERIZED TOMOGRAPHY (CT, CAT)
Tomography (see **Radiography**) is the focusing of X-rays on a specific level or plane of the body (as if one passed a thin piece of photographic paper through, say, the abdomen and recorded only what was in that layer of tissue that the film touched). All other areas above, below, or to either side of that plane are obliterated. With computerized tomography (CT), the extremely narrow X-ray beam passes through a cross section of the body (or the brain) and is picked up by an electronic instrument called a scintillator rather than being exposed on the usual X-ray film. The scintillator then feeds into a computer exactly what density (thickness or thinness) of tissue the X-rays passed through. The computer prints out the densities as an illustration of that cross section of the body. Bone, which is of the highest density, comes out white in

the picture. Liquids and air, which are of the lowest density, come out black. In between are all shades of gray, representing various organs and tissues.

Unlike the typical X-ray exposure, the X-ray camera and scintillator rotate extremely rapidly around the body section being photographed so as to include everything in equal focus. CT is sometimes referred to as transaxial tomography or computerized axial tomography (CAT) because it represents a cross section of the long axis (standing-erect position) of the body. To perform CT on the entire head or a particular body section such as the chest or abdomen takes only one second, and the total amount of X-ray exposure is far less than with one old-fashioned X-ray picture. CT images may be viewed on a television screen or reproduced as photographs for permanent study.

There are two different forms of CT: brain scanning and whole-body scanning. CT scanning is different from **Nuclear Scanning** in that no radioactive chemicals are injected into the body. The machines used for each type of scanning are slightly different. Both types of scanning require that the patient remain absolutely motionless for accurate results.

There has been some controversy over CT scanning within the medical profession and especially within the insurance industry, which must pay the costs of the tests. CT scanning is relatively expensive compared with other techniques such as regular X-ray. Furthermore, only a few physicians can be considered experts in the field, since the device was first used in 1973. At the same time, costly as these new machines are, they have been shown to eliminate the need for a great deal of "exploratory" surgery (operations simply to help diagnose a disease, not to cure it). CT scans have also demonstrated that certain allegedly therapeutic surgery would be ineffective if performed. There is general agreement that CT scanning can eliminate potentially dangerous and not always rewarding tests, such as pneumoencephalograms and arteriography (see **Radiography**).

Positron emission transaxial tomography (PETT or PET) is similar to CT but utilizes radiolabeled substances such as glucose to measure some body functions (metabolic rates in different regions of the body that show the effect of treatment in diseases such as stroke). More recent applications of PETT include demonstrations of brain response to hearing, vision, memory applications, and psychological stimuli. Through the application of PETT structure-function relationships, pathology heretofore unable to be detected has been diagnosed.

One more improvement in CT is called single-photon emission computer tomography (SPECT). This test is much more accurate in diagnosing the exact amount of heart muscle damage caused by a heart attack as well as allowing a more specific evaluation of the heart's pumping effectiveness.

Using a pixel scale (*pixel* stands for a "picture element" that has a specific density), it is sometimes possible not only to pinpoint an area of pathology in the lung but also to quantify the amount, or extent, of the lung damage; this can be of great value for patients with emphysema or lung cancer.

When it comes to CT scanning of specific parts of the body, such as the pancreas (see **Pancreas Function**), most doctors now feel that **Ultrasound** is a better, less expensive, first test when attempting to diagnose the cause of pancreatitis or searching for cancer of that gland. The same principle also applies when diagnosing jaundice and other liver diseases and kidney lesions. CT is preferred when there is a chest lesion, and especially where there is a suspicion of abdominal injuries and when locating and sizing blood vessel disorders.

When performed: The test is performed whenever brain pathology is suspected, especially brain substance deterioration (dementia), as well as after any head injury, especially to detect a subdural hematoma (although this may not show up on a CT scan for several days). It is also used when brain tumors are suspected; sometimes a contrast dye is injected into a neck artery so that the dye will more clearly demarcate the lesion. CT scanning may be used when hydrocephalus (or any increase in cerebrospinal fluid pressure) is suspected.

Body scanning is performed primarily when there are abdominal or chest problems that cannot be diagnosed by the usual tests. A CT cross section can illustrate the size and shape of all the body organs and their relationship to adjacent organs and tissues. Such a test is especially valuable when pancreatic pathology is suspected (tumors, cysts, hemorrhage, edema) and when liver disease is being considered, especially problems with the bile ducts. It is also valuable in detecting kidney masses and how well the kidneys are functioning, particularly when there is suspected disease of the retroperitoneal space, between the abdominal organs and the back muscles and spine (abscesses, hematomas, tumors, diseases of the great blood vessels such as the aorta and large abdominal veins, and lymph node and lymph channel blockage).

Abdominal CT scanning has proved especially valuable when a patient has stomach pains and no evident cause can be found. Many doctors now feel that chest and lung diseases that were once very difficult to diagnose (conditions such as sarcoidosis; old, hidden tuberculosis; enlarged arteries and veins) can be detected by body scanning.

Diseases of the extremities (especially bone and muscle) are being diagnosed by CT more and more often as experience lends itself to greater expertise.

Normal values: A CT scan should show no abnormality in the size and position of organs and tissues.

Abnormal values: Only with extensive experience are doctors able to interpret abnormal findings in a CT illustration and then make a specific diagnosis from that finding. For example, when there is evidence of dementia or physical brain disease, a brain scan will show the convolutions between the brain folds to be much wider than normal—something that cannot be detected by any other test. When CT scans are taken at different levels of the brain, the extent of the disease (along with the possibility of successful treatment) can sometimes be determined. In body scanning, an experienced physician can detect minute pathology such as cysts and tumors that would not be revealed by other tests.

Risk factors: The risk of radiation exposure from a CT scan is less than the risk from a series of routine X-ray exposures. However, there is some X-ray exposure, and repeated CT scans will allow radiation accumulation. The greatest risk in CT scanning occurs when a contrast dye medium is injected in a blood vessel as part of the scanning procedure. In addition to the general risk factors for blood testing and catheter or needle insertion, there is the rare risk of an allergic reaction to the dye substance.

Pain/discomfort: Some patients find it uncomfortable to lie perfectly still on a hard surface for several minutes at a time; a number of the newer machines, however, require the patient to remain still for only a few seconds. See general pain/discomfort factors for catheter and needle insertion.

Cost: A CT head scan averages $150 to $300; the physician who interprets the scan usually charges an additional $50 to $100. A total body scan is $200 to $400, and the physician's charge for interpreting it is $75 to $150. When a contrast dye media is injected, there is an additional $25 to $50 charge.

Accuracy and significance: While CT scanning is considered the most effective means to diagnose almost all forms of brain disease, there have been reports of false-negative tests; a negative result, therefore, should not be considered absolute evidence that brain disease is absent. Total body scans are 95 percent accurate and are of great significance, as they can eliminate the risks that accompany diagnostic surgery. Many doctors consider CT scanning the most effective way to diagnose the cause of low back pain, whether from the vertebrae or the nerves. Of particular significance is the fact that, should the cause of low back pain be demonstrated by CT scanning, it is most often amenable to medical therapy and does not require surgery. (See **Magnetic Resonance Imaging**.)

C-1 ESTERASE INHIBITOR, see *Complement*

C1q SOLID PHASE ASSAY, see *Immunology*

CONGENITAL DISEASE SCREENING, see *Genetic Disorder Screening*

CONGO RED

Congo red is a dye used in testing for amyloidosis (a disease condition in which amyloid, a compound mixture of proteins resembling starch, is deposited in various parts of the body, usually in the connective tissue spaces between body cells). Many physicians feel amyloidosis is an abnormality of the plasma cells that produce immunoglobulins and thus is similar to multiple myeloma (see **Bence-Jones Protein**). The Congo red test is not performed as frequently as it was in the past; today, the diagnosis of amyloidosis is usually made from a **Biopsy** of amyloid-looking tissue. The test is still utilized when a patient has a generalized total-body-reaction disease of a mysterious nature.

The patient is asked to fast for 12 hours before the test. Congo red dye is injected intravenously; two minutes later, the first of two specimens is withdrawn from a vein for examination of the serum. One hour later, a second blood sample is taken, and the serum is tested for the amount of dye still present. The urine is also tested.

When performed: When amyloidosis is suspected; when there is unexplained weight loss or small hemorrhages of the skin; when kidney disease is suspected.

Normal values: After one hour, the serum should still contain at least 60 percent of the Congo red dye. The urine should show no dye.

Abnormal values: In systemic amyloidosis (where the entire body is involved), almost all the dye leaves the serum and is absorbed by the amyloid tissue; from 0 to 10 percent may be recovered after an hour. With kidney amyloidosis, the serum will show about 40 percent of the dye, and the urine will contain large amounts.

Risk factors: Negligible (see general risk factors for blood testing).

Pain/discomfort: Minimal (see general pain/discomfort factors for blood testing).

Cost: The cost for injecting the dye and withdrawing the blood for sampling is $5 to $10. An evaluation of the dye remaining in the blood averages $10.

Some doctors consider this test outmoded, and it is possible that a health insurance company or government-sponsored medical program will not reimburse the doctor or patient for the cost of the test.

Accuracy and significance: Although the test is 70 percent accurate in helping diagnose systemic amyloidosis, its significance has diminished because of the simplicity and reliability of needle **Biopsy**.

CONSENSUAL REFLEX, see *Pupillary Reflex*

CONTACT LENS, see *Fluorescein Eye Stain*

CONTRACEPTION, see *Body Temperature*

CONTRACTION STRESS, see *Nonstress Fetal Assessment*

CONTRAST RADIOGRAPHY, see *Radiography*

COOLEY'S ANEMIA, see *Hemoglobin*

COOMBS, see *Agglutination*

COORDINATION, see *Cerebellum*

COPPER

Copper is an essential nutrient. The body requires approximately 2 to 5 mg of copper a day. There are many dietary sources of copper (liver, oysters, beans, peas, avocado, whole grains), so deficiency is relatively uncommon. Copper is measured in the blood serum. In the body, copper combines with the protein ceruloplasmin, which can also be measured in the serum as an indication of copper content. Copper is sometimes measured in the urine and in hair (see **Hair Analysis**).

When performed: When there is suspicion of Wilson's disease (heptolenticular or liver degeneration); in anemia and pregnancy; in patients taking oral contraceptives.

Normal values: Normal serum copper levels range from 75 to 150 mcg per 100 ml. Normal ceruloplasmin levels range from 20 to 45 mg per 100 ml, or 35 to 65 IU. Normal urine levels of copper range from 15 to 40 mcg in a 24-hour sample.

Abnormal values: Serum copper levels may be increased in cirrhosis of the liver, leukemia, pregnancy, anemia, heart attack, infections, and when oral contraceptive, or birth control, pills are used. Decreased serum copper levels are found in Wilson's disease and sprue. Increased ceruloplasmin is seen in pregnancy, heart attack, infections, cirrhosis of the liver, and patients taking oral contraceptives. Decreased ceruloplasmin is found with kwashiorkor disease and Wilson's disease and in infants with anemia and hypoproteinemia. Increased urine copper values are also found with Wilson's disease.

Risk factors: Negligible (see general risk factors for blood testing).

Pain/discomfort: Minimal (see general pain/discomfort factors for blood testing).

Cost: Whether performed on blood or urine, copper and ceruloplasmin tests range from $14 to $45 for either one.

Accuracy and significance: As almost all the blood's copper is combined with ceruloplasmin, this is the form of copper most commonly measured. Other than its significance in diagnosing Wilson's disease, copper and ceruloplasmin levels vary so much with many different conditions that they are used primarily to confirm diagnoses. About 70 percent accurate.

COPROPORPHYRIN, see *Lead: Porphyrins*

CORNEAL REFLEX, see *Reflex*

CORNEAL STAINING, see *Fluorescein Eye Stain*

CORNELL INDEX

The Cornell Medical Index Health Questionnaire is a medical history test that the patient fills out at home before his first interview with the physician. In the section related to bodily symptoms, the questionnaire covers eyes, ears, respiratory system, cardiovascular system, digestive tract, musculoskeletal system, skin, nervous system, genitourinary system, fatigability, frequency of illness, and habits. There are also questions about family history, past illnesses, and moods and feelings (depression, anxiety, sensitivity, inadequacy, anger, tension).

When performed: The index is used as a preliminary test to aid in diagnosis of the individual patient as well as in mass screening. It is especially valuable in distinguishing between psychological and physical problems.

Normal values: Interpretations are based largely on the physician's assessment, which includes an interview with the patient and a physical examination along with the Cornell Medical Index. In general, there should be fewer than 25 "yes" answers.

Abnormal values: The "yes" answers form a pattern that indicates the patient's medical as well as psychological problem areas. More than 25 "yes" answers indicate a serious problem; answering both "yes" and "no" to the same question, omitting answers on six or more questions, or adding remarks to three questions or more are all considered indicative of a problem.

Risk factors: None.

Pain/discomfort: None.

Cost: Most doctors consider this test a valuable part of the medical history and do not charge a fee for it.

Accuracy and significance: The test is considered 70 percent accurate in helping a doctor confirm any suspicion of a psychological origin for a patient's complaint. It is very significant in directing the doctor's attention to the patient's problem area.

CORONARY ANGIOGRAPHY, see *Radiography*

CORONARY HEART DISEASE RISK, see *Jenkins Activity Survey*

CORTICAL EVOKED (ELECTRICAL) RESPONSE, see *Hearing Function*

CORTICOSTEROIDS, see *Cortisol*

CORTISOL

Cortisol (hydrocortisone) is manufactured from cholesterol. It is the main glucocorticoid hormone (a hormone with anti-inflammatory and metabolic activity) secreted by the cortex (outside layers) of the adrenal glands. Cortisol not only reduces the body's protective reactions to bacteria; it also acts on blood sugar levels by inhibiting insulin, helps control protein metabolism, redistributes fat in the body from the arms and legs to the torso, and regulates body water distribution by directing the excretion of sodium and potassium. The amount of cortisol secreted by the cortex is controlled (1) by the hypothalamus portion of the brain, which reacts to physical and emotional stress as well as to other observations of the senses such as noise, odors, and light and darkness; (2) by the pituitary gland, which reacts to how much cortisol is in the blood; and (3) as a consequence of any abnormalities within the adrenal glands (such as tumors). Cortisol testing is now used to detect congenital adrenal disease in a new baby. An infant with insufficient cortisol can go into shock and die if he contracts any illness, has an accident, or requires surgery. Cortisol measurements may be made from amniotic fluid (see **Amniocentesis**) as a means of evaluating the maturity and effectiveness of a developing fetus's lungs.

The adrenal glands normally produce the greatest amount of cortisol in the early morning and the smallest amount in the evening. When a person's regular hours are changed (as by working nights and sleeping days), the cortisol secretion rates are usually reversed. Thus, when testing for cortisol, it is vital to know the patient's active and sleeping times. It is also important to know the mental state of the patient, since emotions have a strong influence on the adrenal glands. Blood is collected from a vein, and the plasma is tested. Urine is also regularly tested.

When adrenal disease is considered, it is usual to perform an adrenal suppression test. A synthetic glucocorticoid drug such as dexamethasone is given to the patient, and cortisol levels are measured for several days afterward. A patient with normal adrenal glands will show a marked reduction in cortisol secretion the next day and for as long as the drug is administered. With Cushing's syndrome, the adrenal suppression test shows that the adrenals do not stop secreting cortisol; and if cortisol is not even slightly reduced after the first two days, an adrenal tumor is usually indicated. The adrenal suppression test (also called the dexamethasone suppression test or the cortisol suppression test) is also used to confirm the suspicion of organic, or physically caused, depression. If the secretion of cortisol is not decreased after a patient takes a measured dose of dexamethasone (synthetic cortisone), it is considered to be strong evidence that the patient's depression is severe and distinct from neurosis. The adrenal suppression test is further used to help distinguish between senile dementia and depressive states. An opposite approach, called the ACTH stimulation test, while not as accurate, may also be employed. ACTH (the pituitary hormone that causes the adrenals to secrete cortisol) is injected. If there is no increase in plasma cortisol, an adrenal tumor is indicated.

In the metyrapone test the patient is given the drug metyrapone, which prevents direct cortisol production, in order to determine if ACTH will stimulate the adrenals.

The drug is usually given at midnight, and cortisol levels are measured the next morning. Normally, the drug-induced reduction in cortisol will cause the body's ACTH to stimulate cortisol production; failure to produce cortisol indicates that the problem lies within the pituitary gland rather than in the adrenals. In patients taking birth control pills or other estrogens, this test can be falsely positive. On rare occasions insulin is given to provoke cortisol secretions; a normal response is a large rise in plasma cortisol. Cosyntropin, a synthetic chemical that also acts like ACTH, is the most recent way of stimulating cortisol; it requires less time than the other tests and does not provoke the allergic reaction that sometimes comes from pure ACTH.

The Thorn test, sometimes called the adrenal function eosinophil count test, measures adrenal cortical function by noting the effect an injection of ACTH has on certain white blood cells called eosinophils (see **Blood Cell Differential**). The ACTH causes the adrenal gland to secrete cortisol, and when that gland is normal, this hormone decreases the number of eosinophils in four hours—usually by half. If the number of eosinophils stays the same (the count may be repeated after another two to four hours), it is an indication that the adrenal glands are not functioning as they should.

Dehydroepiandrosterone is a related hormone that is increased in the blood when a woman has hirsutism (excessive body hair) from adrenal gland pathology; when it is found in very large amounts, it is usually indicative of a tumor.

Urine testing for pregnanetriol, a hormone metabolic product, is now being used as a confirmatory criterion for adrenal gland pathology and ovary tumors.

There are several other tests to measure adrenal cortex function. Two that are used frequently are the urinary 17-ketosteroids (17-KS) and the urinary 17-hydroxycorticosteriods. The latter measures how much cortisol the adrenals are secreting. The former (17-KS), once the most common adrenal test performed, is no longer considered the most reliable measurement of adrenal activity.

When performed: The test is used primarily to diagnose adrenocortical function such as when Cushing's syndrome (excessive adrenal activity) or Addison's disease (inflammation of the adrenal gland) is suspected. It is also used when there is precocious puberty, hirsutism, and excessive signs of feminization in men. It is performed on newborn infants if there is a suspicion of adrenal disease. Today, it is used quite frequently to aid in the diagnosis of depression.

Normal values: Normal cortisol values in plasma are less than 30 mcg per 100 ml in the morning and less than 10 mcg per 100 ml in the evening. There should be no more than 10 mcg per 100 ml in a 24-hour urine sample.

Abnormal values: Plasma cortisol levels are increased in stress. In Cushing's syndrome, normal night and day variations in cortisol levels are lacking. Cortisol levels are reduced with Addison's disease and with excessive androgenic (masculinizing) hormone activity. Urine levels are increased with Cushing's syndrome and with hyperthyroidism and obesity.

Risk factors: Negligible (see general risk factors for blood testing).

Pain/discomfort: Minimal (see general pain/discomfort factors for blood testing).

Cost: From $20 to $170 for blood measurements; from $25 to $35 for urine measurements; and around $100 when measured with ACTH. For the adrenal suppression test, the doctor usually gives the patient dexamethasone pills at no additional charge. Measurements of 17-ketosteroid average $20. The Thorn test costs approximately $40.

Accuracy and significance: Cortisol measurements are considered 95 percent accurate and very significant in diagnosing Cushing's syndrome and Addison's disease. The adrenal suppression test is considered 80 percent accurate and rarely shows a false-positive result. Although the test requires the patient to take only one dose of dexamethasone the night before blood cortisol is tested, the test is even more accurate when the patient takes dexamethasone four times a day for two days prior to cortisol testing. It is considered valuable in helping to predict the prognosis or outcome following treatment for depression. As with so many other tests, a negative response to the adrenal suppression test does not rule out the possibility of depression.

CORTISOL SUPPRESSION, see *Cortisol*

COSYNTROPIN, see *Cortisol*

COTININE, see *Hemoglobin*

CO$_2$, see *Carbon Dioxide*

COUMARIN, see *Prothrombin Time*

COUNTERCURRENT IMMUNOELECTROPHORESIS, see *Agglutination*

COUNTERIMMUNOELECTROPHORESIS (CIE)

Although there are scores of tests to help diagnose the cause of an infection (see **Agglutination, Complement Fixation, Culture, Gram Stain**) in some instances, counterimmunoelectrophoresis is the fastest way to identify certain disease-causing bacteria. While a culture can take days before the germ can be identified, the CIE test can help supply a specific diagnosis within an hour, allowing the doctor to prescribe the proper antibiotic drug almost immediately. In addition, the CIE test can be performed even if the patient is already taking antibiotics that normally interfere with culture tests. The test, related to agglutination techniques, detects antigens from a patient's blood, urine, and other body fluids—particularly cerebrospinal fluid—and is of particular value in helping diagnose the cause of meningitis.

When performed: Whenever there is a severe, yet undiagnosed, infection—usually serious enough to cause septicemia (blood poisoning); most often when the patient has pneumonia or meningitis, and especially in children with these infections.

Normal values: No evidence of any bacterial antigens, although this result alone is not absolute proof that the bacteria are not present.

Abnormal values: Evidence of bacterial antigens after laboratory differentiation of possible false-positive test.

Risk factors: Negligible when blood is tested (see general risk factors for blood testing). For other body fluid testing, see general risk factors for catheter and needle insertion.

Pain/discomfort: Minimal when blood is tested (see general pain/discomfort factors for blood testing). For other body fluid testing, see general pain/discomfort factors for catheter and needle insertion.

Cost: From $10 to $35.

Accuracy and significance: This can be a significant, even lifesaving, test, despite the fact that it is only considered 70 percent accurate in diagnosing meningitis and pneumonias, as there are numerous reports of both false-negative and false-positive results. Most laboratories know how to cope with false results.

COVER-UNCOVER, see *Strabismus*

COXSACKIE, see *Virus Disease*

C-PEPTIDE

C-peptide (the *C* stands for "connecting") is a portion of the basic material used by the body to manufacture insulin. The test, employed primarily in patients with diabetes, measures how much (if any) insulin the patient's pancreas can manufacture. Commercial insulin contains no C-peptide; thus, a patient taking regular injections of insulin can still be tested to find out if he is producing any insulin of his own. Knowing if a patient is producing natural insulin (even in small amounts) affects the type of treatment for diabetes. Most often, urine is tested; blood serum from a vein may also be measured for C-peptide.

When performed: The test is performed at regular intervals whenever diabetes is known or suspected to ascertain body insulin capability. It is also used to detect if a patient is taking erroneous (usually excessive) doses of insulin and to verify suspected hypoglycemia (low blood sugar). Urine testing is preferred with children when blood specimens are difficult to obtain.

Normal values: There are no specific numerical values for C-peptide. Its presence indicates that the body can manufacture insulin; its absence indicates that there is no insulin production.

Abnormal values: Failure to detect C-peptide after giving a patient glucose to stimulate insulin production usually indicates diabetes. Lack of C-peptide in the blood can also mean that a patient has taken so much insulin that the pancreas has shut down because it has no need to produce the hormone. Large amounts of C-peptide can indicate overactive insulin-producing cells in the pancreas, which can cause hypoglycemia.

Risk factors: Negligible (see general risk factors for blood testing).
Pain/discomfort: Minimal (see general pain/discomfort factors for blood testing).
Cost: From $25 to $30.

Accuracy and significance: The test is considered 95 percent accurate as long as the testing laboratory is aware of the type of insulin a patient is taking (beef, pork, biogenetic). It is of particular significance in helping diagnose hypoglycemia, the excessive use of insulin by a patient who denies it, and the assessment of pancreas secretions after pancreas surgery.

CPK, see *Creatine Phosphokinase*

CPK-MB, see *Creatine Phosphokinase*

CPT, see *Cold Pressor*

CREATINE, see *Creatinine*

CREATINE KINASE, see *Creatine Phosphokinase*

CREATINE PHOSPHOKINASE (Creatine Kinase, CPK, CK)

Creatine phosphokinase (CPK) is an enzyme that is found predominantly in skeletal muscle, heart muscle, and the brain. When muscle is damaged, CPK leaks out into the bloodstream. When heart muscle is damaged, most commonly after a heart attack, CPK blood serum levels will rise within hours after the attack. Of all the different enzymes that are usually liberated when heart muscle is damaged, CPK is increased most rapidly (within six hours). It is believed that the rise in CPK is proportionate to the amount of damaged heart muscle. There are at least three forms of CPK, called isoenzymes, and they are labeled according to where they are primarily found: heart, muscle, and brain. CPK-1 is the brain isoenzyme. CPK-2, also called CPK-MB, is the heart isoenzyme. CPK-3 is the muscle isoenzyme.

Within the past few years, even more sensitive methods have been developed to detect CPK and its isoenzymes. It is now known that an increase in CPK-2 can be found even when total CPK levels are normal. And some patients with known heart attacks have failed to show the expected rise in CPK-2. This has made the use of this test less definitive than previously thought in heart disease diagnosis.

When performed: To verify suspected heart attack; to ascertain muscular disease and to follow the progress of illness; to help discover genetic carriers of progressive muscular dystrophy; to distinguish malignant hyperthermia (abnormally high fever after receiving certain anesthetics) from fever due to postoperative infection.

Normal values: CPK values can vary with different laboratories. Generally, up to 12 Sigma units and up to 50 IU are considered normal in men and up to 80 IU in women. CPK-3 is normally found in serum. No CPK-1 or CPK-2 should be detected.

Abnormal values: Total CPK levels are almost always elevated after a heart attack; CPK-MB is usually present in a patient's blood 6 hours following a heart attack. The CPK-MB isoenzyme usually disappears within 24 to 48 hours, but total CPKs remain elevated for three to four days. When CPK-1 isoenzymes are detected, it usually indicates brain or nervous system disease. Total CPK increases are associated with muscular dystrophy, hypothyroidism, alcoholism, crush injury of the muscles, asthma, and other lung conditions that make breathing difficult. Strenuous exercise and intramuscular injections of medicines can also increase total CPK levels, but these usually disappear within 24 hours. Prolonged bed rest, not related to illness, will lower CPK levels. Recent observations have shown an increase in CPK-2 after undergoing cardiac catheterization (see "angiography," in **Radiography**). There is still medical disagreement as to whether this test for heart muscle damage reflects existing heart disease (heart attack) or is a consequence of the damage caused by the catheter inserted into the heart. CPK-2 also increases after electrical injuries; this could be mistaken for a heart attack.

Risk factors: Negligible (see general risk factors for blood testing).

Pain/discomfort: Minimal (see general pain/discomfort factors for blood testing).

Cost: Total CPK levels range from $8 to $24. Tests to indicate the three different isoenzymes are from $20 to $40. Total CPK measurements are usually included in **Comprehensive Multiple Test Screening** panels, which range from $7 to $42.

Accuracy and significance: Total CPK levels are not too specific because they are elevated in so many conditions. In contrast, CPK-2 (CPK-MB) is considered a significant test to diagnose a heart attack. Recently, the amount of the increase in CPK-2 has been proportionately related to the extent of heart muscle damage. Total CPK measurements are considered about 70 percent accurate; isoenzyme testing is about 90 percent accurate.

Note: More recently, through the use of **Chromosome Analysis** of the blood and **Chorionic Villi Sampling,** it has been possible to identify carriers of Duchenne muscular dystrophy by the third month of pregnancy. This test is said to be more accurate than total CPK measurements.

CREATININE

Creatinine is the end product of muscle metabolism (not from heart muscle, however). It is formed from creatine, which provides energy for the muscles to function. Both creatine and creatinine come from amino acids, which result from the breakdown of dietary protein. Creatinine is often tested along with **Urea Nitrogen,** which is also primarily a measure of kidney function. (Creatinine is considered the better measure of the two.)

Virtually all creatinine is normally excreted by a part of the kidney called the glomerulus, which is the first of six different filter systems the kidney utilizes to retain products the body needs and to dispose of waste material. Although creatinine is frequently measured in blood serum, the most useful measurement is derived from urine.

The creatinine clearance test is performed on a specimen of urine collected over a 24-hour period. (A newer form of the creatinine clearance test requires the collection of urine only over a 5-hour period.) This test measures the glomerular filtration rate (normally about 5 ounces of blood are filtered by the kidneys each minute) and is thus a fairly reliable indicator of how well the kidneys are functioning.

The inulin clearance test is a bit more precise than creatinine clearance but much more difficult to perform. The urea clearance test is less reliable, in that it is affected by diet and how much urine is passed. The **PAH** (sodium p-aminohippuric acid) clearance test is one of many new kidney function tests that work in a similar way to creatinine clearance. Creatine (not creatinine) is sometimes measured in the serum and the urine as a confirmation of creatinine clearance.

When performed: Primarily when there is suspicion of kidney damage; as an aid in the diagnosis of certain muscle diseases, especially those caused by hormone problems; when a liver problem cannot be specifically diagnosed.

Creatinine clearance is especially useful when there is an abnormal urea nitrogen test; the two tests together may help locate the specific area of kidney trouble. It also helps determine if a kidney problem is caused in part by bleeding or by the way protein in the diet affects the kidneys. The creatinine clearance test is of great value in determining the seriousness of kidney disease as well as in measuring the progress of treatment. It is also of special value when compared with the **Amylase** clearance test to diagnose pancreatitis.

Normal values: Blood serum creatinine values range from 0.8 to 1.3 mg per 100 ml. When measured in the urine, creatinine clearance is expressed as the glomerular filtration rate for a 24-hour period. For men, the normal range is between 110 and 170 ml per minute. Women usually have a slightly lower rate (90 ml per minute is still considered normal).

Abnormal values: Elevated serum creatinine along with reduced creatinine clearance indicates a kidney problem. The severity of the disease is indicated by the amount of reduced glomerular flow. When creatinine values are compared with urea nitrogen values, it is sometimes possible to ascertain if the kidney disease is reflecting the blood flow to the kidney or some blockage in the urinary tract between the kidney and the bladder. Serum creatinine is also increased in certain muscle diseases; when there is vomiting or diarrhea; when patients are taking certain drugs such as steroids, barbiturates, and vitamin C; and when large amounts of roast meats (which contain high levels of creatinine) are eaten.

Risk factors: Negligible (see general risk factors for blood testing).

Pain/discomfort: Minimal (see general pain/discomfort factors for blood testing).

Cost: From $4 to $8 when measured in the blood or urine. The creatinine clearance test averages $5 to $24. When creatine is measured with creatinine, the fee is approximately $25. The inulin clearance test averages $30, and the PAH clearance test averages $40. Creatinine alone is usually included in **Comprehensive Multiple Test Screening** panels, which range from $7 to $42.

Accuracy and significance: All the clearance tests measure kidney function with 80 to 90 percent accuracy, but the PAH is the most accurate. Creatinine and the clearance tests are significantly helpful in identifying the damaged area of the kidney and, at times, indicating whether the kidney problem is related to circulation or urinary blockage.

C-REACTIVE PROTEIN (CRP)

C-reactive protein is an abnormal globulin (see **Albumin/Globulin, Complement**) that reacts with certain bacterial substances in many inflammatory conditions. The CRP test is not specific for any one disease. At one time, the test was in widespread use in diagnosing and following patients with rheumatic fever; today, the erythrocyte **Sedimentation Rate** (ESR), a similar but simpler and less expensive test, is often used in place of the CRP. Blood is taken from a vein, and the serum is tested. In a few disease conditions, especially rheumatic fever, CRP may show up in blood serum before the ESR is elevated.

When performed: In conditions causing inflammation and tissue breakdown; to note progress in the treatment of certain illnesses such as rheumatoid arthritis, tuberculosis, and viral infections.

Normal values: C-reactive proteins are not normally found in the blood.

Abnormal values: C-reactive proteins are found in measurable amounts with bacterial and viral infections, rheumatic fever, cancer, arthritis, heart attack, and pneumonia. Aspirin or steroid drugs will mask the appearance of CRP.

Risk factors: Negligible (see general risk factors for blood testing).

Pain/discomfort: Minimal (see general pain/discomfort factors for blood testing).

Cost: From $5 to $45. Usually included in **Comprehensive Multiple Test Screening** panels, which range from $7 to $42.

Accuracy and significance: The test is positive with such a variety of diseases that it can hardly be significant. However, it is still performed to help distinguish infectious from noninfectious conditions. It is considered 70 percent accurate.

Although many doctors prefer the sedimentation rate test (ESR) as a general indicator of some abnormal—usually infectious—process going on in the body, the CRP usually indicates infection sooner than the ESR and reflects the presence of an infection much longer. It is also not affected by a low **Red Blood Cell** count, as is the ESR, and has been reported to be more accurate when used to measure the response of an infection to therapy.

CREMASTERIC, see *Reflex*

CROSS-EYES, see *Strabismus*

CROSS-MATCHING, see *Typing and Cross-Matching*

CRP, see *C-Reactive Protein*

CRYOGLOBULIN, see *Immunoglobulin*

CRYPTOCOCCUS, see *Agglutination*

CST, see *Nonstress Fetal Assessment*

Cs-T (COLOSCREEN SELF-TEST), see *Occult Blood*

CT, see *Computerized Tomography*

CULDOSCOPY, see *Endoscopy*

CULTURE

The purpose of a culture is to isolate and identify the microbes that cause disease by an infectious process. The science of microbiology (microbial culture) was formerly known as bacteriology. The name was changed after many organisms in addition to bacteria—viruses, fungi, rickettsia, parasites—were found to cause disease. Since virtually every part of the body is subject to infection, the test is performed on many tissues, secretions, excretions, and fluids. Blood, urine, spinal cord fluid, joint fluid, feces, bone marrow, and material from an abscess, ulcer, sinuses, eyes, ears, nose, and throat all may be cultured.

Some microbes do damage directly by their presence; others cause illness by giving off a toxic product (**Botulism** toxin). Disease-causing microbes must always be distinguished from nonharmful organisms that normally live in various parts of the body. Thus, while a direct examination on a slide under a microscope may show bacteria, only a culture can positively identify the type of bacteria.

Usually, a sample for culture is placed in two or more containers, each with a different medium (an environment that promotes growth)—one to grow organisms in the presence of air and one to grow them without air. Whenever the specimen is taken, absolute sterility must be observed to avoid contamination. If microbes grow in the sample, many other tests are performed to determine whether the microbes are pathological. Generally, small bits of paper saturated with different antibiotic solutions are placed on the microbes to find out which drugs are most effective in killing them. This is called the antibiotic sensitivity test. Such testing is especially important today because so many microorganisms have become resistant to antibiotics.

Another way of measuring the effectiveness of antibiotic treatment is to measure how well a patient's blood serum will inhibit the activity of the bacteria culture causing the disease. This is called the Schlichter test (named after the doctor who proposed it 40 years ago). Serum is tested before the antibiotic is given and then about a half-hour afterward; the serum should inhibit the bacteria after being diluted at least eight times. This test can also be performed on other body fluids (see **Synovial Fluid**). While it can help show whether a particular antibiotic drug is working, and whether a larger dose is needed, it cannot show whether the larger amount of the drug will be toxic or not. A refinement of the Schlichter test is called the serum bactericidal activity test; here, the destructive effect of an antibiotic on the bacteria causing the disease is measured. Blood serum is taken when the antibiotic's peak activity is believed to occur (30 minutes after an intravenous injection and 1 hour after an intramuscular injection) and when the antibiotic is thought to have little or no activity. To show an effective use of the antibiotic, the serum should destroy at least 99.9 percent of the cultured bacteria (in a special container) in large dilutions. This test can not only show the effectiveness of the antibiotic but can also show if two or more antibiotics will do an even better job. It can also show the doctor when, and if, the dosage of the drug should be changed. Usually, this test is limited to patients with extremely severe infections such as endocarditis (infection of the inside walls of the heart), osteomyelitis (bone infections that are very difficult to treat), critical pneumonias, arthritis, kidney disease, and meningitis.

Because the antibiotic is usually embedded in a paper disk, the test may be called the disk diffusion test or Bauer-Kirby test; the antibiotic-saturated disk should prevent bacterial growth around it, with the degree of effectiveness measured by the area of inhibited growth. More recently, the antibiotics are now diluted to various concentrations and placed in test tubes and thus are called tube dilution susceptibility tests. A positive result, showing the infective agent will be destroyed by the antibiotic on the disk or in the test tube, does not, however, guarantee that the patient's disease—even when caused by the identical microorganism—will automatically respond to the identical treatment.

One test is specific for certain bacteria that are resistant to penicillin products. By testing gonorrhea, influenza, and pneumonia bacteria with penicillinase to see if beta-lactamase is produced, it is sometimes possible to tell whether or not a particular antibiotic will be effective and which one would be the best to use.

When microbial infection is suspected, it is also common to perform **Agglutination** and **Complement Fixation** tests to confirm the identity of the organism. Viruses can now be cultured by using living cells (such as chick embryos in eggs, guinea pigs, suckling mice, or specially cultured cells). Viruses are then identified through electron microscope examination and one of the numerous agglutination or complement fixation tests (fluorescent antibody, enzyme-linked immunosorbent assay, radioimmunoassay). (See **Virus Disease**.) The india ink stain is added to some cultures to help detect cryptococcus.

When performed: Whenever there are symptoms of infection (usually high fever) and no specific diagnosis can be made. To help learn about the microorganisms that might be prevalent in a community, especially when an epidemic is suspected.

Normal values: There should be no growth of microorganisms from the various tissues, secretions, and body fluids (except for the normal bacteria in the intestines, throat, etc.).

Abnormal values: Any evident growth of pathological microorganisms is abnormal. When any disease-causing microorganisms are found in the blood, septicemia is indicated. Tuberculosis is diagnosed only by applying an acid-fast stain to distinguish the bacteria in the culture.

Risk factors: Normally, there is no risk; the patient usually supplies the specimen to be cultured: sputum, urine, pus from a sore, etc. Occasionally, **Endoscopy** is required to obtain a specimen. See also general risk factors for blood testing.

Pain/discomfort: None unless the doctor uses a form of **Endoscopy**. See also general pain/discomfort factors for blood testing.

Cost: A generalized screening culture to identify bacteria is $10 to $100. Special cultures to identify a fungus are $15 to $30; to isolate gonorrhea, $10 to $20; for tuberculosis, $15 to $50; and to isolate microorganisms from the blood, $20 to $50. Once the microorganism is detected, antibiotic sensitivity testing is from $10 to $50, depending on the number of different antibiotics being evaluated for effectiveness.

Accuracy and significance: Culture tests to isolate the cause of an infection are considered 95 percent accurate and equally significant when they are used to select the appropriate drug for treatment of a disease. A negative result (no growth of microorganisms) is important, as it points to a **Virus Disease**. The test can be lifesaving.

CUSHING'S SYNDROME, see *Cortisol*

CUTANEOUS ANERGY, see *Skin Reaction*

CUTLER, see *Sedimentation Rate*

CYANIDE, see *Hemoglobin*

CYCLIC ADENOSINE MONOPHOSPHATE (cAMP), see *Parathyroid*

CYCLOPLEGIA, see *Visual Acuity*

CYSTICERCOSIS, see *Agglutination*

CYSTIC FIBROSIS, see *Sodium; Sweat*

CYSTINURIA, see *Aminoaciduria*

CYSTOGRAM SCANNING, see *Nuclear Scanning*

CYSTOMETRY

Normally, the bladder will hold about 12 ounces of fluid before the urge to urinate is felt. This urge is caused by the pressure of the fluid against the expanding bladder walls. When the exact response to bladder pressure must be determined, or when it is necessary to know if the patient can discriminate between warm and cold temperatures in the bladder, cystometry is performed.

A catheter (very thin tube) is inserted into the bladder through the urethra and attached to a manometer (a graduated glass tube showing the response to pressure measurements). The bladder is then filled, and the patient's response to known pressure (and the amount of fluid) is recorded. A Lewis cystometer produces a graph showing pressure and capacity response. When necessary, the bladder is then alternately filled with warm and cold water, and the patient's response to varying temperatures is recorded.

A particular office test to measure bladder and urethral pressure, especially in women who have difficulty holding urine when coughing or laughing, is called the Robertson test (named after the doctor who invented the special urethroscope [see **Endoscopy**] used in the procedure). Carbon dioxide gas is passed into the bladder while the doctor observes the bladder wall during the patient's activities (e.g., straining, coughing); the test can help the doctor decide whether drugs or surgery will offer the most successful treatment. (Also see **Urine Flow Rate**.)

When performed: Whenever a patient has difficulty urinating (voiding), especially when the patient lacks the normal urge to urinate (usually because of bladder nerve disease); with urinary infections; to test the effect of certain drugs on the bladder, especially when such drugs are to be used to extend the capacity of the bladder or to initiate a response in a bladder that overfills.

Normal values: Until the bladder contains almost a pint of fluid, there should be no uncomfortable sensations. Additional fluid normally causes discomfort, along with sweating and flushing, followed by the urge to urinate.

Abnormal values: Failure to feel pressure after 12 ounces of fluid are instilled in the bladder, along with the inability to distinguish between warm and cold solutions, usually indicates disease of the nerves to and from the spinal cord to the bladder. With infections, the bladder will feel full with only a small amount of fluid.

Risk factors: Negligible (see general risk factors for catheter and needle insertion).

Pain/discomfort: Minimal (see general pain/discomfort factors for catheter and needle insertion).

Cost: In general, the fee for a cystometry is approximately $50. When it is performed in a hospital, there is usually an additional charge.

Accuracy and significance: This test is about 80 percent accurate in determining whether bladder disease is caused by nerve or spinal cord damage, or infection. Many doctors consider it a significant way to measure the effect drugs will have on the urinary system (some drugs, such as codeine and the anticholinergic drugs used to relax the bowel, make it difficult for a patient to urinate).

CYSTOSCOPY, see *Endoscopy*

CYTOGENETICS, see *Chromosome Analysis*

CYTOLOGY

Cytology tests detect and identify both normal and abnormal cells (especially cancer cells) in areas that cannot be easily and directly examined. Specimens to be examined may be obtained from body excretions (urine, feces), secretions (sputum, gastric, eye, peritoneal, breast, prostatic, vaginal, and cerebrospinal fluid), and tissue scrapings (uterus, vagina, mouth, nose, throat, bronchi, rectum, stomach, and cysts). The test can make possible a very early diagnosis and treatment of cancer. It can also indicate hormone activity in the body, as well as specific infections and the effect of radiation. After the smears are collected and stained, they are examined under a microscope.

The "Pap" test (named after Dr. George Papanicolaou, who developed the special stain used to color the tissue under study) is a form of cytology; originally, it was limited to examining the secretions from the vagina as a means of screening for abnormal cells from the cervix that could indicate cancer or precancer. The stain is now used to color secretions from the lung, stomach, and other organs and can even be applied to urine as a means of screening for bladder disease. This test can also give an indication of the phase of a woman's menstrual cycle and thus can also help evaluate certain hormone activities in the body.

In recent years, there have been an increasing number of reports putting the efficacy of the Pap test into question. One study revealed that at least half of all Pap test reports were in error; both false-positive and false-negative test results have been increasing. Most of these erroneous results are from poorly trained—even untrained—pathologists misreading the slides. Other errors have come from carelessness in obtaining the secretions for study; this includes improper technique, failure to obtain specimens from the proper locations, failure to handle the specimens on the slide properly, and the use of out-of-date or defective dyes for staining. Conservatively, it has been estimated that at least 5 percent of vaginal Pap tests have false-positive results; with nearly 50 million of these tests being performed on women annually, this could indicate that more than 2 million women every year may undergo totally unnecessary treatment—even surgery—for a disease that does not exist. A false-negative test could impart an unwarranted sense of security in a woman who is harboring a cancer. Any positive Pap test report, from any body tissue, should be repeated two or three times more—and by different doctors and laboratories—before any therapeutic action is taken; any negative result should be repeated several times—if there are any relevant symptoms. The Pap test in itself is an excellent test when properly performed and interpreted.

A note of caution: Pap tests as such do not screen for cancers in the uterus, as so many people believe. A special "jet wash" of the inside of the uterine cavity must be performed (using the Pap stain) when a uterine problem is suspected.

The **Gravlee method** is a new technique for collecting cells from the uterus; it is also considered an alternative to the routine Papanicolaou (Pap) test as a means of detecting cancer. It is thought to be a more accurate test for women over 35 years of age and for women of any age who have irregular menstrual periods. After the usual Pap smear is taken from the cervix, a very thin tube is inserted into the uterus and the cells are "washed" out with a jet-type spray; usually, a nurse performs the procedure. Most doctors feel this test is more than three times as accurate as the Pap test alone. The test cannot be performed on a woman wearing an intrauterine device (IUD), and it should not be performed if pregnancy is suspected or if the woman has high blood pressure or is taking certain drugs.

The most recent test for cervical disease is called cervicography; here, using a special camera, a distinct photograph is taken of the cervix for study by experts. There is a time delay (up to two weeks) before results are obtained, and the cost is about $15. Used along with a Pap test, it is better than 98 percent accurate.

When performed: As a routine or screening test during a physical examination; whenever cancer is suspected; for hormonal assessment; when there is undiagnosed disease in a particular organ or body system.

Normal values: No abnormal cells should be seen in any stained smear.

Abnormal values: Any cancer cell or even a suspicious cell is considered a positive, or abnormal, result. A positive test is usually repeated. If the second test is still positive, a **Biopsy** (the removal of a minute piece of tissue from the suspected organ), X-rays (see **Radiography**), or other appropriate diagnostic tests must be performed to verify diagnosis. Inappropriate hormone influence on cells or evidence of inflammation is considered abnormal.

Risk factors: Negligible. In addition to the general risk factors for catheter and needle insertion, there are those related to **Endoscopy**. When the Pap test is taken, there is the rare risk of infection, but unfortunately, there is the greater risk that it will be improperly performed and fail to indicate pathology. The possibility of prolonged vaginal bleeding does exist after the Gravlee method test, but in a study of 18,000 women, no serious complications occurred and no emergency treatment was needed.

Pain/discomfort: Minimal. In addition to the general pain/discomfort factors for catheter and needle insertion, there are those related to endoscopy. A Pap smear should cause no pain or discomfort. Some women may have painful contractions when the Gravlee jet washer is inserted; a few may experience vaginal spotting after the test is completed.

Cost: Most doctors do not charge for obtaining most specimens for testing (Pap smear, sputum, and other secretions); when specimens are obtained from other areas, the cost of the procedure (**Endoscopy,** prostate examination, etc.) usually includes the cytological examination. Where cytological staining and examination are not included in the examination or procedure to obtain the specimen, the charge for the microscopic evaluation can range from $1 to $100 (most doctors are charged from $1 to $3 by a laboratory to review and interpret the Pap smear).

Accuracy and significance: When definitive cancer cells are detected, the test is considered close to 80 percent accurate; the problems arise when there are false-positive results implying cancer where no pathology exists. The test is equally significant in evaluating particular hormone activities in the body (Pap test), the effects of X-ray treatment on the body, and the diagnosis of exotic diseases. Aspiration cytology is 90 percent accurate in diagnosing breast cancer. Much depends on use of the proper technique to obtain the sample and on the training and experience of the pathologist who prepares and interprets the specimen under the microscope.

When it comes to the Pap test, it has been reported that a 5 to 20 percent false-positive rate may be usual, as is a 35 percent false-negative rate. Most of the errors are considered to be doctor-technique-caused. A recent survey revealed that half of all doctors who "read" the Pap test slides were not competent to do so.

CYTOMEGALOVIRUS (CMV)

This virus is believed to be part of the **Herpes** virus group that causes cold sores, venereal lesions, shingles, and chicken pox, but cytomegalovirus disease can be far more devastating. Although the signs of a cytomegalovirus infection can resemble those of infectious mononucleosis, more often than not there are no initial symptoms. It is thought that if the population was tested for cytomegalovirus, more than 80 percent of its members would show evidence of exposure to this virus. Although CMV can cause diarrhea, it is most serious when it infects a newborn baby. It is believed that close to 5,000 babies are afflicted with this virus each year and suffer blindness, deafness, blood abnormalities, mental retardation, congenital defects, and encephalitis. It is now known that this virus can be transmitted indirectly through blood transfusions and through bone, heart, and kidney transplants in addition to direct transmission through sexual contact, and it has been found in blood, urine, saliva, semen, and even tears, all of which can be tested by examining a specimen under a microscope or by culture. More often, blood is taken from a vein and examined for antibodies through tests similar to **Agglutination** (fluorescent antibody) and by **Complement Fixation**.

When performed: As part of the **TORCH** screening panel for pregnant women and newborn infants; when infectious mononucleosis is suspected but remains unproven; following open heart surgery and other surgery requiring a number of transfusions; when nerve or eye disease cannot be diagnosed.

Normal values: It is difficult to stipulate a "normal" value, since more than half the population will exhibit a positive antibody test. However, the antibody level should not change if the test is repeated weeks or months later. There should be no cytomegalovirus bodies inside body cells, and no live virus should grow on culture.

Abnormal values: A high titer of cytomegalovirus antibodies in a newborn; a marked rise in the titer (the amount of detectable antibodies) over a period of a few weeks, especially in a pregnant woman; isolation of the virus by culture or its presence inside body cells.

Risk factors: Negligible (see general risk factors for blood testing).

Pain/discomfort: Minimal (see general pain/discomfort factors for blood testing).

Cost: From $25 to $60 for a single test for antibodies; from $50 to $115 for a culture; from $10 to $80 for the microscopic examination of tissue cells.

Accuracy and significance: Unless the antibody titers change markedly, or the culture produces the specific virus, the test, while 90 percent accurate, is of little significance because a positive result is so common.

CYTOTOXIC ALLERGY DETECTION, see *RAST*

D

DACOMED SNAP-GAUGE, see *Impotence*

D&C, see *Dilatation and Curettage*

DAP, see *Pregnancy*

DARK FIELD, see *Syphillis*

DAVIDSON DIFFERENTIAL, see *Mononucleosis*

DEEP REFLEX, see *Reflex*

DEEP-VEIN THROMBOSIS, see *Plethysmography*

DEHYDROEPIANDROSTERONE SULFATE, see *Cortisol*

DELAYED FEEDBACK, see *Hearing Function*

DELTA AMINOLEVULINIC ACID (ALA), see *Lead; Porphyrins*

DELTA HEPATITIS, see *Hepatitis*

DEMENTIA, see *Cognitive Capacity Screening; Facial Recognition; Magnetic Resonance Imaging*

DENSITOMETER CT SCANNING, see *Bone Mineral Density Analysis*

DEOXYURIDINE SUPPRESSION, see *Schilling*

DEPRESSION

Depression is a mental state that can be caused by physical disease, after pregnancy, and with hormone changes, or it can be a personal reaction to an unpleasant situation. It can also come from exposure to heavy metals or other toxic chemicals (see **Toxic Chemical Exposure**) as well as drug abuse (e.g.: cocaine, amphetamines, marijuana, sedatives, etc.). The usual symptoms of depression (tiredness, insomnia, lack of appetite, stomach and intestinal complaints, irritability) can mimic a great many other illnesses. Because of the close association between depression and suicide, it is important to diagnose true depression early.

There are several tests in the form of questionnaires that help to make the diagnosis of depression. In the Beck Depression Inventory, the patient is asked to select responses from several sets of leading statements. A set of statements may range, for example, from "I am dissatisfied with everything" to "I am not particularly dissatisfied." Proponents of this test claim that it aids not only in diagnosing depression but also in measuring the degree of depression.

A somewhat similar test is the Zung Self-Rating Depression Scale. The patient is asked to evaluate a series of self-descriptive statements such as "Morning is when I feel best" by checking off a column headed "none or a little of the time," "some of the time," "a good part of the time," or "most or all of the time." This test also claims to be able to indicate the degree of depression.

All such tests are really only screening devices; a positive diagnosis of depression must be based on in-depth doctor-patient interviews. Additionally, there are biochemical tests to aid in the diagnosis of depression. Among them are the adrenal suppression test (see **Cortisol**); and the MHPG urine test (see **Catecholamines**). Today, **Thyroid Function** testing for hypothyroidism is all but routine for patients suffering from depression. In a recent survey of patients undergoing psychiatric treatment for depression, more than 10 percent were found to have some degree of hypothyroidism. (Also see **Sleep Monitoring**.)

When performed: When patients have vague symptoms, especially tiredness, helplessness, or pessimistic feelings; after a stressful situation in a patient's life (loss of a loved one, loss of a job); when a patient is taking certain drugs, especially tranquilizers; when a patient has marital problems; when suicidal tendencies are suspected by the doctor.

Normal values: Most patients rarely select more than two or three statements that indicate depression.

Abnormal values: Four or more statements associated with a depressed state of mind can indicate mild depression; a greater number of such responses can indicate severe depression and potential suicide. Again, such tests should be used only as screening devices and should be followed by detailed interviews with the patient.

Risk factors: Tests in the form of questionnaires have no risks. See general risk factors for blood testing.

Pain/discomfort: There are no pain/discomfort factors associated with the oral tests. See general pain/discomfort factors for blood testing.

Cost: The Beck Depression Inventory is approximately $25. Usually, there is no charge for interpreting the Zung Self-Rating Depression Scale; a few doctors charge $5 for the form.

Accuracy and significance: While some doctors regard questionnaires as less than 80 percent accurate, they have proved to be 90 percent accurate in helping to determine if depression should at least be considered as a diagnosis; many doctors also use them to evaluate the extent of depression. When followed by biochemical tests and coupled with the doctor's past experience, they become quite significant.

DEPTH PERCEPTION, see *Visual Acuity*

DERMATOME, see *Sensory*

DEXAMETHASONE SUPPRESSION, see *Cortisol; Depression*

DHEA SULFATE, see *Testis Function*

DIABETES INSIPIDUS, see *Vasopressin*

DIABETES MELLITUS, see *Glucose*

DIABETES MONITORING, see *Glycohemoglobin*

DIABETIC ACIDOSIS, see *Ketones*

DIAGNEX BLUE, see *Gastric Analysis*

DIAGNOSTIC CYTOLOGY, see *Cytology*

DIAPHANOGRAPHY, see *Thermography*

DIASTOLIC PRESSURE, see *Blood Pressure*

DIBUCAINE NUMBER, see *Cholinesterase*

DICK, see *Skin Reaction*

DIFFERENTIAL, see *Blood Cell Differential*

DIFFUSING CAPACITY, see *Pulmonary Function*

DIGITALIS TOXICITY

Digitalis and its synthetic substitutes digoxin and digitoxin (called cardiac glycosides) are the most widely used drugs in congestive heart failure. They increase the force of the heartbeat and slow down the initiating impulse that causes the heart muscle to contract, decreasing the heart rate. Before digitalis, digoxin, or digitoxin is administered, it is essential to discover and follow in the patient the fine line between the amount of the drug necessary to achieve a therapeutic effect and the amount that will cause a toxic effect. Too much of one of these drugs can cause nausea, vomiting, and irregular heartbeats (which can be fatal).

The digitalis toxicity test measures the amount of digoxin or digitoxin in a patient's serum (whole-leaf digitalis is rarely used today). The patient should not take the drug for at least 8 to 12 hours prior to the test. Of equal importance, once a therapeutic dose has been established, the patient must not change the brand of drug; it has been shown that different brands of the same drug at the same dose can be toxic because of different dissolving and absorption qualities.

When performed: To follow the course of therapy in patients taking digoxin, digitoxin, and other digitalis drugs in order to prevent poisoning.

Normal values: Normal values are those that produce a therapeutic effect without causing toxicity.

Abnormal values: Digoxin levels above 1.5 ng per ml are often found to be toxic; serum levels below 1.5 ng per ml are not usually toxic but are therapeutic. The therapeutic, nontoxic levels of digitoxin are usually less than 18 ng per ml. These figures are only examples; they vary widely for different individuals. For digoxin, up to 3.5 ng per ml has not been toxic, and for digitoxin up to 40 ng per ml has been safe. In other words, no two people have the same therapeutic, nontoxic blood level.

When digitalis toxicity tests are performed, it is important to test for **Potassium** (elevated serum potassium accentuates digitalis toxicity), **Calcium,** and **Creatinine** clearance (kidney function). Digoxin is excreted by the kidney; digitoxin through the liver; this is important if a patient has kidney or liver disease.

Risk factors: Negligible (see general risk factors for blood testing).

Pain/discomfort: Minimal (see general pain/discomfort factors for blood testing).

Cost: Digoxin analysis is $20 to $25; digitoxin analysis is $25 to $60.

Accuracy and significance: The tests are considered 95 percent accurate and extremely significant in monitoring a patient taking either of the drugs, especially when first prescribed. They are particularly valuable when evaluating a patient's compliance with a prescribed drug regimen. Recent evidence has revealed that many, seemingly unrelated, conditions (e.g., gastrointestinal problems, kidney diseases, high or low blood potassium, calcium and magnesium levels) can cause erroneous serum digoxin results; thus, the test is not as accurate as previously believed unless other blood tests are performed at the same time.

DIGITAL SUBTRACTION ANGIOGRAPHY, see *Radiography*

DIGITOXIN, see *Digitalis Toxicity*

DIGOXIN, see *Digitalis Toxicity*

DILANTIN, see *Drug Monitoring*

DILATATION AND CURETTAGE (D&C)

The D&C is perhaps the most frequently performed test in the diagnosis of gynecologic problems. The examination is usually performed in a hospital or a clinic under general anesthesia. For the dilatation part of the test, dilators of increasingly large circumference are used to create an opening big enough for examination of the cervical canal (the opening in the cervix to the uterus) and the endometrium (lining of the uterus). A curette (spoon-shaped instrument) is used to scrape the endometrial cavity (curettage) for tissue samples, which are then examined under a microscope. Endometrial screening may sometimes be performed by suction collection instead of scraping, and with this method, it can be done in the physician's office, without anesthesia, using a jet irrigation and suction technique. (See **Endoscopy** for hysteroscopy following dilatation.)

When performed: When there is abnormal uterine bleeding or discharge; in infertility; in infections; when there is suspicion of anomaly (uterine abnormality); when there is suspicion of fibroids or cancer of the uterus or cervix; to ascertain the phase of the menstrual cycle; to remove polyps; for therapeutic abortion.

Normal values: Normally, no malformations, blockage of the cervical canal, cancer cells, or polyps are found. The cells that line the uterus usually show hormone activity that conforms to menstrual cycle changes.

Abnormal values: Abnormal findings include tumor, cancerous cells, or cells in the uterine lining that do not match the expected phase of the menstrual cycle.

Risk factors: There is a minor risk of infection and subsequent bleeding following a D&C. When a D&C is used for an abortion, the risk increases, and the procedure can be quite dangerous when attempted on a patient more than four months pregnant. When general anesthesia is administered, there is a moderate risk.

Pain/discomfort: General anesthesia can be followed by nausea and vomiting. After a D&C, there is frequently discomfort in the lower abdomen for a few days; there can also be a menstrual-like discharge lasting up to a week.

Cost: The doctor's and anesthetist's fees are usually the same, each charging from $100 to $200. When a D&C is performed in a hospital, there is an additional charge for use of the operating room. And of course, there is the charge for the hospital stay. If there is a microscopic analysis of the material obtained by a D&C, the pathologist's fee ranges from $50 to $200.

Accuracy and significance: Although the test is considered to be about 80 percent accurate in differentiating cancer from noncancerous pathology, in more than half of all cases, the uterus is not properly scraped—making the test virtually useless. Other studies have shown it to be inappropriately performed almost 90 percent of the time. Suction methods, not requiring anesthesia, are considered more accurate.

DILAUDID, see *Drug Abuse*

DINITROPHENYLHYDRAZINE, see *Phenylketonuria*

DIPHTHERIA, see *Skin Reaction*

DIPLOPIA, see *Strabismus*

DIRECT BILIRUBIN, see *Bilirubin*

DIRECT COOMBS', see *Agglutination*

DIRECT OPHTHALMOSCOPIC, see *Fundoscopy*

DIRECT STREPTOCOCCAL, see *Antistreptolysin O Titer*

DISK (DISC) DIFFUSION, see *Culture*

DISPUTED PARENTAGE, see *Parentage*

DNA HEMOPHILIA PROBE, see *Partial Thromboplastin Time*

DNA MARKER, see *Genetic Disorder Screening*

DOG ROUNDWORM, see *Toxocariasis*

DOLL'S EYE, see *Reflex*

DOPPLER, see *Ultrasound*

DOWN'S SYNDROME, see *Amniocentesis*

DPA, see *Bone Mineral Density Analysis*

DRINK, see *Alcohol*

DRIVING UNDER THE INFLUENCE, see *Alcohol*

DRUG ABUSE

Until recently, it was difficult to test for narcotics such as marijuana, cocaine, codeine, heroin, morphine, methadone, and dilaudid. It was almost as difficult to detect other drugs sometimes used illegally—such as the amphetamines, barbiturates, and some tranquilizers—especially when they were used to produce exhilaration, deliberate delirium, or oblivion. Today, there are quick and simple tests that can reveal the presence of such dangerous drugs in the urine. Requiring no skilled personnel, the tests can be performed in schools, factories, and at home, as well as in the doctor's office or laboratory. Their primary use is to screen, and they have proved extremely effective. When there are legal implications, however, many laboratories resort to biochemical blood or urine analysis, both of which are more complicated procedures. There is a difference between **Drug Monitoring** and testing for drug abuse. Drug monitoring is used to determine the optimum dose of a therapeutic drug in order to avoid adverse effects; it is also employed when there is doubt that a patient is taking the prescribed drug.

When performed: When a doctor suspects a patient is illicitly using drugs that might themselves be the cause of an illness or are producing signs and symptoms that might obscure an underlying disease; to detect criminal activity; to prevent potentially dangerous actions such as driving a car or operating hazardous machinery while under the influence of mind-altering drugs; to explain irrational behavior or sudden personality changes.

Normal values: No evidence of any illegal or unprescribed drug.

Abnormal values: Any evidence of drug abuse. Urine tests are basically qualitative; further technical measurement of the amount of a drug in the body is possible.

Risk factors: None with urine testing (other than possibly providing self-incriminating evidence).

Pain/discomfort: None.

Cost: The average charge for the urine test is $10 to $20 when performed in a doctor's office or clinical laboratory. Biochemical analysis in a laboratory is approximately $40 for each drug search and approximately $100 for a complete drug screening.

Accuracy and significance: Not as accurate as once supposed. Much depends on the laboratory performing the tests and the drugs under suspicion. There have been many false-positive tests—especially in the armed forces—when urine is the specimen tested. And in one survey, 1 laboratory out of 20 failed to detect known marijuana specimens; yet marijuana smoking can cause a positive test for three weeks after use. When properly performed by experienced technicians, the accuracy rate is better than 90 percent; in actuality, however, the overall accuracy rate when screening large groups, such as the military or in industry, has only been about 33 percent.

DRUG MONITORING

Most prescribed drugs are quite potent; the range of safety between the amount of a drug that is therapeutically effective and the amount that is toxic is very narrow. In addition, there are times when a prescribed drug seems to have no effect, either because of some idiosyncrasy in the patient's metabolism or because the patient is not taking the drug as prescribed. It is known that two out of three patients do not properly follow directions for a prescription drug, and one out of three patients never even have the prescription filled.

Anticonvulsant drugs such as Dilantin (for epilepsy) fluctuate greatly in the body, and it takes only a minute overdose to cause severe damage. Gentamicin (an antibiotic) can cause deafness unless it is monitored carefully. Anticoagulant drugs must also be monitored regularly (see **Prothrombin Time**), as must drugs used in arthritis (see **Salicylates**).

Toxicology involves not only testing for overdose of a drug (see **Barbiturates; Bromides**) but also monitoring for the optimal therapeutic effect (see **Digitalis Toxicity**). Antibiotic drugs, psychotherapeutic agents such as tranquilizers and antidepressants, and vitamins are also monitored regularly. In most instances, blood is taken from a vein, and the serum is tested. Urine, body tissues, and even hair or nail shavings are sometimes tested. Drug monitoring is not identical to **Drug Abuse** testing; in most instances, a patient is not unconscious and is able to cooperate.

When performed: To assure that therapeutic blood levels are reached; to prevent toxic reactions from drugs *before* symptoms develop; to detect overdose or abuse of a drug; to determine why a patient does not respond to a drug.

Normal values: Normal values are those that produce a therapeutic effect without causing toxicity. When theophylline drugs (for asthma) are used, they must reach a certain level in the blood before they are effective; less than the required amount in the blood is the same as no drug at all.

Abnormal values: A detectable amount of drug greater than that needed to produce a therapeutic effect is considered abnormal. For example, when Dilantin is prescribed, the drug is given in dosages to produce a blood concentration of from 10 to 20 mcg per ml. Should the blood levels go above 20 mcg per ml, toxicity will occur. Although the therapeutically effective dose of a drug may vary with the size of an individual, the amount of a drug in the blood that can cause toxicity usually remains consistent.

Risk factors: Negligible (see general risk factors for blood testing).

Pain/discomfort: Minimal (see general pain/discomfort factors for blood testing).

Cost: From $20 to $80, depending on the drug being monitored.

Accuracy and significance: While drug monitoring is 90 percent accurate in determining the amount of a drug in the patient's body at the time of blood testing, the significance of the test depends on when the patient took the last dose. The "trough" level of drug monitoring ascertains whether the patient has a therapeutic amount of the drug in his system at all times; the blood sample for testing is taken within 30 minutes before the next dose is due. In contrast, the "peak" level of drug monitoring determines whether the amount of the drug in the patient's system has reached a toxic or dangerous level; the "peak" level is usually tested for immediately after the patient takes the medicine—the exact time depending on the doctor's knowledge of the metabolism of the drug being measured. It should be noted that the blood levels of a drug do not necessarily reflect the amount of that drug taken by a patient. Many variables (absorption, interaction with other drugs, metabolism, kidney function) affect exactly how much of a drug enters, and stays in, the bloodstream. Drug monitoring is also significant in determining a patient's compliance with a doctor's orders.

DRUNK DRIVER, see *Alcohol*

DRY EYE, see *Schirmer's*

DSA, see *Radiography*

DSR, see *Radiography*

DUAL-BEAM PHOTON ABSORPTIOMETRY, see *Bone Mineral Density Analysis*

DUCHENNE MUSCULAR DYSTROPHY CARRIER, see *Creatine Phosphokinase*

DUODENAL BIOPSY, see *Growth Hormone*

DWARFISM, see *Growth Hormone*

D-XYLOSE BREATH TEST, see *Lactose Tolerance*

DYNAMIC ELECTROCARDIOGRAPHY, see *Electrocardiogram*

DYNAMIC EXERCISE CARDIOGRAM, see *Electrocardiogram*

DYNAMIC SPATIAL RECONSTRUCTOR, see *Radiography*

DYNOMOMETRY, see *Electromyography*

DYSLEXIA, see *Learning Disability*

DYSPHAGIA, see *Gastroesophageal Reflux; Nuclear Scanning*

E

EAR BALANCE, see *Caloric*

EARLY DETECTOR, see *Occult Blood*

ECG, see *Electrocardiogram*

ECHINOCOCCOSIS, see *Agglutination*

ECHOCARDIOGRAM

The echocardiogram is considered by many physicians to be almost equal in value to the standard **Electrocardiogram** (ECG). Echocardiography is based on the principles of underwater detection (sonar) that the Navy developed during World War II. When a sound wave is directed into the heart at various locations, the echo, or rebounding sound wave, graphically reflects each part of the heart off which it bounces (see **Ultrasound**). Analysis of the echo images allows a three-dimensional "visualization" of the heart, the heart valves, the muscular structures, and even the blood as it passes through. The technique is similar to fluoroscopy, but with far more detail and with no radiation exposure (the sound waves used to obtain the echoes have never been shown to be harmful).

A transducer (an instrument that can convert energy into sound and also simultaneously receive sound and translate it back into energy that can be visualized) is rubbed over the heart area of the chest. (Usually, a coating of mineral oil is applied to the chest to prevent air from seeping between the instrument and the body.) The transducer can be directed to any specific heart area, and the recorded echo patterns detail the opening and closing and condition of the heart valves. Echocardiograms can also indicate the size of each heart chamber, whether there are any masses in the heart, and especially whether there is excess fluid in the sac around the heart (pericardial effusion)—usually, the result of infection or irritation from disease adjacent to the heart.

When performed: To diagnose heart valve disease, enlarged heart, heart tumors, and especially congenital heart defects in infants; when pericardial effusion is suspected; in instances of chest pain, fever, and fainting that cannot be diagnosed; to follow the progress of patients with heart valve replacements.

Normal values: Extensive experience is required to interpret echocardiograms, and great skill and knowledge of heart anatomy are needed to direct the sound waves properly. Thus, normal values depend primarily on the technique of the test and the ability of the cardiologist to read the results. Multiple layers of thick and thin lines reflect the echoes from the various layers of heart structure that receive the sounds. There are specific measurements in centimeters (cm) for each area—such as the thickness of the heart wall or the heart chamber (when filled and when empty)—as well as normal expectations of how much blood the heart should hold and eject each time it beats. The difference between normal and abnormal may, however, be only a slight variation in the thickness of one sound wave lasting less than 0.1 second.

Abnormal values: A cardiologist can detect a defect in the opening and closing of a heart valve as well as structural defects in all areas of the heart. The picture of an abnormality can help indicate when certain kinds of treatment will be successful.

Risk factors: None.

Pain/discomfort: None.

Cost: From $100 to $250; in many instances, this includes a standard ECG test performed at the same time.

Accuracy and significance: A number of doctors believe the echocardiogram reveals more and is slightly more accurate than the standard ECG. However, most doctors choose to confirm a suspected abnormality appearing on an echocardiogram with a Holter monitoring test or **Nuclear Scanning**. The echocardiograph is particularly significant in detecting fluids in the sac around the heart (pericarditis); fluid should never be found around the heart. Considered to be 80 percent accurate; 98 percent accurate in most chest conditions.

ECHOENCEPHALOGRAM, see *Ultrasound*

ECHOGRAM, see *Ultrasound*

ECHOVIRUS, see *Virus Disease*

EDROPHONIUM

Edrophonium is a chemical that works at the nerve ends to stimulate muscle contractions by inhibiting the action of **Cholinesterase**. One trade name for this product is Tensilon, and the test is sometimes called the Tensilon test. Because the chemical works so rapidly and its activity lasts for so short a time, edrophonium is used to aid in the diagnosis of myasthenia gravis (a condition where the muscles, particularly of the face and neck, tire very quickly to the point of paralysis). It is given as an intravenous injection. Because of the possibility, though rare, that injection of edrophonium will cause nausea, diarrhea, excessive salivation, excessive sweating, and a slowing of the heart rate, atropine is kept ready to use as an antidote (edrophonium's action on the heart allows it to be used on occasion to stop attacks of extremely rapid heartbeat). The drug should be administered with extreme caution in patients with asthma. Just before edrophonium is given, a placebo (an innocuous substance) is injected to make sure that the patient is not simply reacting to the test procedure itself.

If there is no reaction to injection of the drug, a second dose may be given two to three minutes later (a few myasthenia gravis patients need a greater amount of the drug to be effective).

Edrophonium is also used as a means of differentiating chest pain as to whether it comes from the heart or the esophagus (see **Gastroesophageal Reflux**). When this drug is injected, it will reproduce chest pain that comes from the esophagus but not from the heart.

A recent test to aid in the diagnosis of myasthenia gravis is performed by placing a spot of a patient's blood on a piece of special blotting paper and then sending the paper to a laboratory to see if acetylcholine receptor antibody is present. One of the suspected causes of this disease is the destruction of acetylcholine by this antibody. Acetylcholine is a chemical that is necessary to transmit nerve messages to muscles so they will react. (See **Immunology** and **Agglutination** for information on antibodies.)

When performed: Primarily as a diagnostic test for myasthenia gravis; as an indication of overdose of one of the usual medications prescribed to treat myasthenia gravis.

Normal values: In a patient with weakened muscle strength or muscle paralysis (most commonly seen in the eyelids, which cannot be held open), muscle strength returns within one minute after an injection of edrophonium, and the ability to use the muscles lasts for 5 to 10 minutes. Of course, this "normal" value is an indication of disease. Less than .05 nM of acetylcholine receptor antibody is considered within normal limits.

Abnormal values: Weakened or paralytic muscles that respond to one or two injections of the drug indicate myasthenia gravis. On rare occasions, a patient with amyotrophic lateral sclerosis (muscle atrophy) will respond to edrophonium but will not benefit from the usual myasthenia gravis treatment (drugs similar to edrophonium, but much longer-acting). If more than 1 nM of acetylcholine receptor antibody is found, it helps confirm the diagnosis of myasthenia gravis.

Risk factors: In addition to the dangers of administering edrophonium to patients with asthma, there is also a possibility of the drug's causing severe nausea and vomiting.

Pain/discomfort: Many patients on whom this test is performed experience a dryness of the mouth and abdominal cramps; this discomfort usually disappears within an hour.

Cost: As a doctor's presence is required during the test procedure due to the possibility of an adverse reaction, there is generally a charge of $35 to $50.

Accuracy and significance: Most often, a positive reaction to edrophonium (or to neostigmine) can warrant the diagnosis of myasthenia gravis. There are, however, a few people with the disease who do not react to drug testing. About 75 percent accurate.

EEG, see *Electroencephalogram*

EFM, see *Fetal Monitoring*

EJACULATE, see *Semen*

EJECTION FRACTION, see *Electrocardiogram*

EKG, see *Electrocardiogram*

ELECTRIC RESPONSE AUDIOMETRY (ERA), see *Hearing Function*

ELECTROCARDIOGRAM (ECG)

The electrocardiogram, or ECG (formerly known as the EKG because of the original German spelling of the word: *Elektrokardiagramma*), is a graphic measure of the heart's muscular activity and a reflection of the self-generated electrical impulses that pass through the heart muscle, causing contraction and relaxation. Various electrodes, called leads, are placed on the body, usually one on each wrist and ankle and one on the chest, which can be moved over the entire heart area. (The leads are metal contacts capable of detecting electrical activity within the body; they do not give off any electricity or have any activity of their own.)

By employing any two electrodes and greatly magnifying the activity they detect, the physician can obtain a diagrammatic representation of the heart's activity. If, for example, the lead from the right arm and the left leg are used, the ECG will largely reflect the activity of the right side of the heart; the same results will be obtained if the movable chest lead is placed to the right of the sternum (breastbone). Use of the various leads in different combinations offers many different "views" of the heart; 12 different "views" are considered standard or routine.

The recorded electrocardiograph shows the rate and regularity of the heart's rhythm; it can also show the force or effectiveness of each heartbeat; the extent and location of any heart muscle damage (both old and new), and the effect of certain drugs. Unfortunately, the ECG can also give false readings; that is, the graph may show what seem to be abnormalities when the heart is normal, or it may fail to reveal heart damage when present. It is not a perfect test and is usually accompanied by several other tests for confirmation of a diagnosis.

For example, when the ECG appears to be normal but the patient has complaints referable to the heart, a stress ECG (sometimes called a treadmill test, an exercise ECG, or a dynamic exercise ECG) may be performed. With the ECG leads in place, the patient walks on a treadmill at a set speed and incline (or operates a stationary bicycle); the ECG is recorded while exercising. Normally, no change is observed other than an expected increase in the rate of the heart. But in some patients, the extra physical activity cuts down the amount of oxygen reaching the heart muscle, and this may show up on the ECG. The test is stopped immediately if oxygen shortage occurs.

The oldest type of exercise test is the Master two-step (devised by Dr. Arthur Master), in which a patient walks up and down two steps for a specified number of times while the ECG is recorded. This is still an effective test, but it has been replaced by the more impressive treadmills. The stress ECG is considered by a few physicians to be a fair predictor of future heart problems. But many physicians feel that the test has no value. Studies have shown that two out of three patients without symptoms who take an exercise ECG may have a false-positive result; that is, heart disease may be indicated erroneously. Many doctors believe the **Cold Pressor** test to be as effective as the physical exercise stress test in measuring a patient's response to a burden on the heart.

Another form of heart stress testing is the quiz electrocardiogram. While the ECG is being recorded, the patient is asked questions that both threaten his ego and provoke anxiety. Changes in the ECG during the questioning period can indicate emotionally caused heart disease.

A more recent innovation of the ECG is the Holter monitoring test, in which the patient wears a tiny, portable ECG recording machine (sometimes combined with a tiny voice tape recorder) for 24 hours and notes (or records) any unusual stresses during the day as well as all normal activities (eating, going to the bathroom, etc.). This test can isolate previously hidden heart disease and, of even greater importance, can help indicate causative factors such as personality problems. Holter is also called ambulatory electrocardiography monitoring (AEM) or dynamic electrocardiography.

Another method of testing heart function is the SHK-STI (Spodick-Haffty-Kotilainen measurement and calculation of the **Systolic Time Intervals**). The patient wears an earpiece containing a photoelectric cell that measures the velocity of the blood entering and leaving the ear at the same time that chest electrodes are recording the ECG. These measurements of how well the heart is functioning can be made over a 24-hour period and can be correlated with normal physical activity and exercise.

At times, doctors will inject ergonovine (a drug obtained from ergot, and related to lysergic acid, that is used primarily to stop uterine bleeding after childbirth) to see if it will provoke coronary artery spasm as a means of eliciting anginal pains at rest where the diagnosis is in doubt. This is usually done while the ECG is being performed. This test can be quite dangerous—it has caused an irreversible closure of a coronary artery—and should be performed, if at all, only during angiography (see **Radiography**), when lifesaving drugs can be properly administered.

A different test of the heart's efficiency is called the ejection fraction (also see "Cardiac Output," in **Radiography**). This is a measure of how much blood one or more of the heart's chambers can pump with each contraction (pulse); most commonly, the ventricles are tested, with the left ventricle, which pumps blood into the aorta, the most common single chamber measurement. When the test is performed while the patient is exercising, the ejection fraction should increase—even though the heart beats faster and theoretically has less time to fill each chamber. New studies, however, have revealed that when women take this test, they may not show the expected increase and yet still be normal (have no disease that the test is supposed to indicate).

In programmed electrical cardiac stimulation, the doctor reproduces irregular heart rhythms, sometimes called cardiac pacing, to help diagnose the cause of fainting (medically called syncope; see **Carotid Sinus Massage**). It has been claimed that in 70 percent of all patients with unexplained fainting, the cause is an abnormal heart rhythm. The test can also help select the proper therapy (e.g., drugs or a pacemaker).

The newest way to determine the type and cause of irregular heartbeat—and to help uncover those arrhythmias that are of great risk—is called electrophysiologic testing (an intracardiac procedure where the test electrodes are placed inside the heart by a catheter via an artery or vein). At times, the heart may be stimulated (shocked) into a purposefully irregular rhythm by an electrode to measure a drug's effectiveness in controlling the arrhythmia. Some doctors feel this is the most efficient way to help diagnose heart rhythm problems—especially those that cause syncope (fainting or blackouts), but it is still considered a difficult and extremely risky procedure.

When performed: The test is performed whenever heart disease is suspected and often as a routine checkup. (It is advisable to have at least one ECG before the age of 40 in order to note any changes that may occur at a later date.) It is also performed whenever a patient complains of shortness of breath, intermittent chest pain, or "palpitations," and when patients are taking drugs such as digitalis or diuretics (which tend to cause potassium changes that can severely affect the heart's activity).

Normal values: Each lead of the ECG has a fairly normal but slightly different pattern. The rate of the heart should be between 70 and 100 beats per minute (athletes may have normal rates of 50), and the pattern should be regular (no extra or missed beats).

Abnormal values: Extensive training and experience in interpreting ECGs allow the physician to detect even a slight variation from normal and expected patterns. The changes may indicate a muscle defect (either damage or insufficient oxygen), or they may reveal nerve conduction changes, which can come from damage to the heart arteries that bring oxygen to the heart muscle or damage to the muscle itself (from the aging process or from old infections). Enlargement of the heart, congenital defects, and valve disease may also be indicated by the ECG.

Risk factors: See general risk factors for electrical instruments. Although the American Medical Association states that a physician need not be present during a stress electrocardiogram test, the risk of adverse effects associated with the test (collapse, exacerbation of existing heart disease, stroke, and heart attack itself) are such that a patient should insist on the presence of a physician to handle any emergency. For every 10,000 stress ECGs that are performed, at least 4 people have a heart attack—and 1 of them dies—while taking the test. Another study revealed that out of 4,100 people undergoing stress ECG testing, 16 had a heart block.

Pain/discomfort: There should be no pain or discomfort while a standard ECG is performed: some patients find it uncomfortable to lie still for prolonged periods of time. It is possible to have chest pain while undergoing a stress electrocardiogram.

Some people suffer severe skin irritation from the patches used to hold the electrodes on the skin, especially during Holter 24-hour monitoring; if you know you have sensitive skin, tell the doctor and he can prevent the problem.

Cost: A standard ECG, using the 12 standard leads, ranges from $15 to $100. This may or may not include an interpretation of the heart's graphic representations; there could be an additional $10 to $20 charge for "reading" the ECG. The stress ECG is $100 to $500, depending on the type of exercise and the length of time required to obtain satisfactory readings. A Holter monitoring test is $100 to $1,000, depending on the extent of activities measured during the recording period. If additional leads are applied to a patient (sometimes leads are placed on the neck and back for a more detailed ECG), there is often an additional charge of $25 to $50.

Accuracy and significance: When the ECG is used as a screening device to detect heart disease in patients without symptoms, it is only considered 75 percent accurate.

The standard ECG may also miss existing heart disease if the pathology exists in unusual areas of heart muscle or if the problem is related to the heart valves. For patients with obvious heart disease, the ECG is considered 90 percent accurate in locating the problem area. Thus far, the stress ECG is not considered sufficiently accurate to serve as a precise diagnostic technique. There have been a great many studies that show this test can be wrong more than half the time; it is particularly inaccurate when used on healthy people to screen for hidden heart disease. In one instance, the stress ECG test indicated heart disease existed when it really did not 70 percent of the time. The most recent evaluation of the stress test (1985) showed its accuracy rate ranged from only 16 to 21 percent. One indication of the stress test's significance can be deduced from the fact that less than one out of five doctors who prescribe the test will undergo it themselves prior to starting an exercise program. The Holter monitoring test is probably the most accurate ECG test, as it functions for a long enough period of time to reveal heart rhythm abnormalities that could be overlooked in the 10 to 15 minutes of a standard ECG.

Note: See also **Apexcardiogram; Ballistocardiogram; Circulation Time: Echocardiogram; Phonocardiogram; Pulse Analysis; Radiography; Systolic Time Intervals; Vectorcardiogram.**

ELECTROCOCHLEOGRAPHY, see *Hearing Function*

ELECTRODERMAL AUDIOMETRY, see *Hearing Function*

ELECTROENCEPHALOGRAM (EEG)

The electroencephalogram is a graphic recording of the minute electric current given off by brain cell activity. The current is amplified, translated into wavy lines (waves), and recorded on paper. The waves represent intermittent brain cell activity; the height of the waves as well as the distance between each peak depend on body activity (for example, blinking or opening and closing the eyes can create seemingly abnormal waves). The waves can also show hyperactive brain cell activity, as seen with epilepsy, and interference with brain cell activity, as seen with tumors.

From 10 to 24 electrodes are applied to the scalp in specific positions to aid in locating any abnormal lesion that might be reflected on the electroencephalograph. The patient lies quietly with eyes closed and no body movement. At times, the patient is told to breathe fast and deeply, as this seems to amplify EEG waves.

The waves of brain activity recorded on the electroencephalograph are classified by Greek letters (alpha, beta, etc.). The biofeedback machine is essentially an electroencephalograph constructed to detect only alpha waves.

A patient's brain waves may also be monitored continuously over a 24-hour period, using up to 16 electrodes over the scalp, by wearing a very small tape recorder. This test is of particular value in that it can replace the need for hospitalization in patients who report only an occasional seizure-type disorder, such as momentary blackouts. It is especially valuable in helping to detect any environmental provocative factors or determine whether the patient's routine activities are the cause of the convulsions. The cost can run from $100 to $1,000, depending on the number of electrodes employed and the type of equipment used. This test has also been applied to patients who complain of transient episodes of confusion or who have been observed to exhibit moments of peculiar behavior.

A newer application of the EEG is called computerized electroencephalogram mapping; this is another form of brain imaging that demonstrates the effect of certain drugs — such as producing sedation, dulling thought processes, enhancing recognition and thinking, or even increasing alertness. The effect drugs have on the recorded brain waves, along with associated positron emission transaxial tomography (see **Computerized Tomography**), not only affords a study of the drug's actions but also helps identify patients who will show dangerous side effects, such as drowsiness, that could interfere with their work and be dangerous to themselves and others.

Recently, the EEG has been used as a test to predict the health of premature infants, especially the babys' neurological health. It has been suggested that this test be performed routinely on all premature infants as a means of detecting brain problems.

When performed: Whenever any nervous system or brain disease is suspected; whenever there are brief episodes of unconsciousness or fainting; following head injury; whenever a patient has suffered a convulsion; when there are persistent episodes of narcolepsy (falling asleep in the midst of one's usual activities); when alcoholism is suspected.

Normal values: Alpha waves (with a frequency of 8 to 15 cycles per second) and beta waves (with a frequency of 16 to 30 cycles per second) are normally found in all individuals. The strength of the wave (the distance above and below the baseline) is also important in making a diagnosis.

Abnormal values: Theta waves (with a frequency of 4 to 8 cycles per second) may be found in some normal individuals, but they should not make up more than 10 percent of the overall recording. An excess of theta waves can indicate a brain tumor, brain damage following a head injury, epilepsy, or stroke.

Delta waves (with a frequency of less than 4 cycles per second) are indicative of a very serious condition (severe injury, brain abscess, brain tumor, or massive brain hemorrhage). Severe infection (encephalitis) can also cause delta waves.

Other wave patterns are specific for epilepsy; often, the type of epilepsy can be determined by the electroencephalograph. Specific brain wave values can indicate brain tissue atrophy secondary to alcoholism.

Risk factors: None.

Pain/discomfort: Some patients find the tiny needles that are pressed into the scalp quite uncomfortable; newer nonpenetrating electrodes are now available. Many patients find lying still for a prolonged period of time uncomfortable, and some find the necessity to be in an isolated and darkened room somewhat stressful.

Cost: From $50 to $135. When an EEG is performed throughout the night (certain pathology can be detected only while the patient sleeps), the fee can reach $600. If the test is performed in a hospital, there is often an additional hospital charge.

Accuracy and significance: The EEG is 95 percent accurate for the detection of epilepsy and a number of other brain activity disorders. It is considered of particular significance when the recording shows no abnormalities despite a patient's complaints. Some patients seem to have epilepsy but really do not; they have what is known as pseudoepilepsy. Patients suffering from hysteria, or who pretend to have epilepsy as a means of dependence or for whatever other reason, can manifest some of the symptoms of epilepsy (they may complain of losing consciousness or fainting), yet their brain wave pattern recorded by the EEG while they are pretending to show symptoms remains normal. This is how doctors differentiate pseudoepilepsy from actual epilepsy.

ELECTROKYMOGRAPHY, see *Radiography*

ELECTROLYTES, see *Bicarbonate; Chloride; Potassium; Sodium*

ELECTROMYOGRAPHY (EMG)

Electromyography is a diagnostic neurologic test to study the potential (electrically measured activity) of muscle at rest, the reaction of muscle to contraction, and the response of muscle to insertion of a needle. The test is an aid in ascertaining whether a patient's illness is directly affecting the spinal cord, muscles, or peripheral nerves.

The patient lies at rest while the peripheral nerves in various areas are stimulated through electrodes, and the electrical activity in muscles and nerves is recorded. In needle electromyography, a small needle is inserted into the muscle and the patient is observed for electrical activity in the muscle at rest, on insertion of the needle, and during muscle contraction. The test is sometimes employed as a measure of the muscle tension produced by nervous stress; usually, the muscles of the forehead are tested, since they can indicate relaxation or generalized body tension.

Electromyoneurography is the combined use of electromyography and neurography, which applies the procedures of electromyography to nerves instead of muscles. The two tests offer a more precise means of finding the exact location of nerve damage or disorder.

Dynomometry testing uses a dynomometer (most often a dial gauge attached to a spring mechanism that measures the strength of muscles) to ascertain certain physical abilities such as holding an object in the hand. It helps detect diseases of the nerves from the spinal cord to the muscle.

When performed: To aid in the diagnosis of diseases affecting the muscles, peripheral nerves, and spinal cord; to detect "hysterical" weakness and paralysis.

Normal values: Normally, when the muscle is at rest, no electrical activity is observed. When muscles contract, the electromyograph shows a smooth graphic wavelike representation of each contraction; the graph lines are amplified with the increase in strength of each contraction.

Abnormal values: Muscle disease produces a spiked wave pattern; the shape of the spike depends on the particular disease. Muscle weakness produces a diminished wave. With myasthenia gravis, the waves disappear after a few minutes. Nerve involvement, as opposed to muscle involvement, usually shows a decreased frequency of contractions.

Risk factors: Negligible. See general risk factors for catheter and needle insertion and electrical instruments.

Pain/discomfort: Needle insertion, usually performed without local anesthesia, can be quite uncomfortable and, at times, even painful.

Cost: From $100 to $300, depending on how many muscles or nerves are tested. If all extremities are tested, the fee can reach $500. When electromyoneurography is used, the total cost is $300 to $400.

Accuracy and significance: The test is considered 90 percent accurate; it is difficult for a malingerer to pretend to have muscle pathology when muscles respond to electrical stimulation.

ELECTROMYONEUROGRAPHY, see *Electromyography*

ELECTRONEUROGRAPHY, see *Electromyography*

ELECTRONIC FETAL MONITORING (EFM), see *Fetal Monitoring*

ELECTRONYSTAGMOGRAPHY, see *Caloric*

ELECTROPHORESIS, see *Albumin/Globulin*

ELECTROPHYSIOLOGIC (CARDIAC), see *Electrocardiogram*

ELEPHANTIASIS, see *Agglutination*

ELIMINATION DIET, see *Allergy*

ELISA, see *Agglutination*

ELLSWORTH-HOWARD, see *Parathyroid*

ELSBERG, see *Smell Function*

EMG, see *Electromyography*

EMMETROPIA, see *Visual Acuity*

ENCEPHALITIS, see *Complement Fixation*

ENDOMETRIAL SCREENING, see *Dilatation and Curettage*

ENDOSCOPIC BIOPSY, see *Biopsy*

ENDOSCOPIC ULTRASOUND, see *Ultrasound*

ENDOSCOPY

More than 100 years ago, a doctor put an open tube into the esophagus of a patient and, using the light from an oil lamp, was able to inspect the esophagus walls. This was the first instance of endoscopy—direct observation of a body organ or cavity. Since that time, the simple, open tubes have been replaced by far more intricate "scopes"; the latest, called fiberoptic endoscopes, can bend light rays so that the doctor can see around corners and obstacles and pinpoint the exact location of any pathology.

The endoscope is now used to examine the esophagus, the stomach, and even the intestines. The instrument is usually equipped not only to allow for observation but also to pump air into the cavity so as to extend the walls and make observation easier; to wash away anything that may obstruct the view (such as blood when looking for a bleeding ulcer); to suction out suspected material for **Cytology** tests; and to take a

Biopsy specimen for testing. For examination of the upper gastrointestinal tract, the patient usually swallows the tip of the instrument (after the throat has been sprayed with local anesthesia); the swallowed tip carries the narrow tubing along with it. Use of the proctosigmoidoscope in the rectum and large bowel is yet another form of endoscopy. Newer colonoscopes can reach as far as five feet into the lower intestinal tract.

At times, a direct incision is made in the skin and an endoscope is inserted to view the area beneath. When this is done in the portion of the chest just above the breastbone, it is called mediastinoscopy. This form of endoscopy enables the physician to view the bronchi from the outside, the large blood vessels as they enter and emerge from the heart, and the lymph nodes in the area (which are especially diagnostic when looking for certain tumors).

When the incision for an endoscope is made over the abdomen, it is called peritoneoscopy or laparoscopy. Direct examination of the abdominal cavity offers a unique way of testing the liver for size, growth, and clotting defects and for obtaining a tissue specimen. With abdominal endoscopy, it is also possible to see the gallbladder, pancreas, and spleen, along with the ovaries and outer surface of the uterus. A culdoscopy, which uses an endoscope inserted through the posterior vaginal wall, allows a doctor to view all the female reproductive organs (ovaries, tubes, and outside wall of the uterus). A colposcopy, on the other hand, uses a special endoscope fitted with magnifying lenses for a more extensive examination of the cervix and vagina. No incision is made when using a culposcope; in fact, this device rarely enters the body but stays just at the entrance to the vagina and allows the doctor to select suspicious areas for tissue sampling.

A similar type of instrument used to detect lung disease is called a bronchoscope; the bronchoscope is usually equipped with a whirling brush at the tip to pick up bronchial cells under a thick mucous layer for microscopic study. At times, a solution containing the same amount of salt as normal body fluids is instilled into the bronchi and used to wash out (lavage) each bronchus. The fluid is then suctioned back so that the cells it carries can be studied. Diseases such as sarcoidosis, berylliosis (beryllium poisoning), and lung reactions to inhaled organic dusts may be diagnosed this way. The test is called bronchoalveolar lavage.

Hysteroscopy is an endoscopic test that allows direct examination of the inside of the uterus. Cystoscopy refers to direct examination of the inside of the bladder; vaginoscopy offers a more detailed scrutiny of the vagina than can be obtained by the usual techniques. Recently, the endoscope has been adapted to look into joints; knee endoscopy, called arthroscopy, allows a specific test to evaluate meniscus cartilage or ligament tears of that joint. (Doctors can now perform corrective surgery on the knee through the endoscope.) In almost all instances, endoscopy is performed in conjunction with X-rays (see **Radiography**).

Fetoscopy allows an endoscope, called a fetoscope, to be inserted directly through the abdomen and uterus to observe the developing fetus directly. This process is usually performed during the 18th to 20th weeks of pregnancy. While fetoscopy carries with it the greatest risk to the developing infant, it can reveal defects undetectable by other means and can also be used to treat some of those defects prior to birth.

New, ultrathin fiberoptic scopes now allow vascular endoscopy called angioscopy, the direct examination of the inside of blood vessels (arteries and veins). This allows the positive diagnosis of emboli (blood clots that block off the passage of blood and oxygen to tissues).

When performed: When X-rays show suspected lesions in an area that can ultimately be viewed directly by an endoscope (such as bleeding stomach ulcer or liver abscess); when congenital malformations are suspected in various organs, especially the esophagus; when growths, abscesses, or inadequate functioning of an organ is suspected; whenever a biopsy is needed to confirm a diagnosis; when there is abdominal or chest pain that cannot be explained; following trauma when internal injuries are suspected.

Normal values: When an organ (or the surface or lining of an organ) is viewed directly, it should appear normal to the examining physician. Normal values are based primarily on extensive experience (only a trained eye can spot a pinpoint lesion or ulcer).

Abnormal values: Evidence of tumor, abscess, blocked or nonfunctioning ducts, infection, or hemorrhage is considered abnormal.

Risk factors: Generally, when endoscopes are inserted into normal body openings, the risks are minimal. However, there is a possibility of infection because of the difficulty in sterilizing an endoscope. Not only can infections be passed from one patient to another, but bacteria are apt to multiply on endoscopes even when they are not in use. If previously detected pathology is present, there is the slight risk that the endoscope might perforate, rupture, or tear and cause bleeding of the organ being examined. When endoscopes are inserted through a surgical incision, the above risks still apply, in addition to the routine risks of surgery (wound healing, wound herniation, and anesthesia). The more appliances (brushes, biopsy cups, crushing clamps) that are attached to, or manipualted through an endoscope, the greater the risks.

In 1985, it was reported that the greatest number of malpractice actions against gastroenterologists (specialists in esophageal, stomach, and intestinal diseases) were as a result of endoscopy procedures, especially those involving the esophagus. The second greatest cause of lawsuits against these doctors was the use of the sigmoidoscope (an endoscope that is inserted through the anus into the large intestine). Poking a hole through the bowel, hemorrhage, and even shock have occurred during the procedure. The injuries to the patients were attributed primarily to inexperience and carelessness on the part of the physicians.

Pain/discomfort: Most patients find endoscopy uncomfortable, even with local anesthesia. When surgery is part of endoscopy, there is often postoperative pain in addition to the aftereffects of anesthesia.

Cost: Simple endoscopy such as viewing the esophagus, stomach, rectum, sigmoid, or bronchi is $50 to $1,000, depending on the difficulty in reaching the area to be studied and the time involved. If specimens are removed for further testing, such as by biopsy or brushing, there may be an additional charge (if a polyp is removed, for example, there is usually an additional fee of $25 to $500). When hospital surgery is part of the endoscopy, there is often a charge of $100 to $500 for the operative procedure in addition to the anesthetist's fee and the hospital's room charges.

Accuracy and significance: Endoscopy is considered 95 percent accurate when properly performed, because of the opportunity to view the disease site directly. Most doctors consider endoscopy far more significant than radiography. It must be noted, however, that at the present time there are no standards applied to the performance of many forms of endoscopy (e.g.: colonoscopy); a physician may attempt an endoscopic procedure with little (no more than one-half day) or no formal training. Those experienced in such procedures feel it is "ridiculous" for a doctor to perform such a test without adequate, rigid, supervised experience and claim incompetence is the primary cause of inaccuracies.

ENTEROVIRUS, see *Virus Disease*

ENZYME-LINKED IMMUNOSORBENT ASSAY, see *Agglutination*

EOM, see *Strabismus*

EOSINOPHIL, see *Rast*

EOSINOPHIL COUNT, see *Blood Cell Differential*

EPIDEMIC HEPATITIS, see *Hepatitis*

EPILEPSY, see *Electroencephalogram; Manganese*

EPILEPSY DRUG, see *Drug Monitoring*

EPINEPHRINE, see *Catecholamines*

EPSTEIN-BARR VIRUS, see *Herpes; Mononucleosis*

e.p.t. PLUS, see *Pregnancy*

ER, see *Estrogen Receptor*

ERA, see *Hearing Function*

ERECTILE FAILURE, see *Impotence*

ERGONOVINE PROVOCATION, see *Electrocardiogram*

ERYTHROCYTE, see *Red Blood Cell*

ERYTHROCYTE HEMOLYSIS, see *Tocopherols*

ERYTHROCYTE INDICES, see *Red Blood Cell Indices*

ERYTHROCYTE SEDIMENTATION RATE, see *Sedimentation Rate*

ERYTHROCYTE-UNSATURATED FATTY ACID, see *Hot Bath*

ERYTHROPOIETIN, see *Cancer; Red Blood Cell*

ESOPHAGEAL INSUFFLATION, see *Gastroesophageal Reflux*

ESOPHAGEAL pH MONITORING, see *Gastroesophageal Reflux*

ESOPHAGEAL TRANSIT SCANNING, see *Nuclear Scanning*

ESOPHAGEAL X-RAY, see *Radiography*

ESOPHAGITIS, see *Gastroesophageal Reflux*

ESOPHAGOSCOPY, see *Endoscopy*

ESR, see *Sedimentation RateAppendix*

ESTROGEN (Estradiol, Estrone, Estriol)

Estrogens are really several different female hormones comprised of estradiol (the most potent), estrone, and estriol. All the estrogens are manufactured principally by the ovaries, but small amounts can come from the adrenal glands and even, in men, from the testicles, Usually, the total amount of estrogens is measured in the urine; individual components may also be tested. Estradiol can be measured in blood plasma taken from a vein. Estrogen production is controlled by the pituitary gland and responds not only to pregnancy and phases of the menstrual cycle but also to stress (anxiety) situations.

A relatively simple test to detect the presence of estrogen, especially when trying to determine the cause of anovulation (that is, failure to ovulate, which means failure to produce a monthly fertile egg that can be made pregnant) or the cause of unusual menstrual-type bleeding, is called the fern test. It is so named because the doctor, usually during a routine pelvic examination, takes a sample of the mucus from the cervix, puts it on a glass slide and, after it dries (within a few minutes), looks to see if it forms a pattern that resembles a fern leaf, as it will if estrogen is present. Normally, this fern pattern disappears during the last two weeks of the menstrual cycle.

Another test to reveal ovary problems is measuring follicle-stimulating hormone (FSH). This hormone from the pituitary gland (also see the discussion of luteinizing hormone [LH] in **Testis Function**) increases beyond expected normal values when a patient's ovaries become filled with cysts and in cases of precocious puberty, usually associated with adrenal disease (see **Cortisol**). In order to evaluate this test properly, the patient's last menstrual period days must be precisely known.

Both FSH and luteinizing hormone increase at menopause. And these hormones may also show an increase with other conditions that reflect a failure of the ovaries—and even the testicles—to function normally, such as infertility or sexual identification problems. A confirmatory test for menopause is the progestin challenge; here, the drug progestin is given for 10 days to see if it provokes menstrual bleeding. If bleeding does occur, a **Dilatation and Curettage** is usually performed before a definitive diagnosis of menopause is made.

Urine testing for pregnanediol, a progesterone metabolic product, will show increased amounts in girls with precocious puberty that may be due to adrenal tumors (see **Cortisol**) or ovary tumors. Progesterone is a female hormone that prepares the uterus for pregnancy; it, too, is sometimes measured in the blood, but this is a difficult and not-too-accurate test.

When performed: When little or no ovary function is suspected; when pituitary gland dysfunction is suspected; during pregnancy; when certain inherited sexual dysfunctions are under consideration; when a woman has excessive menstruation that cannot easily be explained; in cases of infertility.

Normal values: Nonpregnant women usually secrete from 10 to 60 mcg of total estrogen per 24-hour urine sample during the first two weeks of the menstrual cycle; this amount rises to about 100 mcg per 24 hours of urine during the last two weeks of the cycle. In pregnant women, 24-hour urinary estrogen may rise to 40,000 mcg. Children secrete less than 1 mcg per day. After menopause, 1 to 20 mcg per day is normal. Men normally secrete up to 20 mcg in a 24-hour urine sample.

The normal range of plasma estradiol varies with phases of the menstrual cycle. During the first 10 days, it averages 50 pg per ml; during the last 20 days, it averages 125 pg per ml. Men normally average 20 pg per ml at all times.

Abnormal values: Elevated urinary estrogen levels can result from ovarian tumors, excessive pituitary activity (which can also come from hypothalamic pathology), adrenal hyperactivity, liver disease, and certain inherited chromosomal abnormalities. A decreased amount of estrogens can be found when a patient takes female hormones (which stop body manufacture of estrogens), with problems during pregnancy, with decreased pituitary activity, and with ovarian failure. Severe dieting lowers estrogen levels. Women runners, and other women athletes in training or performing vigorous exercises, may also have reduced estrogen levels.

Usually, when abnormal values of estrogens are discovered, specific tests for the various components of estrogen are performed to ascertain the cause. (When a patient takes diethylstilbestrol, for example, the estriol portion of estrogen decreases.) Recently, estrogen measurements have also been taken in men; an elevated level (especially of plasma estradiol) with reduced testosterone (see Testis Function) seems to be a risk factor in heart disease.

Risk factors: Negligible (see general risk factors for blood testing).

Pain/discomfort: Minimal (see general pain/discomfort factors for blood testing).

Cost: A total estrogen evaluation ranges from $30 to $45. An evaluation of the individual components is $25 to $60 per component. FSH tests average $20.

Accuracy and significance: Estrogen testing, particularly when the various components are measured, is considered 90 percent accurate in evaluating ovary function. It is also a significant test in aiding in the diagnosis of sexual dysfunction and infertility.

ESTROGEN RECEPTOR (ER)

Some cancers of the breast, uterus, ovary, skin, lymph nodes, and stomach "respond" to and can be treated by certain hormones. It is of great advantage to know which cancers will react to hormone therapy. Two out of three cancer tissues that will absorb estrogens (and an even higher ratio of tissues that also absorb progesterones—progesterone receptor) can be treated by various forms of hormonal manipulation and antiestrogen drugs in place of surgery. The estrogen receptor test measures the response of a tumor to estrogen stimulation.

In the estrogen receptor test, a tiny specimen of body tissue (see **Biopsy**), usually breast, is studied to see how responsive it is to estrogens—how it reacts (grows or diminishes) to the hormone's activity in the body. This test is a particular measure of whether a tumor is hormone-sensitive and thus whether it would be of value to have the patient's adrenals or pituitary gland removed (or destroyed by radiation) as part of therapy.

Another evaluation of breast tumors consists of testing for placental protein; when present, it seems to indicate that the tumor will recur within a few years. The protein is called pregnancy-associated plasma protein-A (PAPP-A); when not found, recurrences of breast tumors were minimal. The test is especially valuable in helping decide which form of therapy should be used, and to what extent.

The most recent receptor test as a guide to the best form of breast cancer therapy is measuring the effect of androgens (male hormones). When combined with the estrogen receptor test, it can offer an even better indication of how treatment will work.

Other cancer growths may also be tested for susceptibility to chemotherapy by exposing small bits of the tumor to the drug or drugs. This is called the human tumor stem cell assay.

When performed: To ascertain if a cancer can be treated with hormones; when a patient has a metastatic (spreading throughout the body) cancer whose source cannot be located but the cancer itself can be biopsied to indicate if it is treatable by drugs; to show which cancer patients will not benefit from certain surgical procedures such as removal of the pituitary gland or adrenal glands; to indicate which cancer patients might benefit from chemotherapy.

Normal values: There are no normal values for this test; when more than 3 femtomoles of the protein estrogen receptor are found in a cancer, it is considered positive, or hormone-receptive.

Abnormal values: A negative response, or failure of the tissue to indicate the presence of estrogen receptors, usually means that hormone treatment will not work and that chemotherapy should be tried.

Risk factors: As with any biopsy, there is the slight possibility of hemorrhage and/or infection.

Pain/discomfort: Minimal, as a local anesthetic is commonly used.

Cost: The estrogen receptor test is $100 to $150. When the progesterone receptor test is done simultaneously, the cost is $125 to $160. There is usually a doctor's fee of $25 to $100 to obtain the specimen for testing.

Accuracy and significance: The test is approximately 60 percent accurate in predicting which breast cancers will respond to hormone therapy (only about one out of three breast cancers respond to hormones). Should the progesterone test be positive, the accuracy rate increases to 80 percent. There is, however, the rare patient who has a negative estrogen receptor test yet still responds to hormone therapy.

ETHANOL, see *Alcohol*

ETHYL ALCOHOL, see *Alcohol*

ETHYLENE GLYCOL, see *Methanol*

E-UFA, see *Hot Bath*

EVOKED RESPONSE AUDIOMETRY (ERA), see *Hearing Function*

EXCISIONAL BIOPSY, see *Biopsy*

EXCLUSION OF PARENTHOOD, see *Disputed Parentage*

EXCRETORY UROGRAPHY, see *Radiography*

EXERCISE CARDIOGRAM, see *Electrocardiogram*

EXOPHTHALMOMETER

The exophthalmometer measures the exact amount of eyeball protrusion, called exophthalmos. Most often, "bulging" eyeballs (an excess of the white part of the eye showing) occur in patients with hyperthyroidism. But other diseases can also cause either one or both eyes to protrude. The exophthalmometer (an instrument similar to the device used to measure pupil distance when fitting eyeglasses) is placed in front of the eyes, and the amount of protrusion is measured for each eye.

When performed: When thyroid disease is suspected; when sinus disease, cancer, brain disease, eye infection, or various blood and blood vessel diseases are suspected; when glaucoma is suspected but not found.

Normal values: Eyeball protrusion should not exceed 15 mm.

Abnormal values: Protrusion greater than 16 mm is considered abnormal, especially when one eye protrudes more than the other. Once thyroid disease is eliminated from the diagnosis, special examinations such as X-rays (see **Radiography**), blood tests, and tests for infection are employed. Patients with severe nearsightedness or retraction of the eyelids (either naturally or as a consequence of cosmetic surgery) may appear to have protruding eyes, but this is not an indication of disease.

Risk factors: None.

Pain/discomfort: None.

Cost: There is usually no fee for this test when it is part of a routine examination.

Accuracy and significance: The test does not specifically contribute to any diagnosis; it is more a means to record the amount of eyeball protrusion. It has no accuracy rating.

EXTERNAL OCULAR MUSCLE, see *Strabismus*

EYE, see *Visual Acuity*

EYE SONOGRAM, see *Ultrasound*

EZ-DETECT, see *Occult Blood*

F

FA, see *Agglutination*

FACIAL RECOGNITION

Testing for the ability to differentiate between pictures of unfamiliar faces (and to remember the characteristics of such faces) has been found to be a fairly reliable way to distinguish organic (physical) brain disease from problems of a psychological nature. Patients with real brain pathology cannot discriminate between different unfamiliar faces and have great difficulty remembering an unfamiliar face they have seen several minutes earlier. Patients who pretend to have certain diseases and those with neurotic problems tend to remember faces in such a test and can repeatedly tell one from another. Patients are shown frontal and profile views of unfamiliar faces (photographed under varying light conditions) and are asked to remember them so as to identify other pictures that are of the same person. (Also see **Cognitive Capacity Screening.**)

When performed: To help differentiate between neurological and psychological conditions, especially when brain disease is suspected.

Normal values: Normal test scores range from 36 to 54 (a perfect score).

Abnormal values: A definite abnormal score is 35 or less and usually indicates physical brain damage. Patients with schizophrenia usually have normal scores.

Risk factors: None.

Pain/discomfort: None.

Cost: There is usually no fee for this test when it is part of a routine examination performed in a doctor's office. The fee is approximately $25 when the test is done by a psychologist.

Accuracy and significance: The test is considered 75 percent accurate in helping to distinguish between real brain disease and psychiatric disorders. It is particularly significant in helping to differentiate among physical injury, conversion hysteria, and malingering.

FACT, see *Pregnancy*

FACTOR I (INCLUDING FACTORS II, V, VII, VIII, IX, X, XI, XII, AND XIII), see *Fibrinogen; Partial Thromboplastin Time*

FARSIGHTEDNESS, see *Visual Acuity*

FASTING BLOOD SUGAR, see *Glucose*

FAT CELL SIZE, see *Anthropometric Measurements*

FDP, see *Fibrin Degradation Products*

FEBRILE AGGLUTINATION, see *Agglutination*

FECES EXAMINATION

The average adult excretes approximately 100 to 300 g (3 to 10 ounces) of fecal matter per day, of which about 70 percent may be water. The feces (stool) can offer valuable diagnostic clues to diseases of the bowel, the blood, and the metabolic system, and especially to infectious processes that cannot be diagnosed.

Many tests can be performed on the feces. The usual examination consists of noting the color and the presence or absence of blood and mucus, and then making a microscopic search for parasites (worms, amoeba) and their eggs (ova) and a culture for bacteria. On occasion, the amount of fat is measured after a patient is given a high-fat diet for three days. Patients should not brush their teeth or eat meat for three days prior to the test, since any traces of blood from the gums or from rare meat in the feces can cause a false-positive reaction (see **Occult Blood**).

The Scotch tape test is used to find worms that come out of the bowel at night (particularly pinworms). A piece of Scotch tape is wrapped around a pencil, sticky side out, and touched to the anal area after the body has been warmed, usually under a blanket. The tape is then placed on a glass slide and examined under the microscope.

The **String** test, **Agglutination,** and **Complement Fixation** are also tests to help diagnose parasitic disease. (See **Parasite.**)

The most recent feces examination test is measuring the amount of radioactivity given off after the patient eats a special meal containing a radioactive substance. This is almost always performed with the bile acid breath scan (see **Nuclear Scanning**) as a means of confirming suspected malabsorption (see **Xylose Tolerance**).

When performed: As a routine or screening test to detect unsuspected (very early stage) gastrointestinal disease; in an undiagnosed infection (diarrhea); when there is an undiagnosed metabolic difficulty (weight loss); as a verification of gallbladder disease.

Normal values: The normal color of feces (although a great deal depends on diet) ranges from light to dark brown. Microscopic examination should show a predominance of partly digested foods and only a rare blood cell or shred of mucus. Less than 25 percent of the feces' dry weight should be fat. No parasites or their eggs should be present.

Abnormal values: When there is gallbladder or liver disease, the feces acquire a gray to gray-white color. If there is bleeding high up in the bowel (from the esophagus to the small intestine), the feces have a black, tarry appearance; if the bleeding is near the rectum, red blood may be seen. Yellow-colored feces are seen with certain digestive diseases, especially of the pancreas (sprue). Following a bout of food poisoning, the feces may acquire a greenish hue. Beets can color the stool red. Silver-colored feces, sometimes described as "stainless steel," suggest cancer in or near the pancreas.

Any amount of blood (even occult—that is, not visible but measurable) in the feces is abnormal. Its presence indicates bleeding somewhere in the gastrointestinal system and can mean cancer, infection, anemia, or injury to the bowel.

It is abnormal for more than 25 percent of the solid part of the stool sample to be fat. Increased amounts of fat in the feces are seen with pancreatic disease, biliary tract obstruction, and problems of intestinal absorption.

An increased amount of mucus is seen in many gastrointestinal conditions, especially infection, dysentery, colitis, fistula, and pancreatic disease.

Microscopic examination of the stool sample can show a specific parasite or its egg that may be causing unknown fever, weight loss, and unusual fatigue. Worm infestation can cause asthmatic symptoms.

Risk factors: None.

Pain/discomfort: None. Some people find it disturbing to collect a stool specimen.

Cost: The majority of doctors do not charge for **Occult Blood** examination of feces. If a laboratory performs the test, the fee ranges from $3 to $20. Ova and parasite examinations are $10 to $50; fat measurements, $5 to $30; culture tests for bacteria, $10 to $30. Special tests for tapeworms requiring a collection of feces over a 24-hour period are approximately $30. The Scotch tape test is $6 to $10; the patient usually applies the Scotch tape to the glass slide during the night.

Accuracy and significance: When properly performed, most feces tests are 80 to 90 percent accurate. Parasites can be missed by a careless technician. Any abnormal finding in feces is considered significant.

Note: A new test has been devised to help diagnose a form of colitis due to the use of antibiotics; it is called clostridial toxin and reflects the pathological effect of what is usually a safe bacteria normally found in the intestine called *Clostridium difficile.* Since this disease can be fatal, the finding of the toxin can lead to proper therapy.

FECES RADIOACTIVITY, see *Feces Examination;* "Bile Acid Breath Scan," in *Nuclear Scanning*

FEMALE HORMONE, see *Estrogen*

FEMALE-MALE IDENTITY, see *Chromosome Analysis*

FEMINIZING, see *Cortisol*

FERN, see *Estrogen*

FERRIC CHLORIDE, see *Phenylketonuria*

FERRITIN, see *Iron*

FERTILITY, see *Body Temperature, Estrogens, Rubin, Semen, Testis Function*

FETAL ALPHA GLOBULIN, see *Alpha Fetoprotein*

FETAL HEART DISEASE, see *Ultrasound*

FETAL HEART RATE ACCELERATION, see *Nonstress Fetal Assessment*

FETAL HEMOGLOBIN, see *Hemoglobin*

FETAL LUNG MATURITY, see *Pregnancy*

FETAL MATURITY, see *Pregnancy*

FETAL MONITORING

The use of electronic fetal monitoring (EFM)—originally intended to be limited to high-risk pregnancies (see **Nonstress Fetal Assessment**) and cases where there is a question as to the maturity of the fetus, where amniotic fluid does not appear normal, or where certain drugs are being used—has increased significantly, so that it is now estimated that at least 70 percent of all pregnant women in, or about to enter, labor are so tested. Despite the fact that there has been much criticism as to the need for such testing on an almost routine basis, proponents point out that as its use has increased, the deaths and disabilities related to labor have decreased. In essence, EFM enables the fetal heartbeat to be continuously assessed—either directly, with an electrode placed on the fetus while it is still in the uterus (through the vaginal and cervical canals), or indirectly through the mother, with the electrodes being placed on the abdominal skin over the uterus. At the same time, the test instrument also keeps track of the mother's uterine contractions and their effect on the fetal heartbeat. A slowing of the heart rate of the fetus has always been considered a primary sign of fetal distress, but until the advent of EFM, it had been difficult to follow the fetal heartbeat continuously. In most instances, the electronic monitor and its attachments (usually two small pads in a belt around the mother's abdomen) are applied when the mother begins labor; there may be some situations where the electrodes are put in place prior to labor, depending on the doctor's and nurse's observations. The internal electrodes, when used, are put in place after the membranes around the fetus rupture and amniotic fluid starts to flow. The difference between this test, sometimes called cardiotocography, and the nonstress fetal assessment test (NST)—although both measure the fetal heart rate—is that EFM is primarily to prevent problems during labor, while NST attempts to detect and treat pregnancy problems prior to labor.

When performed: Primarily where a problem is suspected with the fetus just prior to or during labor; to prevent conditions suspected of coming from a decreased oxygen supply to the fetus—especially when caused by uterine contractions (e.g., cerebral palsy; mental retardation; lung, kidney, and nerve damage). More recently, it is being performed almost routinely on all pregnant women when labor starts; it is considered more accurate than the usual sporadic nursing observations. Many doctors feel that its regular use can prevent a low-risk pregnancy from becoming a high-risk one.

Normal values: There should be no slowing of the fetal heart rate, with or without the effect of the contractions of the mother's uterus.

Abnormal values: Any indication that the heart rate of the fetus is slowing or irregular.

Risk factors: When external monitoring is used, the risk factors from the equipment are minimal. With internal monitoring—at times, the only way to detect the fetal heartbeat accurately—there is the risk of infection to both mother and infant, injury to tissues and organs adjacent to the instruments, and bleeding. Some doctors count among the risks the fact that as EFM is more frequently utilized, there has been a corresponding increase in the cesarean section method of childbirth.

Pain/discomfort: With external monitoring, none; some women do feel great anxiety when the electrodes are applied. With internal monitoring, there is normally little pain or discomfort due to the usual discomforts of being in labor, which tend to override the feel of the electrodes.

Cost: On the average, EFM will add about $63 to the total hospital bill.

Accuracy and significance: Obviously, internal monitoring is far more accurate than external; however, it is claimed that both methods are 70 to 80 percent accurate and have markedly lowered the rate of stillbirths and disabilities resulting from oxygen deficiency. At times, blood is taken for **pH** testing to corroborate fetal distress; this increases the overall accuracy of EFM. Again, a significant consequence of the test is the increased incidence of childbirth by cesarean section, considered by some to be an added risk factor.

Electronic fetal monitoring is only as effective as the people who observe the findings. In a recent case of fetal monitoring in a hospital, the doctor present did not know how to read the fetal monitor, and although the monitor showed evidence of fetal distress, the doctor sent the pregnant woman home; she later delivered a brain-damaged child.

FETOSCOPY, see *Endoscopy*

FEVER BLISTER, see *Herpes*

FHRAT, see *Nonstress Fetal Assessment*

FIBRIN (FIBRINOGEN) DEGRADATION PRODUCTS (FDP)

Fibrinogen is one of many proteins made by the liver that allow the blood to clot. Most blood-clotting tests are designed to determine why blood does not coagulate. The fibrin degradation products test, on the other hand, evaluates blood when it clots too much and, in fact, will not unclot, the result of which is usually a thrombosis, such as in a leg vein, or extensive small clotting of arteries throughout the body. It is believed that normal blood fibrinogen turns into separate fibrin particles, which help in the clotting process. Once blood starts to clot, the body attempts to control the degree of clotting by activating an enzyme that serves as a monitor. However, should clotting continue uncontrolled, fibrin degradation products are formed, and it is these that can be measured in blood taken from a vein, or in the urine.

When performed: When a patient has thrombosis, thrombophlebitis (an infected thrombosis), or symptoms or signs of a pulmonary embolus (a blood clot that usually travels from the leg to the lung); during unusual complications of pregnancy; after blood transfusions; in cases of shock; with kidney disease, and especially following a kidney transplant.

Normal values: Less than 10 mcg per ml.

Abnormal values: Greater than 10 mcg per ml; usually, from 40 to 50 mcg per ml; may rise to 100 mcg per ml in instances of extensive and severe clotting.

Risk factors: Negligible (see general risk factors for blood testing).

Pain/discomfort: Minimal (see general pain/discomfort factors for blood testing).

Cost: From $15 to $25; the lower fee usually represents tests simply to determine the presence or absence of FDP; the higher fee represents precise measurements of the amount of fibrin degradation products.

Accuracy and significance: Although the test is used too infrequently to have undergone an accuracy evaluation, it is considered valuable enough to use with patients whose clotting problems are not readily diagnosed, and especially when complications of pregnancy are involved. Some techniques are not as sensitive as others, and the most accurate of the tests is the most difficult to perform.

FIBRINOGEN

Fibrinogen (factor I), a plasma protein manufactured in the liver, is one of the 12 known primary factors essential to the clotting of blood. After a patient suffers an injury that causes bleeding, thromboplastin is given off by damaged tissues and combines with prothrombin and calcium in the body to form thrombin. The thrombin then combines with fibrinogen to make the fibrous substance that allows clot formation. Inability to form fibrinogen may be inherited or acquired from disease. Blood is taken from a vein, and the plasma is tested.

Fibrinogen is but one of the many coagulation factors that can now be tested for individually or as part of an overall assay in clotting disorders. Prothrombin (factor II; see **Prothrombin Time**) and thromboplastin (factor IX: see **Partial Thromboplastin Time**) are described in more detail in separate entries. Other coagulation factors tested for include: the labile factor (factor V); the stabile factor (factor VII); the antihemophiliac, or hemophilia A, factor (factor VIII); the Stuart factor (factor X); the plasma thromboplastin antecedent (factor XI); the Hageman factor (factor XII); and the fibrin stabilizing factor (factor XIII; see **Fibrin Degradation Products**). There is no factor VI; thus, there are only 12 factors in spite of the 13 roman numerals used to designate them. In most instances, these tests are used to help diagnose congenital deficiencies that cause clotting problems, but they are, at times, used to uncover liver diseases, vitamin K deficiencies, and a few rare diseases.

Plasminogen activity assay is a more recent means of testing for the blood's clotting ability; decreased activity is found with certain inherited conditions, severe liver disease, and after surgery or following the use of drugs either to treat excessive clotting (thrombosis) or to treat certain cancers. It has also been used to test for the effect of oral contraceptive pills on blood clotting; these drugs, along with estrogens and some steroid medications, tend to make blood clot more easily—which can be dangerous.

When performed: When a coagulation defect (inability of the blood to clot) is suspected; with excessive unexplained black-and-blue areas or mucous membrane bleeding.

Normal values: Normal fibrinogen levels range from 200 to 500 mg per 100 ml, or 0.2 to 0.5 g per 100 ml.

Abnormal values: Deficiency of fibrinogen (hypofibrinogenemia) may be congenital as well as acquired from liver disease, vitamin B deficiency, and certain bone cancers. Fibrinogen levels may be elevated in nephrosis and multiple myeloma. In pregnancy and in certain severe infections, the levels are slightly higher than normal.

Risk factors: Negligible (see general risk factors for blood testing).

Pain/discomfort: Minimal (see general pain/discomfort factors for blood testing).

Cost: From $10 to $20. Other coagulation factor tests can cost from $20 to $200.

Accuracy and significance: Because abnormal fibrinogen values appear in a variety of conditions, the test is only significant when determining the cause of coagulation problems. In general, factor testing is from 60 to 90 percent accurate.

FIBRIN STABILIZING FACTOR, see *Fibrinogen*

FIELD OF VISION, see *Visual Field*

FILARIASIS, see *Agglutination*

FINE-NEEDLE BIOPSY, see *Biopsy*

FINGER WRINKLE

The autonomic nervous system operates automatically, or without any conscious or willful control. It is composed of two opposing systems: the sympathetic, with more of an excitatory nature, and the parasympathetic, with its antagonistic, or slowing down, actions. Together, the two systems control the heart rate (pulse); blood pressure; rate of breathing; constriction and relaxation of the bronchial tubes; size of the pupils; digestion in, and evacuation of, the gastrointestinal tract; urination; sweating; salivation; the tears of crying; stuffiness in the nose; some physical reactions to sexual stimulation; wrinkling of the skin in water; and even such prosaic activities as yawning. One part of the system, the sympathetic nervous system, causes adrenalin and similar substances to be produced. The functioning of the sympathetic nerves is tested by placing the patient's hands in warm water for at least half an hour and noticing if the skin of the fingers wrinkles after the soaking.

Some other tests used to evaluate the autonomic nervous system include: amyl nitrate inhalation, where the same drug used to treat angina is inhaled to see if it will lower the blood pressure (as it should); the injection of phenylephrine (a drug for treating allergies and similar to those used to curb the appetite) to see if it will raise the blood pressure (as it should); and the injection of atropine, as a test of the parasympathetic system, to cause an increase in the heart rate (which it should).

When performed: When there is suspicion of Raynaud's disease (blockage of artery circulation, usually in the extremities), diabetes, or Guillain-Barré disease (pathology of the nerves).

Normal values: The skin of the fingers will normally wrinkle after being soaked in water.

Abnormal values: With diseases of the sympathetic nervous system, the skin does not wrinkle after soaking. After a sympathectomy (a surgical procedure to sever the sympathetic nerves, usually performed in patients with poor circulation), the skin will not wrinkle on the operated side.

Risk factors: None.

Pain/discomfort: None.

Cost: There is usually no charge when the tests are part of a regular physical examination.

Accuracy and significance: The test serves as a screening technique leading to more specific diagnostic procedures. As such, it is considered to be 70 percent accurate.

FISHBERG, see *Mosenthal*

5-HIAA, see *Serotonin*

5-NUCLEOTIDE PHOSPHODIESTERASE, see *Cancer*

FLOCCULATION, see *Agglutination*

FLOW MICROFLUOROMETRY, see *Lymphocyte Typing*

FLOW-VOLUME CURVE, see *Pulmonary Function*

FLU, see *Virus Disease*

FLUORESCEIN DILAURATE TUBELESS INDICATOR, see *Pancreas Function*

FLUORESCEIN EYE STAIN

Fluorescein, an orange-colored dye, is used in testing for abnormalities of the cornea (the surface over the pupil and lens of the eye). The dye is dropped onto the eye and allowed to spread over the surface. Sometimes, individual sterile strips of paper containing the dye are used instead of liquid fluorescein to avoid the possibility of bacterial growth in the bottled solution. The dye will lodge in any irregularities on the cornea; the rest will wash away with tears. When ultraviolet or "black" light is then directed on the eye, the fluorescein will glow green and so indicate any abnormalities such as scratches, ulcers, foreign bodies (even as small as an eyelash hair), and various infectious diseases that can cause physical damage to the corneal surface.

Most eye injuries and other problems can be observed directly by the physician when the ultraviolet light is directed on the eye; in addition, a biomicroscope or "slit lamp" may be used to obtain a greatly magnified view of the eye surface. The biomicroscope is also used for more detailed examination of the structures of the eye.

At times, the gonioscope (a special instrument to examine the surface of the eye) is used, with or without fluorescein eye stain.

Another test using the fluorescein eye dye can reveal whether the nasolacrimal, or tear, duct is blocked. This duct has its opening in the inner corner of the eye and carries tears to the back of the nose and throat. When it becomes blocked, the eye tears constantly; but because there can be other causes of watery eyes, this test is used to help diagnose the problem. The dye is inserted in the eye, and then the nose and back of the throat are examined with an ultraviolet light in a darkened room. If a green glow is seen, the tear duct is open, and a different cause must be searched for to explain the excessive tearing.

The fluorescein string test is another use of the dye. Here, the patient swallows a string (see **String** test), and when the string reaches that part of the gastrointestinal tract being studied, the fluorescein dye is injected into a vein. After a period of time, the string is removed and examined for traces of the stain; when present, it usually indicates bleeding at that point in the intestine; the distance is measured on the string from the tooth line. Although this test is still in use, it is not considered very accurate. (See "Abdominal Scan," in **Nuclear Scanning**.)

When performed: Whenever any injury to or infection of the eye is suspected, especially when a superficial examination shows no evidence of trauma; during and after the fitting of contact lenses to make sure that tears pass normally under each lens; before applying cortisone to the eye.

Normal values: If there is no break in the surface of the cornea from either disease or injury, the fluorescein stain will wash out with tears and will reflect no damage when subjected to ultraviolet light.

Abnormal values: Any break in the smooth corneal surface will show a greenish fluorescence when viewed under ultraviolet light. From the size, shape, and location of the dye, the physician can usually make a specific diagnosis.

Risk factors: None.

Pain/discomfort: Should the fluorescein stain touch the skin surface around the eye, it might leave a slight discoloration, which is temporary.

Cost: There is usually no charge for application of the stain when it is part of a routine eye examination.

Accuracy and significance: The test is 95 percent accurate in detecting the smallest of eye surface injuries and is particularly valuable in the fitting of contact lenses.

FLUORESCEIN STRING, see *Fluorescein Eye Stain*

FLUORESCENT ANTIBODY, see *Agglutination*

FLUORESCENT TREPONEMAL ANTIBODY, see *Syphilis*

FLUORIDE, see *Mercury*

FLUOROSCOPY, see *Radiography*

FOAM STABILITY INDEX, see *Pregnancy*

FOLATES (Folic Acid)

Folates, of which folic acid is but one version, are essential to prevent anemia. Large amounts are found in beef, green vegetables, liver, nuts, oranges, and yeast. They become reduced primarily from an inadequate diet but also from alcoholism and certain drugs such as birth control pills. The body stores of folic acid last for only a month or two, and folate deficiency can often be diagnosed before anemia is apparent. Blood is drawn from a vein, and the serum is examined.

When performed: When folic acid deficiency, especially in pregnancy, or megaloblastic anemia (abnormally large but undeveloped red blood cells) is suspected; when the tongue is smooth and enlarged.

Normal values: Normal folic acid levels range from 5 to 25 ng per ml of serum.

Abnormal values: Decreased folic acid levels in the serum are found in malnutrition, pregnancy, anemia, alcoholism, and intestinal diseases characterized by malabsorption of folic acid (such as celiac disease and sprue).

Risk factors: Negligible (see general risk factors for blood testing).

Pain/discomfort: Minimal (see general pain/discomfort factors for blood testing).

Cost: From $20 to $30 for blood serum measurements. On rare occasions, the amount of folates is measured in red blood cells; the charge ranges from $25 to $100.

Accuracy and significance: Blood serum folate measurements are 80 percent accurate; however, when there is doubt in relation to clinical findings, folate measurements of red blood cells usually resolve the question. The test is significant in distinguishing the difference between folic acid and vitamin B_{12} deficiency. If anemia is treated without determining this difference, damage to the nerves can occur.

FOLIC ACID, see *Folates*

FOLLICLE-STIMULATING HORMONE, see *Estrogen*

FOOD-COLORING ALLERGY, see *Tartrazine Sensitivity*

FORCED EXPIRATORY VOLUME see *Pulmonary Function*

FORCED VITAL CAPACITY, see *Pulmonary Function*

FORSSMAN ANTIBODY, see *Mononucleosis*

FRANKLINIC, see *Taste Function*

FREE FATTY ACIDS, see *Lipids*

FREE TESTOSTERONE, see *Testis Function*

FREE THYROXINE, see *Thyroid Function*

FREI

A test to diagnose lymphogranuloma venereum, a sexually transmitted disease also know as lymphogranuloma inguinale or bubo, because its most obvious sign is the large, painful lymph node swelling (a bubo) in the inguinal or groin area. It is caused by a microorganism of the chlamydia group (which can also cause trachoma; psittacosis, or parrot fever; newborn pneumonia; and nongonococcal urethritis, which mimics gonorrhea). Although certain chlamydial infections are epidemic in the United States, until very recently, they have been overlooked and hence improperly or inadequately treated. (See also **Chlamydia Identification**.)

The Frei test is performed by injecting a minute amount of killed chlamydia antigen serum just under the surface of the skin, most often on the inside of the forearm, at the same time a like amount of control serum (without the antigen) is injected in the opposite arm. The results are observed after 48 hours.

When performed: When enlarged, swollen glands that cannot be diagnosed appear in the groin or in the axilla (under the armpits). In men with an undiagnosed discharge from the penis and in women with an unexplained discharge from the cervix. Although lymphogranuloma venereum is found primarily in tropical and subtropical countries, it is being seen increasingly in the United States.

Normal values: Neither injection site should show any redness or swelling after the 48-hour period. A normal value may be obscured if the patient is allergic to the diluent serum.

Abnormal values: Any redness or swelling greater than one-quarter inch in size (a control reaction, if present, should be less than the Frei test site and always smaller than one-quarter inch).

Risk factors: There is the possibility of an allergic reaction, especially in patients with other allergies.

Pain/discomfort: Minimal when the needles are inserted into the skin, as they penetrate just under the surface. There can be pain if a positive reaction produces a large swelling.

Cost: About $10, in addition to the doctor's fee for two office visits. Some doctors consider this test outmoded, and it is possible that a health insurance company or government-sponsored medical program will not reimburse the doctor or patient for the cost of the test.

Accuracy and significance: About 50 percent accurate. Most often, the test does not indicate the disease until the patient has had the infection for two to three weeks. Approximately one test in five shows a false-negative response, so it should always be repeated two weeks later. Once a patient has a positive test, it remains positive for life, even after successful treatment. The **Complement Fixation** test is considered more accurate.

FRIEDMAN, see *Pregnancy*

FTA-ABS, see *Syphilis*

FUNCTIONAL RESIDUAL CAPACITY, see *Pulmonary Function*

FUNDOSCOPY

The fundus, or back part of the eyeball, is examined by using an ophthalmoscope. The primary area examined is the retina (which receives images and transmits them to the brain); this is also the only area of the body where blood vessels (small arteries and veins) can be seen directly. The optic disc—the point where the optic nerve enters the brain from the eye—is also examined; the appearance of the edge or margin of this small, circular area is important in the diagnosis of many different diseases. Usually, a tiny beam of light is projected through the pupil onto the back of the eyeball; the area is viewed through a variety of ophthalmoscopic lenses to focus upon the particular object being studied (blood vessel, retina, nerve).

When performed: Usually part of any routine physical examination by a physician as well as any eye exam by an ophthalmologist; when eye disease such as glaucoma is suspected; whenever diabetes, atherosclerosis (artery disease), or hypertension is suspected; when brain lesion or brain disease is considered; following head injury; to corroborate certain infections and malignancies.

Normal values: The optic disc, the retina, and the blood vessels should appear normal to the doctor. Specific terms are used to indicate the presence or absence of disease (such as stages of high blood pressure, diabetes, or the protrusion of the optic disk).

Abnormal values: Abnormal values depend on the degree of disease observed through the ophthalmoscope and are usually rated from I to V, depending on severity.

Risk factors: None.

Pain/discomfort: None.

Cost: There is usually no charge, as fundoscopy is part of every physical or vision examination.

Accuracy and significance: This is one of the most valuable tests a patient undergoes. It is extremely significant, for it can reveal the first signs of heart and blood vessel disease (especially high blood pressure), brain disease, diabetes, and of course, specific eye conditions. Considered to be 90 to 95 percent accurate, but much depends on the experience and ability of the examining doctor to perceive and interpret the normal from the abnormal signs.

FUNGUS

Diseases caused by fungi (molds and yeasts) are called mycotic. They can cause localized problems such as the tiny, itching white patches that sometimes appear in the mouth, throat, or vagina; or they can be the basis for extremely serious, sometimes fatal, systemic body infections such as coccidioidomycosis and cryptococcosis, histoplasmosis, aspergillosis (an allergic-type chest infection often confused with asthma), and blastomycosis (a fungus disease of the skin, bones, and urinary system). Candidiasis is a common fungus infection of moist areas of the body such as the mouth and throat (it may be called thrush) and vagina, although it can occur on the skin—especially between the fingers and toes. Ringworm is a fungus disease; common forms include athlete's foot and, when in the groin, "jock itch."

The easiest way to test for a fungus is to take a scraping, smear, or **Biopsy** from the affected area and examine the specimen under the microscope; each fungus has a characteristic appearance. All take on a blue color when studied with the **Gram Stain** test. Some of the ringworm fungi will fluoresce (give off a greenish or brownish glow) when examined with Wood's light (ultraviolet rays), especially those on the scalp or under the nails.

When systemic illness or a blood infection is suspected, the blood from a vein is cultured to isolate the causative organism; it can sometimes take weeks before definitive growth of the disease-causing organism is seen. In rare instances, specimens thought to contain fungi are injected into animals to observe the effects (fungi develop much faster in animals than in humans). A specimen from the animal can then be tested to determine the kind of fungus growth (see **Culture**). After a fungus is cultured, a periodic acid Schiff smear may be applied to a sample and examined under the microscope. This smear demonstrates the shape of the spores and fungi for better identification.

A recent, simpler way of obtaining a specimen of skin or hair to test for the presence and kind of fungus utilizes the new cyanoacrylate glues (Bondini, Instant Krazy Glue, etc.). Here, a drop of the glue is placed on a glass slide. The slide is then pressed against the suspected area, carefully peeled away from the skin or hair, stained, and then examined with a microscope. The test can eliminate the need for a biopsy, with its associated expense and discomfort. Special care must be taken when removing the slide from the body to prevent any scar formation.

One other way of diagnosing fungus disease is through **Complement Fixation**; when this method is employed, several blood samples are taken two weeks apart.

When performed: Most commonly on areas of itching skin, especially the scalp; with persistent vaginal discharge; with persistent lung infections; with undiagnosed generalized infections, especially meningitis.

Normal values: Normally, fungi are not found in or on the human body. On occasion, a non-disease-causing fungus may be isolated from the mouth or vagina. Such infestations usually do not last very long.

Abnormal values: The isolation of any pathological fungi from the skin, hair, or blood or under the nails is considered abnormal. Fungus diseases may be confirmed by **Skin Reaction, Agglutination,** and **Complement Fixation** tests.

Risk factors: Negligible (see general risk factors for blood testing; also see **Biopsy**).

Pain/discomfort: Minimal (see general pain/discomfort factors for blood testing).

Cost: Culture tests average $15 to $80. Blood agglutination or complement fixation studies are $10 to $40. Skin tests are commonly performed in a doctor's office; there can be a $5 to $50 charge for the smear examination.

Accuracy and significance: Culture tests for fungus are considered 90 percent accurate, but there is a prolonged wait for results. Blood testing, while limited in its accuracy (many people with an infection do not show a positive blood test; some people who have undergone prior skin testing for fungus can show a positive blood test without having the disease), is valuable when time is of the essence. Many doctors do not consider skin testing a valuable aid to diagnosis.

FUROSEMIDE RENOGRAM, see "Pyelography," in *Radiography*

FUROSEMIDE STIMULATION, see *Renin*

G

GALACTOSE, see *Galactosemia*

GALACTOSEMIA

Galactosemia is an inherited defect in one part of carbohydrate metabolism. Galactose is a form of sugar found in milk, sugar beets, and seaweed. There are two forms of the disease, both due to the lack of an enzyme needed to change galactose either to glucose or to some other substance. One form causes vomiting and diarrhea in the newborn baby, followed by liver disease, mental retardation, and cataracts if not diagnosed and treated early enough. The second form causes cataracts only. Once diagnosed, the treatment is to eliminate galactose from the diet.

Blood is taken from the infant, usually from the umbilical cord at birth.

As opposed to testing the blood for the presence or absence of the necessary enzyme, galactose itself may be searched for in urine; if present at all, it should be in extremely low quantities. While a somewhat simpler test, it is not considered as accurate as blood testing.

When performed: When newborn infants show nutritional problems or gastrointestinal symptoms. Galactosemia testing of newborn babies is required in most of the United States; the exceptions are: Alabama, Alaska, Arkansas, Hawaii, Indiana, Kansas, Missouri, Nebraska, North Carolina, North Dakota, Oklahoma, Pennsylvania, South Carolina, South Dakota, Tennessee, and Washington. Some states waive the regulation if the parents object to such testing.

Normal values: Detection of the appropriate enzymes.

Abnormal values: Failure to detect the appropriate enzymes.

Risk factors: Negligible when blood is tested (see general risk factors for blood testing).

Pain/discomfort: Minimal when blood is tested (see general pain/discomfort factors for blood testing).

Cost: From $6 to $10.

Accuracy and significance: The routine screening tests are about 90 percent accurate; however, some techniques are so sensitive that they may show a rare form of galactosemia that causes no symptoms.

GALLBLADDER SCANNING, see *Nuclear Scanning*

GALLBLADDER VISUALIZATION, see *Radiography*

GALLIUM SCAN, see *Nuclear Scanning*
GAMMA CAMERA, see *Nuclear Scanning*
GAMMA GLUTAMYL TRANSFERASE, see *Alcoholism*

GASTRIC ANALYSIS

Gastric analysis is performed primarily to determine whether the stomach secretes hydrochloric acid (as it normally should); the test also shows whether the stomach produces the necessary digestive enzymes and whether it contains any cancer cells. Water, electrolytes, hydrochloric acid, mucin, pepsin, **Gastrin,** and a substance called intrinsic factor (which is necessary to absorb vitamin B_{12}) are all components of gastric secretions. When a patient is at rest, only small amounts of acid are secreted. The sight and smell of food, as well as actual food intake, can cause the stomach to secrete acid.

A tube is passed through the nose or mouth and into the stomach. The gastric fluid is withdrawn by suction continually for one hour. (The patient should not eat or take any medication for 12 hours prior to the test.) If, at the end of one hour, there is still doubt about whether acid is being secreted, an injection of histamine may be given to stimulate maximal acid production. One hour later, the gastric fluid is again tested. A tubeless method of analysis (which is not as exact but is more comfortable for the patient) may be performed by having the patient swallow a dye (Diagnex Blue) and noting the color of the urine.

The stomach fluid of newborn infants is sometimes examined within six hours after birth to help diagnose the respiratory distress syndrome (breathing difficulty). The presence of lung fluid in gastric contents is considered positive for the disease.

When performed: Whenever there is an undiagnosed anemia or repeated stomach infections (gastritis); when certain vitamin deficiencies are suspected; when searching for stomach cancer; when tuberculosis is suspected but the tuberculosis bacteria cannot be found.

After ulcer surgery, insulin is sometimes injected into a patient to see if stomach acid is still being secreted. Normally, insulin causes acid to appear, and absence of acid is a measure of the success of the surgery, which should have prevented acid formation. This is called the Hollander test.

Normal values: The average gastric hydrochloric acid output is 1.25 to 4 mEq per hour, but it can go as high as 12 mEq per hour and still be normal. Normal gastric secretory volume (all components) is between 50 and 100 ml per hour.

Abnormal values: Acid secretion is elevated in duodenal ulcer and in Zollinger-Ellison syndrome (gastrin-secreting tumor). In gastric cancer and anemia, less than the normal amount of acid (or no acid) is secreted. A new finding indicates that an increased amount of **Lactic Dehydrogenase** in the gastric fluid seems to be a sign of stomach cancer.

Risk factors: Virtually none; even the passage of the tube into the stomach rarely causes any complications. A histamine injection may cause asthma, headache, low blood pressure or a rash.

Pain/discomfort: Some patients find the insertion of the tube into the stomach quite uncomfortable.

Cost: There is usually a charge of from $50 to $200 for insertion of the tube into the stomach and the intermittent removal of gastric fluid for a one-hour period of time. Should the time extend to two hours, the cost is usually doubled. If the test is performed in a hospital, there is usually an additional charge. When the Hollander test is included as part of gastric analysis, the fee averages $300. Laboratory analysis of gastric fluid (pH, acidity, and amount) averages $30; enzyme and hormone studies are $30 to $50; cytological studies looking for cancer cells are $10 to $100. Some doctors consider the Diagnex Blue test outmoded, and it is possible that a health insurance company or a government-sponsored medical program will not reimburse the doctor or patient for the cost of the test.

Accuracy and significance: Although gastric analysis reveals the presence or absence of stomach acid, the test is not definitive and does not differentiate among the numerous stomach disorders. However, it can be extremely significant if cancer cells are found. It is considered to be about 75 percent accurate.

Note: Gastric analysis should not be confused with a stomach contents examination. A stomach contents exam is occasionally performed (after washing out the stomach) to ascertain a poison or drug. It is commonly performed on a deceased person to help determine the time of death based on food contents and the degree of digestion.

GASTRIN

In addition to acid and enzymes, the stomach produces a hormone called gastrin. This hormone, first provoked by eating food, causes the stomach lining to secrete hydrochloric acid. Gastrin also causes the pancreas to produce insulin and enzymes and the liver to produce bile, all of which aid in digestion. Finally, gastrin increases stomach and intestinal muscle activity, helping to move food down the intestinal tract. There are several other stomach hormones, but gastrin is the only one regularly tested for at this time. Blood is taken from a vein, and the serum is measured.

When performed: When there are severe, seemingly incurable ulcers of the stomach and intestine; in cases of suspected pernicious anemia.

Normal values: Normal values range from 0 to 300 pg per ml; the amount seems to increase naturally as a person gets older and may reach 700 pg per ml.

Abnormal values: With the occasional exception of the elderly, any test value over 500 pg per ml is considered a sign of disease. When a stomach ulcer is responding to treatment, gastrin levels will be normal; but in patients with Zollinger-Ellison syndrome (tumors that secrete gastrin and cause multiple ulcers), gastrin levels may rise to 300,000 pg per ml. To confirm the diagnosis, a trace of very dilute hydrochloric acid is given. With Zollinger-Ellison syndrome, the gastrin level stays the same; with anemia, it decreases markedly after the acid reaches the stomach.

Risk factors: Negligible (see general risk factors for blood testing).

Pain/discomfort: Minimal (see general pain/discomfort factors for blood testing).

Cost: From $20 to $40.

Accuracy and significance: There is some question as to normal gastrin values, since patients with certain anemias and peptic ulcers not located in the stomach can show a slight rise in gastrin levels. In fact, the test is significant only when confirming Zollinger-Ellison syndrome. This is a classic example of how a test's accuracy can depend on the selection of patients. It is considered to be about 70 percent accurate, but only if the right patient is tested at the right time and when the patient's symptoms perfectly match what the test is supposed to show.

GASTROESOPHAGEAL REFLUX

It has been reported that more than 1 out of 10 people suffer from gastroesophageal reflux, or acid reflux as the condition is also known. When stomach acid regurgitates or flows back into the lower portion of the esophagus, it causes a burning sensation in the chest just behind the sternum or breastbone. This is commonly called heartburn or pyrosis, and the pain can be so severe that sometimes it is mistaken for a heart attack. The two conditions must be differentiated in order to provide proper treatment. It is thought that the lower esophageal sphincter (LES) — a sphincter is a band of muscles that opens and closes entrances to body cavities — loses the ability to stay closed under pressure from the stomach's contents; this allows the acid to enter the esophagus and irritate the lining, which is insufficiently coated (as is the stomach) to protect itself from the acid's effect. If the burning symptoms, sometimes described as cramping, sharp pain, or simply as pressure, are due to gastroesophageal reflux, they seem to be aggravated by lying down and relieved by standing up, seem to be more frequent at night, and usually occur within an hour after a heavy meal. Furthermore, the regurgitation of stomach acid can produce a cough or difficulty in breathing should the acid seep into the windpipe. Another term for the condition is *hiatus hernia*, where an ostensible defect in the diaphragm allows the upper portion of the stomach to enter the chest area.

There are a variety of tests to diagnose gastroesophageal reflux. The most common is the standard acid reflux test (SART). For this, a measured dose of hydrochloric acid (approximating normal stomach acid) is put into the stomach and a **pH** measuring electrode placed in the lower esophagus. The patient is asked to cough, take very deep breaths, and bear down as if having a bowel movement; the patient repeats this process in different positions (standing, sitting, reclining). If acid is detected in the lower esophagus, gastroesophageal reflux is considered a good possibility. Another, somewhat similar, test is 24-hour esophageal pH monitoring, where the electrode is left in place day and night to observe the esophageal reaction to eating and other usual activities. This test is almost always performed in a hospital so the patient can be observed each time there is pain. Scintiscanning (see **Nuclear Scanning**) is a means to observe the esophageal spincter in action. The patient swallows radioactive liquid, which is then scanned in the sphincter as pressure is put on the abdomen. **Endoscopy** and **Biopsy** of the esophageal surface are other tests to measure the direct effect of acid on the esophageal lining. **Radiography,** in which barium is swallowed and observed in the stomach while the patient is placed in an upside-down position, is one of the older diagnostic techniques.

One of the most frequently used tests for gastroesophageal reflux is called manometry. In essence, this involves directly measuring the pressure inside the esophagus, and especially of the LES, while swallowing with and without drinking water. In particular, peristalsis, or the wave of contractions of the esophageal wall that carry food from the back of the throat to the stomach, and the constriction or relaxation of the LES are recorded. Recent reports have called this test useless as a means of diagnosing heartburn—albeit it costs $250—although it may be helpful in patients with unexplained chest pain.

Some doctors will give their patients a dose of bethanechol (a drug that accelerates the motility or contractions of the gastrointestinal tract and also increases bladder tone and may provoke the immediate need to urinate). The patients are then given food, and it is noted if the LES constricts or relaxes, as a means of arriving at a diagnosis when "heartburn" symptoms cannot be explained.

Another, older test, not as efficient but still in use, is the acid infusion, or Bernstein, test. For this, a weak dilution of hydrochloric acid—similar to normal stomach acid—is instilled into the esophagus. The onset of pain similar to the heartburn originally complained of reveals the esophagus's abnormal sensitivity. However, the test does not prove the existence of gastroesophageal reflux. When acid is placed farther down the gastrointestinal tract, usually by a tube just past the stomach, it is the Palmer test, designed to help diagnose ulcers. In the past, when doctors operated on patients to cut the vagus nerve that controls stomach acid secretions, insulin was injected into the patients to determine if the surgery was successful. Insulin made the acid flow again if all the vagus nerve fibers were not severed. This is known as the Hollander test. Today, many of these tests have been replaced by the **String** test. A new device, called the Medilog 1,000 system allows a patient to swallow a small capsule anchored to a tooth by a string that, through radio waves (telemetry), monitors the pH of the lower esophagus while the patient goes about daily and nightly activities; hospitalization is no longer necessary. (Also see **Edrophonium.**)

The simplest test of all, at the lowest cost, is a trial period of taking antacid preparations to see if they bring relief—both before eating, with discomfort, and after meals. Another part of this "trial therapy" includes raising the head of the bed while sleeping; this, too, may bring nighttime relief and help substantiate the diagnosis.

A test of esophageal function is called esophageal insufflation. Here, pressure is applied inside the esophagus, and the response can help reveal how well a patient will be able to speak after the larynx (voice box) is removed.

When performed: To diagnose heartburn; to differentiate among the possible causes of chest pains (usually by performing the test along with the **Electrocardiogram, Radiography,** and **Endoscopy**); to help determine the cause of anemia (the reflux irritation sometimes causes internal bleeding); where repeated bouts of a pneumonialike condition cannot be diagnosed; in infants who do not develop normally.

Normal values: A pH measurement greater than 4 in the esophagus at all times; no evidence of a weak lower esophageal sphincter; no visible evidence of stomach contents (radioactive or radioopaque material) seen in the esophagus; no evidence of ulceration or erosion when viewed by endoscopy.

Abnormal values: A pH measurement less than 4 (showing extreme acidity) in the esophagus at any one time, especially if apparent after eating greasy or spicy foods, after the consumption of alcohol, after having pressure applied to the abdomen, while lying down or during sleep; X-ray evidence of hiatal hernia; direct, endoscopic evidence of irritation to the esophageal lining.

Risk factors: Aside from the usual risks associated with radiography, biopsy, endoscopy, and nuclear scanning (all of which are noted in the entry for each test), there is the slight risk that the acid solution will precipitate the perforation of an existing ulcer or cause a hemorrhage should the esophageal lining be sufficiently eroded. Then, too, there is the remote possibility that the swallowed electrode may break or become detached, possibly necessitating surgery for recovery.

Pain/discomfort: Some people find it difficult to swallow the electrode, but this is usually overcome by anesthetizing the back of the throat. There may be some discomfort when pressure is applied to the abdomen or when the body is positioned upside down. Should the tests cause pain, it is similar in intensity to the heartburn for which the tests are performed.

Cost: About $50 for the standard acid reflux test performed over a period of one-half to one hour; about $100 in addition to a day's hospital charge for 24-hour esophageal monitoring; about $100 for nuclear scanning tests; from $75 to $100 for radiography (an upper gastrointestinal series); approximately $100 for endoscopy and biopsy. A Bernstein test can cost $150.

Accuracy and significance: While the 24-hour esophageal pH monitoring test is considered the most accurate, nearing a rate of 95 percent, the standard acid reflux test, performed over a much shorter period of time, is only about 80 percent accurate. Nuclear scanning is about 75 percent accurate, while X-rays—using barium—are reported to be only 60 percent accurate. The standard acid reflux test is said to be 80 percent accurate, but many doctors disagree; some think it worthless. Endoscopy and biopsy, even though they allow a direct view of the esophagus and a microscopic view of esophageal tissue, are only a little more than 80 percent accurate. Despite the many different tests, and their alleged accuracy, there are doctors who doubt that gastroesophageal reflux is the single, direct cause of heartburn. Any one of these tests, however, becomes significant if it leads to pain relief.

GASTROINTESTINAL ENDOSCOPY, see *Endoscopy*

GASTROINTESTINAL SERIES, see *Radiography*

GC, see *Gonorrhea*

GDH see *Alcoholism*

GELLE, see *Tuning Fork*

GENE PROBE, see *Genetic Disorder Screening*

GENERAL VOLATILE (TOXIC CHEMICAL) SCREENING, see *Toxic Chemical Exposure*

GENETIC DISORDER SCREENING

A gene is the basic unit of heredity (determining the color of one's eyes, height, and other physical characteristics as well as the control of various enzyme activities, body and mind functioning, hormone regulation, and even physiological reactions to food and drugs—to name but a few). At this time, it is estimated that from 50,000 to 100,000 genes are in the 23 chromosomes each parent carries and transmits to the child (see **Chromosome Analysis**).

A genetic disorder is a disease, disability, or physical deformity usually caused by some deviate gene formation. It may be the absence of a gene or part of same; it may be a mislocation of gene substance; it may be an excess of gene material; or it may be a defect or break in the gene substance. In some instances, only one gene—or a part of one gene—can cause the disorder; at other times, two or more genes must be affected before a disorder becomes obvious.

Genes are composed of a long helix (like two spiral staircases intertwined) of deoxyribonucleic acid (DNA) segments, and it is the various combinations of these DNA units that impart function as well as hereditary characteristics to the cells that make up body organs, tissues, and even appearance. It is also believed that damage to DNA following excessive exposure to chemicals (see **Toxic Chemical Exposure**), drugs, and ionizing radiation (see **Radiography**) plays a critical role in cancer as well as many inherited genetic disorders. DNA is also, in essence, the infecting material of bacteria and viruses; they insert their DNA into the body's cells and then reproduce themselves, causing disease.

At present, it is estimated that there are 15 million people in this country suffering from some form of genetic disorder. Thus, the advantage of genetic screening (sometimes called genetic counseling) should be obvious, especially if there is the knowledge—or even the vaguest hint—of a genetic-type illness in the family tree. It has now been predicted that within the next two to five years, routine gene mapping will be commonplace; all laboratories will be able to help determine an individual's susceptibility to a great many inherited diseases, including the tendency to heart attacks and cancer.

The testing for a DNA marker for a specific disease is also entering the diagnostic field. It is possible to identify the marker for Huntington's disease (persistent, involuntary jerky movements called chorea) years before the symptoms and signs appear. This is a form of gene probing that constitutes predictive testing for hereditary disease. And in 1985, another such test was announced: a gene probe that can predict whether a child will develop an inherited eye cancer called retinoblastoma (prior to this time, it was only possible to give an individual—one of whose parents had the disease—a warning that any offspring of those parents would have a 50 percent chance of being born with the condition). Genetic disorder screening has also been used to offer vital information to the individual and the family, and it has been used as well to provide information to indirectly related parties (insurance companies, employers or potential employers, governmental agencies such as health departments and motor vehicle bureaus, etc.). The availability of such data brings up the matter of confidentiality. There is always the risk of such information's reaching the wrong hands and causing almost as much disruption of one's life as the disease itself. Those who submit to such testing must be assured of the privacy of the results.

Another application of genetic screening is employed by industry. Several companies conduct tests on employees—and on applicants—to determine if individuals have a particular trait that might make them ill from one of the chemicals used in the company's production processes or from one of the company's products. They may also test for traits that could make an individual harmful to self or coworkers. While there are arguments on both sides—invasion of privacy and possible discrimination vs. the welfare and safety of the public—it seems to make good sense not to allow someone who is inherently susceptible to a danger to work in an environment known to be dangerous. At the same time, genetic monitoring during and after employment could reveal genetic damage that occurred after being on the job.

At the present time, almost 6,000 different inherited diseases or traits (exhibited by carriers of genetic diseases who do not usually show signs of the disease) are known. Many of these disorders reveal themselves as metabolic defects that interfere with normal body enzyme chemistry; they may also be the consequence of the lack of one or more enzymes necessary for the proper development or function of organs or tissues. Genetic screening tests try to uncover individuals who have a greater-than-average risk of passing on an inherited condition. Prior to the wide application of genetic disorder screening by doctors and the passage of state laws requiring prenatal testing of pregnant women, more than 100,000 children with congenital defects or genetic disorders were born each year in the United States alone.

Genetic screening may be performed on either parent-to-be (or even on a relative of a parent-to-be) prior to pregnancy; on the mother-to-be or on the fetus during pregnancy; and on the newborn infant before an inherited disorder can take effect. Sometimes, a detailed family history can offer clues leading to the discovery of a potentially dangerous genetic disease or trait, the confirmation of which, through testing, can help prevent a subsequent birth defect or disorder and even allow future normal childbearing.

In addition to genetic defects that are metabolic, abnormalities of the fetus can also come from hormonal disorders, infectious diseases, toxic drug influences, and even certain kinds of malnutrition suffered by a mother during pregnancy. Chromosomal disorders may arise from exposure to X-rays, excessive use of drugs, and infections; in some instances, genes are missing or present in excess, located at the wrong site within the chromosome, or defective in some way.

There are a great many different tests to uncover genetic or prenatal disorders. Some are required by law; others are available upon request. The most common ones are described under their own names:

> **Alpha Fetoprotein**
> **Aminoaciduria**
> **Amniocentesis**
> *Amniography* (see **Radiography**)
> **Bilirubin**
> **Chlamydia Identification**
> **Chorionic Villi Screening**
> **Chromosome Analysis**
> **Cortisol**
> *Cystic Fibrosis* (see **Sodium; Sweat**)
> **Cytomegalovirus**
> *Fetoscopy* (see **Endoscopy**)
> **Galactosemia**
> *German Measles* (see **Rubella**)

Hemophilia (see Partial Thromboplastin Time)
Herpes
Measles (see Virus Disease)
Muscular Dystrophy (see Creatine Phosphokinase)
Phenylketonuria
Sickle-Cell Anemia (see Hemoglobin)
Syphilis
Tay-Sachs Disease
Thalassemia (see Hemoglobin)
Thyroid Function
Toxoplasmosis
Ultrasound

A computerized system containing information on more than 1,000 known birth defects has been established at the Massachusetts Institute of Technology/Tufts New England Medical Center at Boston. Its services are available to any physician who desires diagnostic techniques, treatments, and prognostic information.

GENETIC MARKER TYPING, see *Semen*

GENETIC SEX IDENTITY, see *Chromosome Analysis*

GERMAN MEASLES, see *Rubella*

GESELL DEVELOPMENTAL SCHEDULE, see *Motor Development*

GGT, see *Alcoholism*

GGTP, see *Alcoholism*

GHb, see *Glycohemoglobin*

GIARDIA, see *Parasite*

GIEMSA, see *Malaria*

GIGANTISM, see *Growth Hormone*

GI SERIES, see *Radiography*

GLA-PROTEIN, see *Bone Mineral Density Analysis*

GLAUCOMA, see *Tonometry*

GLOBULIN, see *Albumin/Globulin*

GLOMERULAR FILTRATION RATE, see *Creatinine*

GLUCAGON

Glucagon, a hormone produced by the pancreas (which also produces insulin), converts protein and fat molecules into blood sugars to be used as energy. Glucagon also causes insulin to be released into the body. Blood is taken from a vein, and the plasma is tested. Glucagon is sometimes injected into a patient to help diagnose excess glycogen (stored glucose). Glucose is the body's chief energy substance; it is stored primarily in the liver but also in muscles. Normally, after a patient receives glucagon, blood glucose will increase markedly.

When performed: When hypoglycemia (low blood sugar) is suspected; to assess the control of diabetes (whether a patient is well regulated); to aid in the diagnosis of a type of pancreatic tumor that occurs primarily in women after the menopause and causes a distinctive skin rash and weakness.

Normal values: Glucagon levels in plasma range from 60 to 100 pg per ml.

Abnormal values: Glucagon values are greatly increased with tumor of the pancreas, uncontrolled diabetes, and inadequate amounts of insulin. On occasion, glucagon is decreased with certain forms of hypoglycemia. It is also decreased after eating a large amount of carbohydrates.

Risk factors: Negligible (see general risk factors for blood testing).

Pain/discomfort: Minimal (see general pain/discomfort factors for blood testing).

Cost: From $25 to $50.

Accuracy and significance: The test is about 75 percent accurate in confirming diseases related to the pancreas, but for the most part, it is not significant enough to pinpoint a diagnosis. (See **Pancreas Function.**)

GLUCOSE (Sugar)

The glucose test measures the amount of glucose floating free in the blood or excreted by the kidneys into the bladder. The test is really a measure of how well the body handles carbohydrate metabolism (the breakdown of starches such as vegetables as well as all the various sugar products in the foods we eat). Glucose is the primary fuel, or energy source, for all the body tissues. It may be burned directly or converted into fat and stored for later use as fatty acid energy. Glucose is stored primarily in the liver and, in small amounts, in other tissues. A uniform blood glucose level is generally maintained in the body through insulin secretion (which decreases it), despite variations due to dietary increase in sugar and energy expenditure. Blood is taken from the vein to assess the level of glucose in serum; glucose may also be tested in whole blood or plasma, in urine, or in spinal fluid.

In preparing for the glucose tolerance test (GTT), the patient eats his usual amount of carbohydrates for several days. Then he fasts for 8 to 12 hours prior to the test. First, a fasting blood glucose and urine glucose are measured. Then the patient is given 100 g of glucose in water or soda to drink. Thirty minutes afterward, both the blood and urine are again examined for sugar levels. Glucose testing after eating is called postprandial. Every hour thereafter for the next five hours, urine and blood samples are taken to determine how long it takes the body to metabolize the 100 g of glucose. Sometimes, the spinal fluid and joint fluids are tested for glucose. (Before more sophisticated methods of medical laboratory testing were developed, doctors used to taste their patient's urine for sugar.)

Today, an increasing number of physicians no longer require their patients to fast for 8 to 12 hours prior to the glucose or glucose tolerance test. The results seem no less accurate as long as food is not ingested for 2 hours prior to the test.

When performed: The fasting blood glucose is performed when there is dizziness, weakness, excessive thirst, excessive urination, or any other symptoms and signs suggesting diabetes. The test also helps diagnose hormone disorders, pancreatic disease, certain brain and spinal cord diseases, and many hereditary conditions. A single postprandial test may be performed as a confirmatory measure.

The glucose tolerance test is performed when the fasting and/or postprandial glucose determinations are borderline and diabetes or other disease is still being considered.

The urine examination for sugar is a routine screening test for diabetes as well as for suspected kidney, liver, or hormone disease.

Normal values: Fasting blood glucose levels normally range from 80 to 120 mg per 100 ml of serum, 60 to 100 mg per 100 ml of whole blood. Postprandial levels should not exceed 180 mg per 100 ml.

During the entire five to six hours of the glucose tolerance test, the peak should remain below 180 mg per 100 ml, and after two hours, the levels should return to the same as for fasting.

In the urine sugar test, normally no sugar or only an insignificant trace should be detected, even after a high-carbohydrate meal. However, in some individuals who have a low kidney threshold, sugar may be detected in the urine without the presence of disease.

Abnormal values: The fasting blood glucose level is increased (hyperglycemia) with diabetes, Cushing' syndrome (pituitary disease), many endocrine problems, liver disease, and many drugs including diuretic therapy. The level is decreased with pancreatic disorders, excessive insulin, and glycogen storage disease.

In order to justify a diagnosis of hypoglycemia as a disease condition, blood glucose levels must be less than 40 mg per 100 ml of serum in at least three different instances at the identical time the patient is having symptoms (sweating, palpitations, weakness, bizarre behavior). Alcohol intake may cause temporary hypoglycemia, as will fasting, liver disease, and certain cancers.

In the glucose tolerance test, levels are elevated for more than two hours with diabetes mellitus and decreased with pancreatitis, excess insulin production, and hypoglycemia. In contrast, in 1984, many doctors came to the conclusion that if a patient had a blood glucose level greater than 140 mg per 100 ml on more than one occasion after fasting (the patient takes no food for at least 12 hours prior to testing), this also justifies a diagnosis of diabetes. To confirm the diagnosis, a blood sugar level greater than 200 mg per 100 ml 2 hours after drinking a measured amount of sugar is sufficient; the glucose tolerance test is not considered necessary.

Elevated levels of glucose in the urine may be caused by diabetes mellitus, liver disease, hyperthyroidism and other hormone disorders, pregnancy, brain injury, and excessive ingestion of sugar. In meningitis, spinal fluid glucose is decreased; with joint infections, joint fluid sugar is decreased.

Risk factors: Negligible (see general risk factors for blood testing).

Pain/discomfort: Minimal (see general pain/discomfort factors for blood testing).

Cost: A blood glucose test ranges from $4 to $24. The test is usually included in **Comprehensive Multiple Test Screening** panels, which range from $7 to $42. When several glucose tests are measured—the glucose tolerance test, for instance—the cost for six to eight tests is $15 to $105. Urine glucose testing averages $5; there is usually no charge if chemical dipsticks are used. Glucose measurements from other body fluids, such as joint or spinal fluid, average $10.

Accuracy and significance: Although glucose measurements can be affected by numerous foods and drugs (oral contraceptives may alter glucose values for several days), the test is considered 90 percent accurate as the diagnostic test for diabetes. Although the glucose tolerance test can be significant in determining hypoglycemia, its accuracy only has meaning if the overt symptoms of hypoglycemia occur at very low blood glucose levels. The most recent studies disclaim any value for the GTT as a hypoglycemia test; the preferred tests being fasting glucose, **C-peptide** and **Insulin**.

When spinal fluid is tested for glucose, it can help distinguish the type of brain or meningeal infection. The accuracy of the glucose tolerance test, however, can depend more on the values a doctor decides are normal and abnormal than on the biochemical measurements. Many doctors now believe a value greater than 180 mg per 100 ml is not necessarily abnormal and is actually a false-positive result. They contend that normal values can reach 270 mg per 100 ml and that only when values exceed that amount should a diagnosis of diabetes be made. Using these new upper limits of normal, false-positive tests that may occur when a patient is under emotional stress are almost always eliminated.

At the present time, it is considered sound medical practice to confirm a suspected diagnosis of diabetes with the **C-Peptide** test. Further confirmation is obtained through the **Glycohemoglobin** test.

GLUCOSE 6-PHOSPHATE DEHYDROGENASE (G6PD)

Glucose 6-phosphate dehydrogenase is an enzyme normally found in red blood cells. In people with a deficiency of this enzyme (an inherited condition), red blood cells are no longer protected from oxidation, causing hemolysis (destruction of red blood cells and subsequent separation of hemoglobin), which can lead to anemia. The deficiency is more frequent in blacks, Orientals, and Caucasians from the Mediterranean area and more serious in men than in women. Blood is taken from a vein and tested. It may simply be screened for the presence of G6PD, or the quantity of G6PD may be measured precisely. Either test can still miss the deficiency in some women.

An indirect test for G6PD is to note the autohemolysis (self-destruction) of **Red Blood Cells** after a 48-hour period. Normally, less than 1 percent of the cells will destroy themselves, but with a G6PD deficiency, at least 5 percent will disintegrate; if the cells are mixed with glucose, however, patients with the deficiency will stop autolysing.

When performed: In undiagnosed hemolytic anemia; before administration of certain antimalarial drugs, some sulfonamides, and nitrofurans.

Normal values: Glucose 6-phosphate dehydrogenase should normally be found in significant amounts in red blood cells: 120 to 280 units per billion cells.

Abnormal values: Glucose 6-phosphate dehydrogenase deficiency, while not usually serious or chronic, can at times be fatal. It does not show itself until the patient ingests drugs or foods that precipitate the hemolytic anemia, which can then cause hemoglobinuria, jaundice, fever, and renal failure. Some of those drugs are Primaquine (for malaria), aspirin, sulfa products, nitrofurans, vitamin C, certain antibiotics, some worm medicines, inhalation of naphthalene (moth repellent), and eating fava beans—but only in people born with a G6PD deficiency.

Risk factors: Negligible (see general risk factors for blood testing).

Pain/discomfort: Minimal (see general pain/discomfort factors for blood testing).

Cost: From $10 to $25 for a general screening test. For specific measurements of G6PD, the fee ranges from $30 to $40.

Accuracy and significance: The test is very accurate and will detect approximately 90 percent of those who have an inherited deficiency of this particular enzyme. It can be significant in screening individuals who should take prophylactic drugs against malaria and those who persistently suffer from anemia after taking a variety of medicines, but it is not precise in this regard.

GLUCOSE TOLERANCE, see *Glucose*

GLUTAMATE DEHYDROGENASE, see *Alcoholism*

GLUTAMIC OXALACETIC TRANSAMINASE, see *Aspartate Aminotransferase*

GLUTAMIC PYRUVIC TRANSAMINASE, see *Aspartate Aminotransferase*

GLUTAMINE, see *Ammonia*

GLYCEROL LYSIS (GLT), see *Hemoglobin*

GLYCOHEMOGLOBIN (GHb), GLYCOSYLATED HEMOGLOBIN

The glycohemoglobin test measures the percentage of hemoglobin molecules that have glucose (sugar) attached to them. The greater the amount of glucose in the blood, the greater the percentage of glycosylated hemoglobin (also known as HBA_{1a-c}). The test is of particular value in monitoring a patient with diabetes to ascertain that the patient's blood sugar level is properly controlled; thus, it is also a measure of the success or failure of treatment.

Initially, the glycohemoglobin test is usually performed along with the **Glucose** tolerance test, but it may be substituted for that test after a treatment regimen has been established, since it requires far less time and far fewer blood samples from the patient and since the patient need not fast beforehand. Glycohemoglobin measurements indicate blood sugar activity during the six to eight weeks prior to the test, whereas the glucose tolerance test measures only blood sugar levels at the moment. At the present time, the glycohemoglobin test is usually performed every two months in order to provide the physician with data to help control the diabetic patient. Blood from a vein is examined.

Note: Today, glycohemoglobin may also be called GHB or GhB, HbA_{1a}, HbA_{1b}, or HbA_{1c}; it is now known that there is more than one form of this hemoglobin. Increased use of, and experience with, this test has decreased its overall value for well-controlled diabetics, and some doctors now feel that standard **Glucose** tests are still preferable. Certain forms of anemia, not related to diabetes, have produced lower-than-normal blood levels, as have certain kidney diseases.

When performed: The test is used primarily to measure the control (proper treatment) of a patient with diabetes; it not only helps reveal difficulties in sugar utilization but can also reveal patients who ignore their prescribed treatment. Sometimes, the test is used to measure the body's carbohydrate metabolism.

Normal values: Patients without diabetes, and patients with the disease who are responding to treatment average from 2 percent to 7.5 percent glycohemoglobin.

Abnormal values: Patients who have uncontrolled diabetes or who are receiving inadequate treatment will have glycohemoglobin values greater than 7.5 percent. Values in excess of 9.2 percent indicate definitely improper control of a diabetic condition. Rarely, a patient with a known hemoglobin disease, but without diabetes, will have elevated values.

Risk factors: Negligible (see general risk factors for blood testing).

Pain/discomfort: Minimal (see general pain/discomfort factors for blood testing).

Cost: From $13 to $45.

Accuracy and significance: Some doctors believe that the test is 90 percent accurate and that it will replace **Glucose** as a way to follow the progress of patients with diabetes. False-positive results have been known to occur, although these are primarily due to laboratory carelessness or failure to measure all forms of GHb.

GLYCOPROTEIN p30, see *Acid Phosphatase*

GLYCOSIDES, see *Digitalis Toxicity*

GLYCOSYLATED HEMOGLOBIN, see *Glycohemoglobin*

GONADOTROPIN, see *Pregnancy; Testis Function*

GONIOSCOPE, see *Fluorescein Eye Stain*

GONORRHEA (GC, CLAP)

Gonorrhea is primarily an infection of the urethra (the passageway that carries urine from the bladder to outside the body) and is one of the most common communicable diseases in the United States. (By law, all instances of gonorrhea must be reported.) Other parts of the body that can become infected with gonorrhea are: the rectum, the throat, the eyes (the disease can cause ulcers on the eye surface), and any and all of the genital or reproductive organs (a common cause of infertility or sterility). Arthritis is the most common late complication of gonorrhea; heart disease, meningitis, and skin lesions are also known to follow this disease. In men, the most frequent symptom is a burning during urination followed by a cream-colored or yellow discharge from the end of the penis; the onset of pain is usually 24 to 72 hours after being infected. Although women can have similar symptoms, more often than not they are unaware they are infected. Gonorrhea must be differentiated from nongonococcal urethritis, a similar condition caused by Chlamydia. (See also **Chlamydia Identification**.) While the incidence of chlamydial infection is probably greater than that of gonorrhea, it is not required that chlamydial infections be reported to health authorities. The diagnosis of gonorrhea is usually made by the **Gram Stain** test of the discharge from the male urethra; the bacteria that cause the disease are easily seen inside **White Blood Cells** and appear as distinct pairs resembling tiny bookends. **Culture** helps to confirm the diagnosis; although there are a few **Complement Fixation**–type tests, they are not thought to be too accurate. Today, many forms of the gonorrhea germ are resistant to a number of different antibiotics, making culture sensitivity tests particularly important to successful treatment. Patients with gonorrhea must be tested monthly for **Syphilis** for a minimum of six months after the infection is diagnosed.

A new test that can offer a presumptive diagnosis of gonorrhea within 30 minutes is the limulus amebocyte lysate (limulus testing is one way of diagnosing many infectious diseases; see **Synovial Fluid**); it is considered useful only for male urethra specimens and not of real value in uncovering rectal or pharyngeal gonorrhea. And a recent enzyme immunoassay test, called gonozyme, has been introduced that has been reported to be as accurate as culture. It is said to be especially valuable in detecting a carrier of this disease who has no symptoms or signs (discharge); it requires less than an hour's time.

When performed: When a man has any penile discharge, undiagnosed throat or rectal infection, or pain in or near the testicles; on women with an undiagnosed vaginal discharge or undiagnosed abdominal pains. On patients known to have had sexual contact with suspected carriers of the disease. When a patient has arthritis, especially in only one joint, that cannot be diagnosed (see **Synovial Fluid**).

Normal values: No gonorrhea bacteria should be found.

Abnormal values: Any evidence of the gonorrheal bacteria on a gram stain or culture.

Risk factors: None.

Pain/discomfort: None.

Cost: From $5 to $15 for a Gram stain; from $10 to $50 for a culture. The new immunoassay tests that can be performed in the doctor's office average $12.

Accuracy and significance: The Gram stain alone is considered to be about 80 percent accurate; much depends on who studies the specimen under the microscope. A culture test is 95 percent accurate, assuming the specimen was properly obtained from the correct place. The newer tests are said to be from 80 to 90 percent accurate.

GONOZYME, see *Gonorrhea*

GOUT, see *Uric Acid*

GRAM STAIN

The Gram stain test (named after Dr. Hans Christian Gram, a Danish physician) is used primarily to distinguish various bacteria under the microscope that would otherwise be impossible to identify. Sputum, joint fluid, spinal fluid, urine, sinus discharge, urethral discharge, vaginal fluid, and exudates (ooze) from infections can all be examined in this manner. When the specimen takes a gentian violet (bluish purple) or safranin (red) stain, the morphology (size, shape, and form) of bacteria is more easily visualized, which aids in both diagnosis and treatment. (Certain bacteria such as tuberculosis germs will not show up on the Gram stain and need special dyes.)

When performed: The test is used primarily to evaluate and distinguish infectious organisms in various body fluids and to aid in the precise choice of therapy. Certain antibiotics are effective only against Gram-positive organisms; other antibiotics are effective only against Gram-negative organisms.

Normal values: Normally, no pathological bacteria are observed after staining.

Abnormal values: Gram-negative organisms stain an orange-red color and are usually representative of coliform-type (intestinal and urinary tract) diseases. Gram-positive organisms stain a bluish purple and are usually representative of streptococcal and staphylococcal (upper respiratory tract and abscess) diseases.

Risk factors: Negligible. If joint or **Cerebrospinal Fluid** is withdrawn for examination, see general risk factors for catheter or needle insertion. In most instances, the patient furnishes the specimen to be examined.

Pain/discomfort: None if the patient furnishes the specimen. See general pain/discomfort factors for catheter and needle insertion if joint or cerebrospinal fluid is to be examined.

Cost: Most doctors perform this simple test in their offices, and they may charge from $5 to $15. If the microscopic slide is obtained and examined in a commercial laboratory, the charge is approximately $5. When cerebrospinal and joint fluid are examined, there can be an additional $40 to $50 charge for obtaining the specimen.

Accuracy and significance: Although the test is valuable as a rapid differentiation among bacterial infections, it is basically only a screening procedure that helps the doctor select an antibiotic before receiving the results of a **Culture** test. In many instances, instability of the chemical solutions used to stain the specimen causes up to 40 percent false-positive results. When the Gram stain is used to diagnose bacterial pneumonia, about half the tests show false-negative results. About 60 percent accurate.

GRAVLEE METHOD, see *Cytology*

GROWTH HORMONE

A pituitary gland hormone called somatotropin or human growth hormone (HGH) controls the height an individual attains. It is, of course, essential for normal growth. Testing for growth hormone offers the earliest indication of generalized pituitary problems. Blood is taken from a vein, and the serum is tested. Several tests must be taken at different times before true values can be determined. At times, it is necessary to give the patient a large amount of insulin (to produce hypoglycemia, or low blood sugar) to obtain accurate results. Today, drugs are available to stop excessive growth hormone secretion (preventing gigantism, or abnormally tall individuals) as well as drugs to allow normal growth hormone secretion (preventing dwarfism).

Another test for the cause of growth failure is duodenal **Biopsy.** Here, a small piece of the lining of the duodenum (the first part of the small intestine connected to the stomach) is examined for celiac disease (sprue), a malabsorption condition (see **Xylose Tolerance**). It is thought that celiac disease is more likely to be a cause of short stature than pituitary gland dysfunction.

Measuring levels of somatomedins, insulinlike growth factors controlled by the growth hormone, may also offer a clue as to why children are not growing properly; normal amounts usually indicate sufficient growth hormone, but decreased amounts can point to a pituitary gland problem. Increased amounts usually indicate acromegaly (excessive growth).

More recently, drugs other than insulin have been used in growth hormone provocation studies; these include premarin (a synthetic form of estrogen) with L-dopa (a drug used to treat parkinsonism), clonidine (see **Catecholamines**), and an arginine-insulin mixture.

Knemometry, a special way of measuring the length of the lower leg, is used as a test to evaluate the effect of growth hormone after it is injected in children.

When performed: The test is used whenever gigantism (acromegaly) or dwarfism is suspected. The earlier the test is performed and the abnormality revealed, the easier and more effective the treatment. The test is given, too, when hyperactive children take stimulant drugs such as dextroamphetamine or methylphenidate (Ritalin); these drugs seem to retard growth.

Normal values: New born infants usually have higher levels of somatotropin than adults (over 30 ng per ml); children generally average from 1 to 15 ng per ml; women average up to 30 ng per ml; and men usually range below 10 ng per ml. It is normal for growth hormone levels to increase after insulin is given and to decrease to near zero after a large amount of glucose (sugar) is consumed.

Abnormal values: Lower-than-normal values are found with dwarfism; elevated values appear with gigantism. Values may also be elevated with diabetes, in stressful situations, following surgery, and with infections. Taking female hormones will cause a rise in growth hormone levels.

Risk factors: Negligible (see general risk factors for blood testing).

Pain/discomfort: Minimal (see general pain/discomfort factors for blood testing).

Cost: From $15 to $35.

Accuracy and significance: The test is considered to be 80 percent accurate in conditions that raise growth hormone levels. There are times, however, when conditions that reflect little or no secretion of growth hormone may make it impossible to evaluate the level of growth hormone in the blood. When this occurs, other hormones and/or chemicals can be injected into a patient to see if they will stimulate production of sufficient growth hormone for measurement. The accuracy of the growth hormone test can be affected by the time of day the blood is taken, and the test may thus require multiple samples for greater significance.

G6PD, see *Glucose 6-Phosphate Dehydrogenase*

GTT, see *Glucose*

GUAIAC, see *Occult Blood*

GUANASE, see *Hepatitis*

GUTHRIE BACTERIAL INHIBITION ASSAY (GBIA), see *Phenylketonuria*

H

HAGEMAN FACTOR, see *Fibrinogen*

HAIR ANALYSIS

Although the analysis of hair—especially for the detection of such toxic minerals as arsenic, lead, cadmium, and mercury—is increasing, there are still many doctors with reservations about the efficacy of this kind of test. So many variables affect the hair sample that medical history is as important as the hair sample itself. Before an accurate analysis can be made, certain information must be gathered: the part of the body the hair comes from, how close to the root of the hair was the sample located, the activities, such as swimming, that had been engaged in before the hair sample was taken, the materials—shampoos, dyes, dryers, etc.—that had been used on the hair. In most instances, if a hair sample reveals traces of body poisoning, the doctor examines the blood, urine, and other body tissues (see **Biopsy**) for confirmation. Although there is no general agreement on the analysis of hair for nutritional problems, its use in the field is increasing, and many health insurance plans now pay for the test when it is designated as one to reveal mineral deficiencies. A hair sample is usually taken from the nape of the neck; the sample must be the first inch of new hair. Hair that has been bleached, dyed, or given a permanent wave is not used for testing. It is also important that the testing laboratory be aware of any vitamin and mineral pills being taken.

When performed: Primarily in surveys to ascertain increases in toxic minerals in people; as a screening test when exposure to harmful metals is suspected (at times, it is used to evaluate children whose learning disabilities are thought to result from poisoning by lead or other metals); to help ascertain some nutritional deficiencies.

Normal values: Toxic metals should not be detected in properly obtained, uncontaminated hair samples, although some studies stipulate that minute amounts—5 mg per kg (2.2 lbs.)—may be normal.

Abnormal values: Evidence of toxic metals; evidence of decreased amounts of such nutritive metals as calcium or zinc, although such evidence is not accepted by all medical professionals.

Risk factors: None.

Pain/discomfort: None, if the scissors are used carefully.

Cost: From $30 to $50 for a total analysis (covering some 12 metals that might well be found in hair); from $4 to $8 for an analysis of a single, rarely isolated metal such as lead, aluminum, or lithium. Some doctors consider this test unproved, and it is possible that a health insurance company or a government-sponsored medical program will not reimburse the doctor or patient for the cost of the test.

Accuracy and significance: Although hair samples can show the presence of various minerals, the test is not considered particularly accurate; too many extraneous factors can interfere with hair analysis. For instance, a child whose green-colored hair showed copper levels four times above normal was found to be swimming in a pool contaminated by copper from the pipes. Blood, urine, and tissue studies are more precise.

When two portions of a hair sample from one individual were sent to 2 different commercial hair analysis laboratories, the test results were so dissimilar that they were totally useless; mineral and vitamin interpretations, in most instances, were at extreme opposite ends of the test value ranges. In a 1985 report in a medical journal, samples of the same hair were sent to 13 different commercial laboratories, and here, the reported results from each laboratory were markedly different; they were even called "bizarre." The Federal Trade Commission has barred at least one laboratory from making false advertising claims about its hair analysis testing.

HAM

Ham, named after Dr. Thomas Ham, is a test for paroxysmal nocturnal hemoglobinuria, a disease that occurs in certain people after middle age. Symptoms include attacks of anemia, generalized aches and pains, chills, fever, and excessive amounts of hemoglobin in the urine as a consequence of hemolysis (destruction of defective red blood cells) and usually occur during sleep. It is believed to be caused by a defect in the membranes surrounding red blood cells. The red blood cells, it seems, are unusually sensitive to the blood's **Complement,** which causes them to self destruct. Because the condition is so insidious, it can take years before a diagnosis is made. Blood is taken from a vein, and the serum is tested in an acid solution. A somewhat similar but less definitive test is the sugar water test (sucrose hemolysis test), in which the defective red cell, if present, dissolves in the presence of sucrose.

When performed: When paroxysmal nocturnal hemoglobinuria is suspected (usually because of an excess of hemoglobin in the urine on awakening); when a patient has repeated, severe infections that cannot be diagnosed; when there are undiagnosed pains, especially in the lower back or legs.

Normal values: Normally, red blood cells do not hemolyze (dissolve and release their supply of hemoglobin) when mixed with a very mild acid solution or when exposed to a sugar (sucrose) solution.

Abnormal values: In patients with paroxysmal nocturnal hemoglobinuria, red blood cells break down when exposed to an acid solution with a **pH** of 6.7 or less or when placed in a sucrose solution.

Risk factors: Negligible (see general risk factors for blood testing).

Pain/Discomfort: Minimal (see general pain/discomfort factors for blood testing).

Cost: From $30 to $40 for the Ham acid hemolysis test. From $24 to $31 for the sugar water, or sucrose, hemolysis test.

Accuracy and significance: While there is some controversy as to which of the two tests is the more accurate (acid hemolysis or sucrose hemolysis), both tests are considered to be about 80 percent accurate and are sufficiently significant to justify a diagnosis when positive.

HAMSTER ZONA-FREE OVUM, see *Semen*

HAPTOGLOBIN

Haptoglobin, a plasma globulin (see **Albumin/Globulin**), is a direct measure of hemolysis in the body. Hemolysis means a markedly increased breakdown of red blood cells and the liberation of **Hemoglobin** into the plasma; it can come about from disease, from certain inherited conditions, from certain drugs, and after snakebite. When hemolysis occurs, the red blood cells do not last as long as they should, and this usually (but not always) results in anemia. Blood is taken from a vein, and the serum is tested.

A somewhat simpler test, especially when searching for the cause of an **Iron**-deficiency anemia in infants, is the hemosiderin stain applied to a urine specimen. This pigment is not normally found in urine, and its presence is usually an indication of a disease process; it may, however, be found after transfusions.

When performed: When anemia is present, especially when it is thought to be from an inherited condition such as thalassemia (Mediterranean or Cooley's anemia) or from Rh problems; when it is suspected that certain environmental factors (chemicals, drugs, or physical injury) are causing anemia; in severe infections; with liver disease.

Normal values: Normal haptoglobin levels range from 50 to 150 mg per 100 ml of serum.

Abnormal values: As red blood cells are destroyed, the hemoglobin that is released combines with haptoglobin; thus, reduced levels of haptoglobin indicate hemolysis, no matter what the specific cause. Decreased values of haptoglobin are also found in liver disease and with infectious mononucleosis. Certain severe infections, tissue damage such as with heart attack, and cancers cause increased haptoglobin levels.

Risk factors: Negligible (see general risk factors for blood testing).

Pain/discomfort: Minimal (see general pain/discomfort factors for blood testing).

Cost: From $35 to $46.

Accuracy and significance: Although the test is 90 percent accurate in indicating the breakage of the body's red blood cells, its significance is not great enough to allow a specific diagnosis. The value of the test lies in confirming the susceptibility of red blood cells to breakage.

HARDY-RAND-RITTLER, see *Color Blindness*

HARTNUP'S DISEASE, see *Aminoaciduria*

HAV, see *Hepatitis*

HB, see *Hepatitis*

HbAla-c, see *Glycohemoglobin*

HBD, see *Hydroxybutyric Dehydrogenase*

HBsAg, see *Hepatitis*

HCG, see *Pregnancy; Testis Function*

HCO$_3$, see *Bicarbonate*

HCS, see *Placental Lactogen*

HDL, see *Cholesterol; Lipoproteins*

HEARING FUNCTION

Sound is heard in two ways: by its intensity or volume (loudness) and by its tone, which depends on how fast or how slowly the sound waves vibrate. In tests of hearing ability, both factors are measured. In addition, patients are tested for the ability to hear sound by two different means of conduction: air conduction (sounds heard through the ear canal) and bone conduction (sounds detected by the bones around and behind the ear).

The simplest measures of hearing ability are the whisper and voice tests, in which the doctor, sitting about 20 feet away from the patient, whispers and then says numbers out loud while the patient listens with one ear covered. In the ticking-watch test, the physician notes how far away from the ear the watch is still heard.

The most precise hearing test is measured by the audiometer, a machine that puts out sounds of various tones and intensities (volumes). Pure tones vary from 64 cycles per second, or cps (very low, bass-type tones), to almost 12,000 cps (extremely shrill or high-pitched tones). The human ear can usually detect sounds from 16 to 16,000 cps (although some people can hear up to 20,000 cps). Many animals can hear tones of 50,000 cps, beyond the range of human hearing.

The intensity (volume) of sound is expressed in decibels (db). A whisper measures about 20 db. Background noise in the average home runs about 50 db; in an office, about 60 db. Loud classical music rates 80 db; rock music is more than 120 db; and a jet engine ranges from 140 to 180 db. Usually, sounds greater than 130 db will cause pain; sound greater than 85 db can cause hearing loss in a few hours.

For the air conduction part of the test, the patient wears earphones from the audiometer and listens to sounds of designated tones and intensities or to spoken words (sounds may also be broadcast through a speaker in a soundproof room). An attachment from the earphones is then applied to the bone behind the ear, and hearing is tested via bone conduction. How well the patient hears sounds through air conduction is an indication of eardrum and middle ear function as well as ear-nerve disease. Bone conduction ability tests the function of the inner ear. **Tuning Fork** tests may also be used to survey hearing problems and to confirm bone or nerve deafness.

Most doctors recommend that an audiometer test be performed *before* any ototoxic drug (ear-nerve-damaging) is administered in order to detect any deafness that might result from the medication.

The Lombard test helps to detect faked hearing loss. While wearing audiometer earphones, a patient reads from a book; after a minute or two, a noise from the audiometer is sent to each ear. If hearing is normal, the reader's voice will become louder. Patients with true hearing loss will not raise their voices while reading.

The very latest form of audiometry is called evoked response audiometry (ERA), sometimes known as electrical response audiometry. In essence, this involves utilizing the **Electroencephalogram** as a means of detecting the ability to hear sounds. There are at least 15 different variations of this test, distinguished mostly by the part of the body on which are recorded the electrical impulses that result from sound stimulation. At the present time, however, only three are in regular use. The most commonly applied version of ERA is called auditory brain stem response (brain stem audiometry or brain stem electrical potential); it records brain wave reactions to sound (most often clicks) through electrodes placed on the skin at the top of the head and over the mastoid bone. Because the brain wave response is so small, it is electrically magnified and fed through a computer, where it is recorded on a graph. The cortical evoked response version of ERA measures the reaction of the brain above the brain stem to perceived sound. (The brain stem is that part of the brain that connects the upper areas of the brain—the cerebrum and cortex, where thinking and voluntary body directions arise—to the spinal cord.) It is alleged to be a test of the entire hearing system. The third version of ERA is called electrocochleography. Here, a needle electrode is passed through the eardrum into the cochlea (the snail-shaped bone of the inner ear that houses the delicate hairs that normally detect noise) to assess the nerve that goes from the ear to the brain.

These tests are particularly useful when the usual hearing tests fail to offer any diagnostic clues. They allow the testing of infants—even newborns—and mentally retarded individuals; they are also used when a brain tumor is suspected, when Meniere's disease is under consideration (this is a condition where dizziness accompanies hearing loss), and when there is unexplained hearing loss in only one ear. Because these tests are considered objective, they are applied to people who seek compensation for hearing loss, usually related to employment or military service, and in fact, are described as a "lie detector" in medical-legal cases. The incidence of monetary claims as a consequence of claimed hearing loss has grown tremendously in recent years, justifying the use of such tests.

A different form of audiometry is called impedance audiometry. In regular audiometry, the sound goes through the external ear (ear canal) to the eardrum and vibrates it; the sound bouncing back from the eardrum is not taken into account. The impedance audiometer measures the reflected sound and can help detect whether a hearing problem comes from the middle, rather than the inner, ear. Then there is Békésy audiometry; here, the patient, in a sense, performs the test by controlling the sound volume through the earphones while the tones change. This test helps determine if a hearing loss comes from the middle ear, the inner ear, or the nerve from the inner ear to the brain.

Certain additional tests for hearing loss, some of which are also used to uncover malingering, include: swinging voice, where, as a story is read to the listener through earphones, part of the story is sent first to one ear and then to the other to see whether it makes sense and whether or not all the words were heard; the delayed feedback test, where a recording is made of the individual reading a story that is then played back, through earphones, a fraction of a second later while the person tries to read the story again, to see if it causes confusion—which it will in someone trying to fake a hearing loss; the Stenger test, which may, by projecting the same volume of sound to both ears, reveal whether one ear's hearing really is bad and to what degree when there is a question of one ear's hearing less than the other; psychogalvanic skin resistance audiometry (sometimes called electrodermal audiometry), which is a unique way of unmasking malingerers as well as being a way of testing very young children who cannot cooperate with plain audiometry by giving the examinee a very slight electrical shock a second after making a sound through an earphone to see if he becomes "conditioned" to both sound and shock while a skin galvanometer measures sweat and temperature changes associated with the shock, for after several minutes, someone pretending to be deaf will show signs of sweating after the sound but prior to the shock.

When performed: Whenever there is difficulty in hearing, usually due to ear infection, an inherited condition, or excessive exposure to loud noises (as in certain occupations); following head injury.

Audiometer tests are now being performed in schools to screen out children with hearing loss at an early age.

Whenever ototoxic drugs are administered (antibiotics such as kanamycin, neomycin, ganamycin, and streptomycin; diuretic drugs such as Lasix; and even when large doses of salicylates are administered).

Normal values: For screening purposes only, two pure tones of 256 cps and 4,096 cps (encompassing the range of normal speech sounds) at 5 to 10 db are transmitted through the earphones (air conduction). Should the patient have difficulty in hearing either of these sounds, a more detailed audiogram is performed. Normally, an individual can hear lower tones (64 cps) at 1 to 2 db, higher tones (11,584 cps) at about 10 db, and all pure tones in between at 10 db or less. Air conduction hearing is usually better than bone conduction hearing.

Abnormal values: The inability to hear pure tones below 10 db indicates inner-ear or nerve damage. There are many different kinds of deafness; some people lose only the ability to perceive high tones or low tones; some lose only air or bone conduction hearing. Following injury or excessive noise exposure, high-tone hearing is usually lost. When deafness is inherited, hearing for the entire range of tones is missing. Following infection, the speech range is most commonly lost. Certain antibiotic drugs cause nerve deafness; if the drugs are not used over too long a period of time, hearing may return, but in some instances the medication can cause permanent deafness.

Risk factors: None.

Pain/discomfort: None.

Cost: Audiometry screening that uses only a few frequencies is $10 to $15. When the complete range of tones and volumes is employed, the cost is $40 to $50. The Lombard test is often used as a supplement to comprehensive audiometry; it averages an additional $10. Evoked response tests can cost from $100 to $300.

Normally, bone and air conduction tests are part of diagnostic audiology. When audiometry is used for hearing aid evaluation, the fee is $25 to $35.

Accuracy and significance: Hearing function tests, when properly performed with properly calibrated equipment, are 95 percent accurate in diagnosing the degree and specific location of a hearing problem. The Lombard test is particularly significant in revealing malingerers.

Note: There are literally scores of hearing function tests, from simple **Reflex** reactions such as the Moro response (where a loud noise is used to produce a "startle" embrace—the arms, hands, and fingers assume the position of an embrace—in an infant if the ability to hear is present) to tone decay testing, where it is noted if a continuous tone must be made louder in order to be heard—as a means of differentiating an inner-ear from an ear nerve problem. Today, most doctors can evaluate hearing function at the same time they examine the ears; the Audioscope (a special otoscope) allows a simple screening test that takes only a moment.

HEARTBURN, see *Gastroesophageal Reflux*

HEART-DISEASE-PRONE PERSONALITY, see *Jenkins Activity Survey*

HEART SCAN, see *Nuclear Scanning*

HEAVY METAL SCREENING, see *Mercury*

HEINZ BODY STAIN, see *Hemoglobin*

HEMA-CHEK, see *Occult Blood*

HEMATOCRIT

The hematocrit shows the percentage of blood cells (mostly red blood cells) comprising the total blood volume. A blood sample from a vein is centrifuged (the solid matter is forced to the bottom of a specially marked tube, leaving the clear plasma in the upper section). In a sense, the test measures the viscosity (thickness) of the blood as well as the amount of fluid in the blood. Many doctors feel the hematocrit test is a better measure of anemia than the **Hemoglobin** test, especially if the patient's diet includes normal amounts of iron.

At times, the total blood volume is measured; this includes the hematocrit plus the plasma volume. This test is usually performed following surgery, where there has been a large loss of blood, after severe heart failure, and especially when a patient is in shock; it also helps confirm abnormal hematocrit values.

When performed: In diagnostic screening for anemias and dehydration; to follow the course of therapy for anemias and hemorrhage.

Normal values: Normal hematocrit readings range from 40 percent to 55 percent (slightly lower in women).

Abnormal values: Low hematocrit readings (decreased percentage of total cells) are found in red blood cell anemias, immediately after hemorrhage, and whenever there is excessive fluid intake. High hematocrit readings are found in severe dehydration and polycythemia, angina, and after surgery, trauma, or burns and in heavy smokers.

Risk factors: Negligible (see general risk factors for blood testing).

Pain/discomfort: Minimal (see general pain/discomfort factors for blood testing).

Cost: from $3 to $7; most laboratories automatically include a hemoglobin level with the hematocrit report. It is usually included in **Comprehensive Multiple Test Screening** panels, which range from $7 to $42.

Accuracy and significance: Basically, the test screens for indications of anemia. The patient's fluid intake for several hours prior to the test must be considered, as either dehydration or an excess of liquid can produce false values. An abnormal result should be followed by more appropriate tests; on its own, a hematocrit value has no real significance. Considered to be about 80 percent accurate.

HEMIANOPIA, see *Visual Field*

HEMOCCULT, see *Occult Blood*

HEMOCHROMATOSIS, see *Iron*

HEMOGLOBIN

There are many different forms of hemoglobin in the blood; these forms are usually measured together as the total hemoglobin. Hemoglobin is an iron protein substance manufactured inside newly forming red blood cells and stored there for the life of the cells. Because of its unique affinity for oxygen, its task is to pick up oxygen as the red blood cells pass through the lungs and deliver that oxygen to tissue cells throughout the body.

The amount of oxygen the blood can carry depends not only on the amount of hemoglobin present but also on its effectiveness. Exposure to toxic substances can alter the hemoglobin molecule; carbon monoxide gas will easily replace oxygen attached to hemoglobin and form carboxyhemoglobin, preventing any vital oxygen from reaching tissue cells. Carboxyhemoglobin turns the blood (and sometimes the skin) a brilliant red. The Katyama test distinguishes between carboxyhemoglobin and hemoglobin. Testing for **Carbon Monoxide** in the blood can also be performed by measuring its content in the breath; there are several instruments that do this. The test results are considered as accurate as blood testing and are less expensive. Incidentally, it is possible to measure the effect of passive smoking (simply being near someone who is smoking can cause carbon monoxide damage in an adjacent person's lungs and blood) by testing for cotinine (a metabolic product of nicotine) in the urine of a nonsmoker.

Methemoglobin forms when the red blood cells are exposed to certain drugs (especially nonprescription ones such as phenacetin and other aspirin substitutes) or to large amounts of nitrates that are used to treat heart disease and as food preservatives. Methemoglobin picks up oxygen but will not release it to the tissues, making the skin appear bluish. Aspirin-substitute drugs and certain laxatives containing sulfur can cause sulfhemoglobin; this differs from methemoglobin only in that it cannot be treated and stays in the blood until the red blood cells break down. Because of the many drugs that can result in the formation of methemoglobin, a condition that can be fatal if not treated immediately, a new, rapid test to detect this form of hemoglobin consists of diluting the blood cells with water in order to break them and then adding potassium cyanide to the solution. If the brown-colored blood (usually present with methemoglobin) turns red, it confirms the diagnosis.

Hemoglobin S is associated with sickle-cell anemia; when detected, it usually indicates an inherited inability of red blood cells to carry sufficient oxygen to body tissues. There are several specific screening tests to help diagnose sickle-cell anemia (Sickledex, Sickle-I.D. System, Sicklequik); these tests may also uncover a sickle-cell trait in carriers of the disease (while it is believed that more than 50,000 people in the United States have sickle-cell anemia, it is also estimated that more than 2.5 million Americans carry the sickle-cell trait without showing any signs of the disease). Sickle cells may also be observed through the microscope during the **Red Blood Cell** test; they resemble a farmer's sickle. Abnormally shaped sickle cells can also plug up tiny arteries in the hands, feet, and abdomen, causing inadequate circulation and producing excruciating pain.

There are some popular misconceptions about sickle-cell disease. The disease exists where there is sickle-cell anemia; here, both parents have passed on a sickle-cell gene to the child, and almost all the hemoglobin is hemoglobin S. At times, only one sickle-cell gene can be paired with another abnormal hemoglobin gene called hemoglobin C; this, too, can cause the disease. If a sickle-cell gene and a thalassemia gene (hemoglobin A) are passed on to the child, sickle-cell-thalassemia disease usually results. In contrast, if only one sickle-cell gene is inherited, from one parent, and a normal hemoglobin gene is inherited from the other parent, disease rarely exists; instead, the child has sickle-cell trait and should he mate with someone also carrying a sickle-cell gene, it could result in sickle-cell disease in the offspring.

Hemoglobin A or A-2 may be increased or decreased in the presence of one of the two forms of thalassemia (sometimes called Mediterranean anemia, because it was first discovered in people living adjacent to the Mediterranean Sea, or Cooley's anemia, after Dr. Thomas Benton Cooley), a form of erythroblastic anemia, indicating the type of red blood cells involved. The condition, an inherited disease in which hemoglobin is not properly or adequately formed, can cause stillbirth and severe blood problems in later life.

A Heinz body stain is sometimes mixed with blood to help confirm the diagnosis of an anemia, especially **Glucose 6-Phosphate Dehydrogenase**. A Dr. Heinz, of Germany, discovered the stain that would reveal unusual attachments to **Red Blood Cells** in the presence of certain anemias.

Note: A new test, called the glycerol lysis test, first proposed in 1974, has recently been shown to be more than 95 percent accurate in differentiating between the thalassemia trait and ordinary iron-deficiency anemia; it is considered to be a simple, inexpensive way of screening for thalassemia.

Fetal hemoglobin is the oxygen-carrying iron in the fetus; it almost disappears in adulthood but remains in large quantities when there are various blood diseases.

Iron in the diet is the primary source of hemoglobin; replacement iron is necessary when there is blood loss such as with injury or menstruation.

Whenever there is a decreased amount of hemoglobin in the body (the blood carries less oxygen), the heart usually compensates by increasing its effort to circulate blood (the pulse rate becomes more rapid). Only one drop of whole blood—which can be taken from the fingertip, earlobe, or heel—is needed for the test. Hemoglobin can, of course, be evaluated from blood taken for any other procedure. It is also looked for in urine as an indication of bleeding or poisoning.

At times, especially after a muscle injury—or even after excessive exercise—myoglobin, a protein molecule similar to hemoglobin, is released into the blood and ultimately is found in urine. This product may be tested for when muscle damage—even heart muscle damage—is suspected; it is usually performed along with **Creatine Phosphokinase**.

When performed: Primarily when there is suspicion of anemia, no matter what kind or what the cause; to aid in the diagnosis of many inherited conditions; to distinguish certain poisonings from disease; as an indication of how much blood has been lost after injury or surgery. A few states require newborn babies to be tested for sickle-cell anemia; these include Arizona, Colorado, Georgia, Louisiana, New Mexico, New York, North Carolina, Texas, and Wyoming (see **Red Blood Cell**).

Normal values: Total hemoglobin levels for men range from 14 to 18 g per 100 ml; for women, 12 to 15 g per 100 ml. Up to 1 percent carboxyhemoglobin or fetal hemoglobin may be present, but no more than 0.1 percent of methemoglobin or sulfhemoglobin should be detected. The urine should contain no hemoglobin.

Abnormal values: Serum hemoglobin is sometimes increased when red blood cells are suddenly damaged or destroyed, as with sickle-cell disease or the Rh anemia of infancy. Polycythemia (a disease characterized by excessive red blood cells) may result in increased hemoglobin.

Hemoglobin values are decreased in almost all forms of anemia, especially those associated with iron deficiency. Symptoms of anemia usually do not appear until the hemoglobin level goes below 8 g per 100 ml. Hemoglobin is decreased in leukemia, after hemorrhage, and in pregnancy (especially after delivery, when there is loss of blood).

Heavy cigarette smoking may cause carboxyhemoglobin values up to 20 percent, markedly reducing the amount of normal hemoglobin. Thus, the test is often used as a check on people who smoke but who deny the fact.

Risk factors: Negligible (see general risk factors for blood testing).

Pain/discomfort: Minimal (see general pain/discomfort factors for blood testing).

Cost: An undifferentiated hemoglobin test ranges from $3 to $38; often, there is no charge when the doctor performs the test in the office from fingertip blood. It is usually included in **Comprehensive Multiple Test Screening** panels, which range from $7 to $42. When the multiple forms of hemoglobin are differentiated, the fee is $7 to $80, depending on the type of hemoglobin that is isolated and measured.

Accuracy and significance: Total (undifferentiated) hemoglobin is simply a screening test for anemia and, on its own, has no specific significance. However, tests for particular forms of hemoglobin are 90 percent accurate and can be lifesaving.

HEMOGLOBIN A_1, A_{1c}, see *Glycohemoglobin*

HEMOGRAM, see *Blood Cell Differential; Hematocrit; Hemoglobin; Red Blood Cell; Red Blood Cell Indices; White Blood Cell*

HEMOLYSIS, see *Haptoglobin*

HEMOPHILIA, see *Partial Thromboplastin Time; Fibrinogen*

HEMOQUANT, see *Occult Blood*

HEMOSIDERIN, see *Haptoglobin*

HEPARIN, see *Coagulometer; Partial Thromboplastin Time*

HEPATIC COMA, see *Number Connection*

HEPATITIS

Hepatitis is an acute and extremely serious infection of the liver primarily caused by several liver-specific viruses. It can also come from parasites, bacteria, drugs, alcohol, and some metabolic disorders. Different viruses, such as those that cause infectious mononucleosis and those known as **Cytomegaloviruses** that produce congenital defects and encephalitis, can also cause hepatitis. Depending on which strain of hepatitis-specific virus inflames the liver, the condition is called type A, or infectious, hepatitis or endemic hepatitis, when type A virus is at fault; when type B virus is the culprit, the disease is usually referred to as type B, or serum, hepatitis. There is a third form of hepatitis, called non-A, non-B, that seems to occur largely after blood transfusions. (It is not labeled type C because it is thought that more than one new virus is responsible.)

Type A hepatitis is commonly spread by contaminated feces that pollute water supplies and foods, particularly shellfish that are eaten raw. It can also be communicated from person to person, but it is rare to find a type-A hepatitis carrier similar to the typhoid carrier. Type A, which strikes children and young adults most frequently, is not as serious a disease as type B. One injection of type-A-specific immune serum, gamma globulin, prior to possible exposure to the virus can prevent the illness. Type-

B hepatitis, on the other hand, is a very severe disease that can occur at any age. Although symptoms may not appear for months following exposure and infection, they can be so slight they are easily overlooked. Most often, the disease is acquired from contact with infected blood (or from improperly sterilized needles or other medical instruments that have had contact with infected blood). Type-B hepatitis is easily transmitted through sexual contact. There is now a vaccine to help protect against hepatitis-B.

It is easy to have hepatitis and not know it. At first, the signs and symptoms resemble influenza. If there is no evidence of jaundice and the urine does not turn dark, the condition can come and go without being diagnosed. This is potentially dangerous, as even a mild case of hepatitis can lead to severe liver damage months or even years later. There are several specific antigen and antibody tests for hepatitis (to understand the antigen-antibody testing principles, see **Agglutination**). When the tests are performed as a panel, they reveal whether the patient has been exposed to hepatitis; the specific type of hepatitis virus; whether the infection exists at that moment; whether the disease is in an early or late stage; whether the patient is a carrier; whether recovery is taking place. The tests examine blood from a vein for:

HAV (hepatitis A virus)
HAVAb (hepatitis A antibody)
HAVAb-M (the specific immunoglobulin M hepatitis antibody)
HBcAb or Anti-HBc (hepatitis-B core antibody)
HBeAg (hepatitis-B core antigen)
HBsAb or Anti-HBs (hepatitis-B surface antibody)
HBsAg, formerly called Australian antigen, or AU (hepatitis-B surface antigen)

The terms *core* and *surface* refer to the body and the outer layer of the hepatitis virus. Tests for the specific virus in the feces are also performed.

Recently, a new hepatitis virus has been discovered; it is called the "delta" virus, and it seems to cause an infection only in the presence of the hepatitis-B-type virus. It occurs primarily among drug abusers who inject their drugs—as opposed to those who take drugs orally or inhale them. A test to diagnose this new, severe form of the disease is expected to be available in 1986.

When performed: When undiagnosed flulike illness persists; when unexplained jaundice and/or dark urine is observed; to distinguish between the various types of hepatitis; to protect against subsequent chronic liver disease such as cirrhosis or cancer; to detect carriers of the disease (food handlers, blood donors, medical staff personnel, and patients with certain inherited metabolic defects).

Normal values: No antigen or antibodies of the hepatitis virus should be present; when antibodies alone are detected, it is usually indicative of an inactive hepatitis infection, but additional tests must be performed to ascertain if the patient is a symptomless carrier. No virus particles should be found in the feces examination.

Abnormal values: The detection, along with the quantity, of hepatitis antigens and/or antibodies reveals that the disease is, or was, present; the specific type of causative virus; the stage of the disease (even if in the incubation period before symptoms appear); and whether a carrier state exists. Virus particles are most often found in the incubation period.

Risk factors: Negligible (see general risk factors for blood testing).

Pain/discomfort: Minimal (see general pain/discomfort factors for blood testing).

Cost: From $15 to $50 for any one antigen or antibody test; $50 to $70 for each screening panel or diagnostic profile of four different tests. Viral cultures, usually from the feces, range from $50 to $90. The HBsAg antigen, formerly called the Australian antigen, is occasionally included in **Comprehensive Multiple Test Screening** panels, which range from $7 to $42.

Accuracy and significance: The tests, when performed as a panel, are considered 95 percent accurate. The HBcAb test has since been shown to be only about 12 percent accurate. However, as with many tests to diagnose infection, failure to detect any hepatitis antigen or antibody is not conclusive evidence that the disease is not present. The test can be especially significant in light of the fact that between 5 and 10 percent of all patients who receive transfusions contract hepatitis, usually of the subclinical (not obvious) variety, and that 25 percent of these develop subsequent liver damage.

Note: In 1984, the guanase test was introduced to help differentiate hepatitis from cirrhosis. While a positive result is a fairly accurate indicator of liver disease (a negative test is considered to eliminate the possibility of a liver problem), it did not prove very reliable in distinguishing between the different types of liver involvement.

HEROIN, see *Drug Abuse*

HERPES

There are several different but related herpes viruses. The first, and probably the best known, is herpes simplex I (or herpes virus hominus type I). It is the cause of the common cold sore (fever blister) that frequently appears on the lips, in and around the mouth, and sometimes in the throat. Most often, those who acquire a herpes simplex I infection do so before the age of 5 and then have recurrences throughout their lives. In most instances, the sores heal within a week or two. Herpes simplex II (herpes virus hominus type II) causes sores similar to cold sores but they are almost always in, on, and around the genital organs and urinary passageways. Today, herpes genitalis, as herpes simplex II is also known, is considered one of the most potentially dangerous sexually transmitted diseases (formerly called venereal diseases). Not only can it cause spontaneous abortion, especially in the first months of pregnancy, but it can also cause terrible damage to the newborn infant (congenital malformations, nerve and brain infections, skin conditions of such severity that they are usually fatal, and myriad eye problems). It is also believed that herpes simplex II may cause cancer of the cervix. The third herpes virus, varicella-zoster virus (VZV), is the cause of chicken pox as well as herpes zoster, better known as shingles because of the narrow layers of blisterlike skin eruptions that appear around the trunk or extremities of the body when the virus travels down the nerves to the skin surface. While chicken pox is commonly a disease of childhood, herpes zoster is largely a disease of late middle age. Next, there is herpes virus simiai, primarily the cause of a disease in monkeys in captivity, but a condition that can bring on encephalitis and herpes zoster–like symptoms in humans if they are bitten by infected monkeys. Other viruses thought to be part of the herpes family include **Cytomegalovirus** and the Epstein-Barr virus, which causes **Mononucleosis.**

While scrapings from skin lesions can be examined under the microscope to reveal specific cell characteristics, and it is also possible to culture and identify the virus, the most common tests to aid in diagnosis are those blood tests (usually on blood drawn from a vein) related to **Complement Fixation** and **Agglutination** that detect specific antibodies for each type of virus.

When performed: When a patient has blisterlike lesions around the genitals; when there is undiagnosed fever, lymph gland swelling, or an unusual pattern of skin eruptions; as part of the **TORCH** screening panel for pregnant women and newborn infants; in instances of unusual nerve or eye disease.

Normal values: No, or very low amounts of, herpes antibodies. No change in antibody amounts (titers) when the test is performed in two stages two to three weeks apart, the second test being conducted well after the onset of suspicious signs and symptoms. No isolation of the virus.

Abnormal values: Large amounts of the specific antibodies, especially an increased amount after several weeks; any physical evidence of the virus, such as its culture.

Risk factors: Negligible (see general risk factors for blood testing).

Pain/discomfort: Minimal (see general pain/discomfort factors for blood testing).

Cost: A single antibody test for each virus averages $30 to $80; cultures are $22 to $90; microscopic examination of the blisters is $10 to $50.

Accuracy and significance: Considered 90 percent accurate if antibodies are found, and particularly if the antibody level increases within a few weeks, Skin lesion examinations are considered about 80 percent accurate when the virus is isolated from a cell culture and almost as accurate when cell changes induced by the virus are seen. (See **Tzanck Smear.**)

HETEROPHILE AGGLUTINATION, see *Agglutination*

HETEROPHILE ANTIBODY, see *Mononucleosis*

HETEROTROPIA, see *Strabismus*

HGH, see *Growth Hormone*

HIAA, see *Serotonin*

HIATUS HERNIA, see *Gastroesophageal Reflux*

HIGH BLOOD PRESSURE, see *Blood Pressure*

HIGH-DENSITY LIPOPROTEIN, see *Cholesterol; Lipoproteins*

HINTON, see *Syphilis*

HIRSCHBERG, see *Strabismus*

HISTAMINE, see *Cancer*

HISTAMINE ACID, see *Gastric Analysis*

HISTIDINEMIA, see *Aminoaciduria*

HISTOCOMPATIBILITY ANTIGENS, see *HLA*

HISTOPLASMOSIS, see *Agglutination; Skin Reaction*

HIVES, see *Tartrazine Sensitivity*

HLA (HL-Antigen, Histocompatibility Antigens)

Some white blood cells (leukocytes) and platelets contain antigens (disease-causing material) that initiate the formation of antibodies (disease-fighting material). These antigens are called human leukocyte locus A, or HLA, antigens. (Originally, only one antigen location was discovered on a gene, and it was called "A"; since then, additional HLA antigens have been found on locations other than "A.") Antileukocytic antibodies can be tested for by **Agglutination** or **Complement Fixation** or by combining the suspected blood serum with lymphocytes (a particular type of **White Blood Cell**) and noting if the lymphocytes are destroyed, indicating the presence of an HLA antibody.

The test is also used to determine histocompatibility, or whether the cells of tissues and organs from one person will "take" when transplanted into another person. There are many different HLA antigens (approaching 100 at present), and the closer the donor-recipient agreement of HLAs, the better the chance that a transplant will not be rejected. Blood is taken from a vein for testing.

When performed: Primarily prior to any organ transplant operation (kidney, heart, or skin grafting); prior to some blood transfusions; with undiagnosed high-fever illnesses, arthritis, and anemia; as part of the many **Disputed Parentage** tests (each person inherits four basic HLA antigens).

Normal values: There are no specific normal values; either the various HLA antigens are present or they are not.

Abnormal values: The greater the number of HLA typing dissimilarities, the less the chance that an organ transplant will take or that a skin graft will heal properly.

Different HLA antigens have been associated with certain diseases. HLA-B27 is found in almost all cases of ankylosing spondylitis (an arthritic condition primarily of the sacroiliac joint and the spine); Reiter's syndrome (a disease, primarily found in men, that is characterized by an infection of the urethra with a discharge from the penis and an infection of the eye and the joints); in certain forms of arthritis in children prior to adolescence; and in a particular form of joint pain that occurs along with an infection of the bowels. A positive HLA-B27 is rarely found with true rheumatic disease. HLA-B13 and HLA-B17 (and occasionally, HLA-B27) are usually found in patients with the arthritis of psoriasis. HLA-B7 is increased in patients with pernicious anemia. HLA-A2 is increased in patients with myasthenia gravis. HLA-B8 seems to be associated with dermatitis herpetiformus and systemic lupus erythematosus; it is also positive in many hormone disorders (thyroid, adrenal, and diabetes). Recently, it has been found in patients with myasthenia gravis and hepatitis.

Risk factors: Negligibile (see general risk factors for blood testing).

Pain/discomfort: Minimal (see general pain/discomfort factors for blood testing).

Cost: From $30 to $50 for each HLA antigen detection. Detection of four or more HLA antigens ranges from $200 to $300.

Accuracy and significance: While HLA detection and typing can be of considerable value in tissue transplant matching and in helping solve disputed parentage cases, it has no real significance in the specific diagnosis of any one disease. Some 20 percent of the population seems to have a positive HLA-B8 test without any evidence of disease. However, there are doctors who believe a positive HLA-B27 is better than 80 percent accurate in diagnosing ankylosing spondylitis and Reiter's syndrome, albeit it is not as accurate in black people.

HOLLANDER, see *Gastric Analysis; Gastroesophageal Reflux*

HOLTER MONITORING, see *Electrocardiogram*

HOLTZMAN INKBLOT TECHNIQUE, see *Rorschach*

HOMATROPINE, see *Tonometry*

HOMOCYSTINURIA, see *Aminoaciduria*

HOMOVANILLIC ACID, see *Catecholamines*

HOT BATH

Multiple sclerosis is a difficult disease to diagnose. Although **Immunoglobulins,** when tested for in cerebrospinal fluid, can help to confirm the diagnosis, the hot bath test is more a clinical—or direct-observation—means of determining the cause of suspicious neurological manifestations such as eye muscle and vision changes, weakness, skin tingling, and speech difficulties. Knowing that most patients with multiple sclerosis experience an increase in the severity of their symptoms, along with an increase in muscle problems observable by their doctors, when their body temperature increases, the hot bath test is used to deliberately raise the patient's body temperature. Initially, the patient lies in a bath with the water temperature at 100° F (38° C). The temperature is then raised about a degree at a time while the arms, legs, and especially the eyes are closely observed. Within 15 minutes, the temperature reaches 110° F (43° C), at which point it is cooled to the starting temperature. **Blood Pressure** and **Pulse** measurements are also recorded.

When performed: When multiple sclerosis is suspected; to help evaluate the cause of various eye, especially eye muscle, problems together with other difficult-to-diagnose muscle weakness in the extremities; when the patient has speech difficulties that might be linked to the speech muscles.

Normal values: Normally, a person shows no muscle or vision changes when immersed in a hot bath, even when the water temperature is raised.

Abnormal values: When the water temperature is raised more than 1°, multiple sclerosis patients experience various signs and symptoms of the disease—either for the first time or, if they had been present before, to a much worse degree. Vision becomes impaired; the eyelids may be difficult to hold open; the eyeball may suddenly move from side to side; one or more of the extremities may become extremely weak and seem paralyzed; speech may be difficult. Usually, the appearance or exaggeration of the patient's symptoms occurs when the temperature is increased 1° to 2°.

Risk factors: Usually none, although some patients undergo changes in pulse and/or blood pressure that can produce weakness or palpitations. There have been reports of a few patients whose exacerbated symptoms persisted for more than 24 hours after cooling of the bath water; this rare phenomenon must be kept in mind. In 1985, there were new reports of permanent or prolonged neurological complications in some patients after undergoing the hot bath test.

Pain/discomfort: Minimal unless the hot water exacerbates latent symptoms to the point of discomfort.

Cost: It depends on where the test is performed. If the neurologist's office is equipped with a bathtub, there is usually no charge over and above the examination fee. If performed in a hospital, there is usually a charge of $25 to $50 in addition to the doctor's fee.

Accuracy and significance: Because a multiple sclerosis diagnosis is commonly made by observation, this test is considered significant in assisting the doctor to come to a conclusion. It has been reported that more than 60 percent of patients with multiple sclerosis will show abnormal values when hot-bath-tested, while only 1 percent of "normal" people will show an abnormal value. But the test is not considered standardized, and some doctors regard it as a poor test.

Note: A more recent laboratory test for multiple sclerosis is called the E-UFA test (the letters stand for erythrocyte-unsaturated fatty acid), where **Red Blood Cells** are tested by electrophoresis (see **Albumin/Globulin**) to note changes in their motility. Some doctors feel that multiple sclerosis is an inherited inability to metabolize unsaturated fatty acids.

HOT CALORIC, see *Caloric*

HPL, see *Placental Lactogen*

HPRL, see *Prolactin*

HRR, see *Color Blindness*

HTLV-III ANTIBODIES, see *Acquired Immunodeficiency Syndrome*

HUHNER, see *Semen*

HUMAN CANCER MARKERS, see *Cancer*

HUMAN CHORIONIC GONADOTROPIN, see *Pregnancy; Testis Function*

HUMAN CHORIONIC SOMATOMAMMOTROPHIN, see *Placental Lactogen*

HUMAN GROWTH HORMONE, see *Growth Hormone*

HUMAN LEUKOCYTE LOCUS A, see *HLA*

HUMAN PLACENTAL LACTOGEN, see *Placental Lactogen*

HUMAN T-LYMPHOTROPIC VIRUS TYPE III, see *Acquired Immunodeficiency Syndrome*

HUMAN TUMOR STEM CELL ASSAY, see *Estrogen Receptor*

HVA, see *Catecholamines*

HYDROCHLORIC ACID, see *Gastric Analysis*

HYDROGEN BREATH, see *Lactose Tolerance*

HYDROGEN ION CONTENT, see *pH*

HYDROXYBUTYRIC DEHYDROGENASE (HBD)

Alpha-hydroxybutyric dehydrogenase is one of the many enzymes that appear in increased amounts in the serum subsequent to tissue damage. The HBD test is similar to the **Lactic Dehydrogenase** test in that it is supposed to be specific in diagnosing a heart attack, although the enzyme also increases slightly with liver disease, leukemia, and some cancers. It usually shows an abnormal rise within 12 hours after a heart attack and persists in an elevated state for up to a month. Blood is taken from a vein, and the serum is tested.

When performed: Primarily as a confirmatory measure when a heart attack is suspected.

Normal values: Levels of 150 to 300 units per ml are considered normal.

Abnormal values: Levels usually rise to over 300 units per ml within 24 hours after a heart attack, reaching a peak, sometimes as high as 1,000 units per ml, in three days and then returning to normal during the next three weeks.

Risk factors: Negligible (see general risk factors for blood testing).

Pain/discomfort: Minimal (see general pain/discomfort factors for blood testing).

Cost: From $10 to $20.

Accuracy and significance: A fairly insignificant test (accuracy less than 50 percent); used only to confirm a heart attack when other enzyme tests are equivocal. It has no other real significance in medicine.

HYDROXYPROLINE

Hydroxyproline is an amino acid (one of the basic building blocks of proteins). It is unique in that it exists mostly in collagen, a substance found in bone and in slightly smaller amounts in the skin. While hydroxyproline levels are primarily an indication of a bone condition or bone disease, the test can also be used to search for certain inherited conditions. Although hydroxyproline can be found in the blood, the test is most often performed on urine.

When performed: When defects of bone metabolism are suspected (usually increased production or increased reabsorption of bone substance); after bone fractures; to follow the treatment of Paget's disease (an inflammation of the bones that causes deformation and bowing of arm and leg bones); to help diagnose rickets (vitamin D deficiency) and to follow the results of treatment; to aid in the diagnosis of certain inherited conditions such as Marfan's syndrome (a disease whose major feature is abnormally long bones).

Normal values: Total hydroxyproline levels range from 10 to 75 mg in a 24-hour specimen of urine.

Abnormal values: Increased amounts of hydroxyproline in the urine are found in most conditions where excessive bone structure is being made or repaired (fractures in children during normal growth, Marfan's syndrome, Paget's disease, and certain hormone problems). A decrease in hydroxyproline levels during treatment for certain bone diseases indicates successful therapy.

Risk factors: Negligible (see general risk factors for blood testing).

Pain/discomfort: Minimal (see general pain/discomfort factors for blood testing).

Cost: Total hydroxyproline tests are $15 to $80. At times, free hydroxyproline is also measured at a charge of $50 to $60.

Accuracy and significance: Only in the first few months of life is a blood test more accurate than a urine test. After that period, urine tests are 90 percent accurate in detecting abnormal levels of hydroxyproline. The test is quite significant in helping diagnose inherited defective metabolic diseases.

HYDROXYTRYPTAMINE, see *Serotonin*

HYPERGLYCEMIA, see *Glucose*

HYPERHIDROSIS, see *Sweat*

HYPERLIPIDEMIA, see *Lipids*

HYPERMETROPIA, see *Visual Acuity*

HYPEROPIA, see *Visual Acuity*

HYPEROXALURIA, see *Oxalate*

HYPERPARATHYROIDISM, see *Parathyroid*

HYPERTENSION, see *Blood Pressure*

HYPERTHYROIDISM, see *Thyroid Function*

HYPNOTIC DRUG, see *Barbiturates*

HYPOGLYCEMIA, see *Glucose*

HYPOGONADISM, see *Testis Function*

HYPOPARATHYROIDISM, see *Parathyroid*

HYPOTHERMIA, see *Body Temperature*

HYPOTHYROIDISM, see *Depression; Thyroid Function*

HYSTEROSALPINGOGRAPHY, see *Radiography*

HYSTEROSCOPY, see *Endoscopy*

I

ICD, see *Isocitric Dehydrogenase*

ICE CUBE, see *Allergy*

ICE WATER, see *Cold Pressor*

ICG, see *Bromsulphalein*

ICTERUS INDEX

Icterus means jaundice. The icterus index measures the color of the blood serum as a gauge of its **Bilirubin** (yellow-brown bile pigment) content. Blood is drawn from a vein, and the serum is compared with a standard solution of a normal serum color; the index is comparative density. While this test is considered outmoded by many physicians, it is still being performed; in most cases, direct bilirubin is used as a more specific measurement.

When performed: When there is enlarged liver, tender liver, or a suggestion of jaundice of skin or eyes.

Normal values: An index of 3 to 5 is considered normal.

Abnormal values: An elevated index, between 6 and 15, indicates latent jaundice (jaundice that may not be apparent by examining skin or eyes), as with early hepatitis. An index above 15 indicates both clinical jaundice and a nonspecific form of liver and/or gallbladder disease. An index below 3 indicates decreased bilirubin, as in malaria and anemias.

Risk factors: Negligible (see general risk factors for blood testing).

Pain/discomfort: Minimal (see general pain/discomfort factors for blood testing).

Cost: From $5 to $10.

Some doctors consider this test outmoded, and it is possible that a health insurance company or government-sponsored medical program will not reimburse the doctor or patient for the cost of the test.

Accuracy and significance: The test is seldom used, as so many superior liver-function tests are now available. However, it is performed occasionally for medical-legal purposes when it is necessary to record the biochemical and numerical progress or regression of jaundice. Considered to be 50 percent accurate.

ILLEGITIMACY, see *Parentage*

IMMUNE BODIES, see *Antinuclear Antibodies*

IMMUNE DEFICIENCY, see *Acquired Immunodeficiency Syndrome*

IMMUNITY

Immunity is a generalized term that indicates the body's ability to defend itself against disease. One type is called humoral (pertaining to body fluids, particularly blood and lymph), where antibodies (see **Immunoglobulin**) are specific—having been acquired from previous contact or immunization. Another type, cellular immunity, involves resistance to infectious diseases, cancers, allergies, and autoimmune conditions (see **Antinuclear Antibodies**). In addition to the antibodies that come from lymphocytes (see **Lymphocyte Typing**), substances in the skin and mucus from the respiratory and gastrointestinal tracts may also offer protective factors against disease-causing antigens (see **Agglutination** and **Complement**). Also see **Acquired Immunodeficiency Syndrome, Immunology, RAST, Skin Reaction,** and **White Blood Cell.**

IMMUNOGLOBULIN (Ig)

Immunoglobulins are the blood protein antibody particles (gamma globulins) of the body. They react with, protect against, and help destroy antigens, which can cause illness. An antigen may be a microorganism (bacteria, virus, fungus), a chemical, or a toxin given off by an invading microorganism. Usually, antibodies are specific; that is, they react only to a particular disease-causing substance (either a new substance or one that has previously attacked the body). Antibodies come from lymphocyte (white blood) cells.

Five major immunoglobulins can be tested for in the blood (a sixth disappears after birth); they are known by letters of the alphabet. IgG (immunoglobulin G), the most abundant type, responds to any foreign-body invasion and can also cause Rh anemia problems. IgA protects against virus and bacterial infections and can cause transfusion reactions. IgM is another response to infection; it also reacts to arthritis and is the primary complement antibody (see **Complement Fixation**). IgE is involved in allergic reactions such as asthma, hay fever, and skin rashes (see **RAST** and **Skin Reaction**). IgD can be isolated, but its action is still not understood.

The presence of immunoglobulin is the basis on which **Agglutination** tests determine specific diseases. Immunoglobulins are measured individually primarily for purposes of research; they can, however, confirm diagnostic suspicions. Blood is taken from a vein, and the serum is tested. Immunoglobulins are also tested in **Cerebrospinal Fluid**.

Note: Cryoglobulins are immunoglobulins that precipitate only in cold temperatures and are present primarily with blood vessel diseases.

When performed: When excessive gamma globulins (hypergamma-globulinemia) are found, as with leukemias, certain cancers, kidney problems, parasitic infections, and chronic infections; after surgery for cancer as a guide to progress; when multiple sclerosis is suspected (see **Albumin/Globulin**).

Normal values: Normal serum levels for the five major immunoglobulins are as follows:

IgG: 500 to 2,000 mg per 100 ml
IgA: 50 to 400 mg per 100 ml
IgM: 50 to 200 mg per 100 ml
IgE: 0.01 to 0.10 mg per 100 ml
IgD: 0.5 to 5 mg per 100 ml

Abnormal values: Immunoglobulins are increased as a result of infection, allergy, and various autoimmune conditions, in which the body in essence turns on itself and causes illness (as in systemic lupus erythematosus). After cancer surgery, an increase in immunoglobulins is usually a good prognostic sign. Immunoglobulins may be decreased with certain leukemias, cancers, and other conditions where immunity is lacking.

Risk factors: Negligible (see general risk factors for blood testing).

Pain/discomfort: Minimal (see general pain/discomfort factors for blood testing).

Cost: Total immunoglobulins range from $10 to $25. The test for IgE, which is usually performed separately, is $20 to $40. Tests for the individual immunoglobulins range from $15 to $54.

Accuracy and significance: Immunoglobulins exist in such minute quantities that they are difficult to measure. Furthermore, they respond to such a variety of infections and other diseases that, at present, their significance is of more academic than practical value. Yet in certain conditions, they help confirm diagnoses of suspected illnesses. Immunoglobulins, when measured in the spinal fluid, are considered 90 percent accurate for the early diagnosis of multiple sclerosis; however, the same immunoglobulins can also appear with several other diseases.

IMMUNOLOGICAL REACTIVE TRYPSINOGEN (IRT), see *Sweat*

IMMUNOLOGY

Freely translated, the word *immune* means to be "safe" (it literally means to be "free or exempt from something"). In medicine, it means to be safe from the adverse effects of bacteria, virus, pollen, etc., that can cause a disease. Immunology pertains to the study of immunity—be it natural or artificial (e.g., immunizations, allergy shots)—and now more so to the way the body responds to, and protects itself from, an antigen (see **Agglutination**) by producing antibodies to destroy the antigen. With the advent of new technology in laboratories, many doctors now order *immunological testing*. This is a general term for a variety of tests designed to help diagnose three categories of disease. First, there are the tests to uncover the cause of an infection, such as **Agglutination** and **Complement Fixation**; the immunological process is to detect the antibodies the body makes to attack the disease-causing antigens. (Such microorganisms as bacteria and viruses contain antigens.) Next are the immunology tests that encompass allergies—to food, pollen, dust, animals, chemicals, and drugs (see **RAST**). Last are the tests for those diseases doctors label autoimmune, in which the body tissues or cells produce their own "antigens," followed by antibodies that attempt to heal but may, in fact, cause greater damage than good. The **Antinuclear Antibodies** (ANA) test is a classic example of this immunological phenomenon, and systemic lupus erythematosus is considered the archetypal disease consequence.

As diagnostic skills become more sophisticated, scores of symptoms once attributed to viruses and unknown causes are now understood to be the consequences of immunological deviations. Bone aches, nerve pains, joint pains (some forms of arthritis are considered common immunological conditions), a multitude of skin conditions, especially mysterious rashes, rare forms of thyroid gland inflammation, certain kidney failures, unusual susceptibility to infections, a few anemias, odd muscle weaknesses, and even inexplicable stomach pains are but a few of the bodily manifestations that can now be attributed to immunological conditions. Today, it is incumbent upon the doctor to search for the immunological cause of disease when no other diagnosis is possible.

There are any number of immunology tests to ascertain if any circulating immune complexes are at work within a patient's body; the Raji-cell assay, the polyethylene glycol (PEG) assay, and the C1q solid-phase assay are among the terms used to describe exotic testing for autoantibodies (those manufactured by the body that then attack the body and cause illness). Other immunology tests described elsewhere in the book include:

Acquired Immunodeficiency Syndrome
Agglutination
Antinuclear Antibodies (ANA)
Complement
Complement Fixation
C-Reactive Protein
HLA
Immunoglobulin
Lymphocyte Typing
Macroglobulin
RAST
Rheumatoid Factor
Skin Reaction
Thyroid Function

Immunological tests are proliferating so rapidly it is difficult to keep abreast of them; many are tried and proved useless. However, if immunology testing is ordered, it is reasonable to assume a doctor is considering one of the autoimmune diseases as a diagnosis or is looking for a condition in which the body actually turns on itself and attacks certain of its organs, just as if some outside cause of disease were doing the same thing. Circulating immune complex tests range from $20 to $100.

IMPEDANCE AUDIOMETRY, see *Hearing Function*

IMPEDANCE PLETHYSMOGRAPHY, see *Plethysmography*

IMPOTENCE (Male)
Although most male impotence (inability to achieve an erection of the penis) is thought to be of a psychological nature, in a substantial number of instances, the problem has an organic (physical) basis or is caused by taking certain drugs. Alcohol, many medicines that treat high blood pressure, many tranquilizers, and most hormones can cause impotence and/or loss of libido. Specific drugs reported to cause loss of sexual desire and impotence in men and frigidity in women include guanethidine (Ismelin), methyldopa, clonidine (Catapres), rauwolfia and reserpine compounds, phentolamine, tolazoline, phenoxybenamine, propranolol (Inderol), Aldactone, and thiazide diuretics (for treating blood pressure and circulatory problems); the benzodiazepines and other minor tranquilizers such as Dalmane, Librium, Valium, Serax, and Tranxene; the phenothiazines and other major tranquilizers such as Mellaril; monoamine oxidase inhibitors, tricyclic drugs, and lithium (for treating depression); anticholinergic drugs (for treating and relaxing irritable stomach, bladder, and bowel as well as for glaucoma and parkinsonism); certain antibiotic drugs such as nitrofurantoin and ethionamide and parasite-killing drugs such as thiabendazole; drugs used to attack cancer cells; almost all narcotics; marijuana; and methadone.

Most tests for impotence are based on the principle that it is normal for a man to have penile erections during deep sleep and that the ability to do so is a fairly reliable indication that failure to achieve erection when awake is probably psychogenic. Before therapy can be administered for impotence, it must be determined if the cause is physical or psychological. While this is obviously important for education regarding human sexuality, it is particularly important subsequent to injuries to the genital area. After "straddle"-type accidents, many men feel the obvious physical damage has left them impotent; once they are made aware that they still have erections, albeit during sleep, they usually recover completely. Other situations necessitating some form of impotency test include a potential lawsuit in which the wife of a patient claims the doctor's treatment—be it surgery or medication—caused the couple to suffer "loss of consortorium," or the inability of the spouse to perform sexually.

One specific test requires the patient to spend at least three consecutive nights in a laboratory that has facilities for measuring REM (rapid eye movement) levels of sleep (the deepest stage) as well as nocturnal penile tumescence (swelling). Electrodes are placed on the head and are attached to silicone rings around the penis; measurements are made throughout the night during sleep. (See also **Plethysmography** and **Thermography**.)

Recently, a penile tumescence monitor has been introduced that allows a patient to take the portable typewriter-sized machine home, place the sensor rings around the penis at bedtime, and detect the number, size, and duration of any erections that occur during the night. The erections are recorded on a graph, which is sealed inside the machine. Later, a doctor can present the observations to the patient, together with appropriate explanations and reassurances. Some doctors use the machines in their offices to evaluate the effects of drugs on erectile failure. Many doctors, when faced with impotent patients, use a simple screening test prior to involved laboratory measurements. They advise the patient at bedtime to encircle the flaccid penis with a strip of postage stamps perforated along the side of the stamps and fasten the first and last as an overlap. The test is usually carried out for three successive nights. If the stamps come apart at the perforations during sleep, it can be assumed an erection occurred and there is no organic or physical basis for impotence. Alcohol or sleeping medications must not be used prior to performing the postage stamp test; these drugs tend to prevent REM levels of sleep, during which nocturnal erections are most apt to occur. A more precise, more scientific, stamp substitute device is now available. Called the Dacomed Snap-Gauge, it is a padded, Velcro-closed band that fits around the penis and can also reveal the degree of rigidity or intercourse capability. It is available from a doctor at a cost of from $25 to $30, and health insurance companies will usually reimburse you.

There is a new test to determine if impotence is caused by vascular, or blood flow, problems; these can accompany many other diseases such as diabetes and atherosclerosis. It is called the penile xenon washout because the radioactive gas xenon is injected into the base of the penis and then monitored by a scintillator (see **Nuclear Scanning**) to see how quickly it passes through the penile circulation. Normally, the gas rapidly disappears; with impotence caused by circulation problems, the gas remains four to five times longer. Patients are said not to find the test uncomfortable, and it is relatively inexpensive; the cost averages about $100. (Also see **Body temperature.**)

When performed: When impotence cannot be diagnosed; prior to surgical penile prosthesis implant insertion; following head, spinal cord, or back injuries; during the rehabilitation of some sex offenders.

Normal values: Most men have several penile erections during the night when in deep stages of sleep, especially while dreaming. Such a response indicates that there is no physical pathology or disease causing impotence.

Abnormal values: Failures to show any penile response after three days of testing indicates some physical basis for impotence. Normally, the number of nocturnal sleeping erections decreases in men over 50, but total absence indicates a drug, nerve, blood vessel, or spinal cord problem.

Risk factors: Most measuring instruments operate on such low voltage that no real risks are involved.

Pain/discomfort: Some men find it embarrassing to participate in all-night laboratory situations. Other men undergo extreme anxiety prior to, and during, the test.

Cost: When the tests are performed in a laboratory setting, the fee can reach $900 a night. When the portable machine is used at home, the cost ranges from $100 to $250 a night.

Some health insurance companies and government-sponsored medical programs will not reimburse the doctor or patient for some penile tumescence monitor tests because the technique is still considered to be of an experimental nature.

Accuracy and significance: The tests are about 80 percent accurate in detecting nocturnal erection. Their significance lies in helping to differentiate between physical and psychological impotence.

INCISIONAL BIOPSY, see *Biopsy*

INCOMPATIBLE TRANSFUSION, see *Typing and Cross-Matching*

INDIA INK STAIN, see *Culture*

INDICAN, see *Xylose Tolerance*

INDIRECT BILIRUBIN, see *Bilirubin*

INDOCYANINE GREEN, see *Bromsulphalein*

INFANT BOTULISM, see *Botulism*

INFECTION, see *Agglutination; Complement Fixation; Counterimmunoelectrophoresis; Culture; Gram Stain*

INFECTIOUS HEPATITIS, see *Hepatitis*

INFECTIOUS MONONUCLEOSIS, see *Mononucleosis*

INFERTILITY, see *Body Temperature; Estrogens; Rubin; Semen; Testis Function*

INFLUENZA, see *Virus Disease*

INFRARED INTERACTANCE, see *Anthropometric Measurements*

INHERITED DISEASE SCREENING, see *Genetic Disorder Screening*

INKBLOT, see *Rorschach*

INSECTICIDE POISONING, see *Cholinesterase*

INSECT STING, see *RAST*

INSULIN

Direct measurement of insulin in the blood is primarily an indication of the ability of the pancreas to secrete this hormone (the stomach can also secrete a very small amount) in response to carbohydrate foods, certain amino and fatty acids, and certain other hormones and drugs.

The patient is asked to fast for 12 hours before the test. Blood is taken from a vein, and the serum is tested. At times, the patient is then given a measured amount of glucose (sugar), and the blood insulin is measured every half-hour for 3 to 4 hours. The test cannot be performed on a patient taking insulin injections. The **C-Peptide** test can distinguish naturally produced insulin from injected, commercially produced insulin. (Also see **Glucose.**)

It is now possible to test for insulin antibodies (these are **Immunoglobulins**) to determine if a patient is inherently resistant to insulin and requires an unusually large amount of injected insulin.

When performed: When diabetes is suspected; when physical growth problems are evident; as an indication of whether certain oral antidiabetic drugs will work; when pancreatic disease, especially tumor, is suspected; to rule out hypoglycemia.

Normal values: After a 12-hour fast, the amount of serum insulin normally measures from 5 to 30 μU per ml. After glucose is given, blood insulin levels usually rise to more than 200 μU per ml within an hour and return to normal after 4 hours.

Abnormal values: Insulin levels are increased with an insulinoma (a tumor of insulin-producing cells), obesity, liver disease, and acromegaly (abnormally enlarged bones). Certain hormone drugs will also raise insulin levels, Insulin is lower than normal with diabetes, following surgery, after a heart attack, and when certain other hormones are absent from the body. Patients under emotional stress will also have reduced amounts of insulin secretion.

Risk factors: Negligible (see general risk factors for blood testing).

Pain/discomfort: Minimal (see general pain/discomfort factors for blood testing).

Cost: From $15 to $25. Insulin antibody testing is from $25 to $100.

Accuracy and significance: The test is 80 percent accurate in helping diagnose an insulinoma (pancreatic cancer). Its particular significance is in helping a doctor differentiate among the various types of diabetes (juvenile, adult-onset). Insulin antibody tests are of particular value in patients whose diabetes is unstable.

INSULIN ACIDITY, see *Gastric Analysis*

INSULIN ANTIBODY, see *Insulin*

INSULIN-CORTISOL SECRETION, see *Cortisol*

INSULIN PRODUCTION, see *C-Peptide*

INTELLIGENCE QUOTIENT (IQ)

The first mass use of the intelligence test was in France around 1900 as part of an effort by the government to distinguish children who could benefit from going to school from those who were considered too dull for an education. Today, there is little agreement on a universal definition of intelligence. It is generally recognized as an ability to make use of learning, reasoning, and memory in problem solving.

Most intelligence tests measure an individual's ability to learn in comparison with the ability of the general population. The IQ (intelligence quotient) is expressed by dividing the mental age (as determined in the test) by the chronological age (the actual age in years and months) and then multiplying the result by 100. Thus, a 10-year-old with average mental ability for that age would have an IQ of $10/10 \times 100 = 100$.

Numerous forms of IQ tests are in use today. The Stanford-Binet relies heavily on verbal ability in its scoring and is therefore considered deficient in recognizing an individual's strengths and special abilities. The Wechsler Intelligence Scale for Children (WISC) and the Wechsler Adult Intelligence Scale (WAIS) include both verbal and physical performance tests; it is felt that the combined verbal and performance scores offer a better individual profile than verbal scores alone. Performance measurements are especially valuable in testing the handicapped, young children, and people of foreign background with a limited knowledge of the language in which the test is given. Performance tests are considered better than verbal tests as predictors of adjustment, while verbal tests are considered better predictors of educational achievement.

Group intelligence tests used in schools and the military are not considered to yield results as accurate as individual tests. The group tests determine whether a subject is performing up to ability and is capable of taking on more advanced work. A few of the many group tests include the Army General Classification Test, the Otis Self-Administering Test of Mental Ability, the Kuhlmann-Anderson Intelligence Tests, and the Terman-McNemar Test of Mental Ability.

When performed: To assess the mental skills and learning ability of different individuals or groups; to discern dementia (physically caused mental deterioration).

Normal values: In general, IQ scores of 90 to 110 are considered average; a score of 140 or more is referred to as the genius level. On the average, the Wechsler scale results are about seven points below the Stanford-Binet scores. Other tests may vary slightly in scoring.

Abnormal values: IQ scores of 20 to 35 are considered indicative of severe mental retardation; 36 to 51, of moderate mental retardation; 52 to 67, of mild mental retardation; and 68 to 83, of borderline mental retardation. A person with a definite psychosis will have spotty responses (missing simple questions yet answering difficult ones). Senility due to arteriosclerosis will give a lowered score.

Risk factors: None.

Pain/discomfort: None.

Cost: In most instances, the fee depends upon the time required and ranges from $50 to $100.

Accuracy and significance: The results of any of the IQ tests should be evaluated with caution, especially if only one test is performed. Experience has shown that the patient's background and environment are important considerations. The tests are about 75 percent accurate and are no longer thought to be as significant as they once were. In certain instances, the courts have held that a person suffering embarrassment due to errors in the interpretation and reporting of an IQ can be compensated with a monetary award.

INTESTINAL ABSORPTION, see *Xylose Tolerance*

INTESTINAL DISACCHARIDASE DEFICIENCY, see *Lactose Tolerance*

INTRAATRIAL PACING, see *Radiography*

INTRACARDIAC ELECTROPHYSIOLOGIC, see *Electrocardiogram*

INTRACUTANEOUS, see *Skin Reaction*

INTRACUTANEOUS PROVOCATIVE, see *RAST*

INTRADERMAL, see *Skin Reaction*

INTRAOCULAR PRESSURE, see *Tonometry*

INTRATHECAL SCAN, see *Nuclear Scanning*

INTRAVENOUS PYELOGRAM, see *Radiography*

INTRINSIC FACTOR, see *Schilling*

INTRINSIC FACTOR BLOCKING ANTIBODY ASSAY, see *Schilling*

INULIN CLEARANCE, see *Creatinine*

IODINE, see *Thyroid Function*

IOWA TEST OF EDUCATIONAL DEVELOPMENT, see *Learning Disability*

IQ, see *Intelligence Quotient*

IRON

While the iron test is performed primarily to measure the amount of iron in the body, it is more a measure of the total iron-binding capacity, or the iron's availability to pick up oxygen from the lungs and deliver it to body tissues. Body iron is affected by pregnancy, blood loss, hemoglobin destruction, anemia, deficient iron in the diet, and poor intestinal absorption of iron even when dietary amounts are adequate. An average, balanced diet supplies about 10 mg of iron each day, but no more than 10 percent of that iron is normally absorbed by the intestines to be utilized. At the same time, the body loses about 1 mg of iron a day (through urine, feces, and sweat). Fortunately, the body usually has a large store of excess iron. Blood is collected from a vein, and either the serum or plasma is tested. When repeated iron tests are performed, it is essential that the blood samples be taken at the same time of the day. Iron values are usually highest in the morning, after sleep, and may be half the morning's value by evening. These findings are reversed for people who work nights and sleep days.

Other measures of blood and body iron are the serum iron-binding capacity (transferrin), or the specific amount of iron that can be carried in plasma; and the ferritin level, or the amount of iron stored in the body (primarily in the bone marrow). A patient can have a normal amount of iron, but that iron may not carry and deliver a sufficient amount of oxygen to the tissues.

A new way to help detect iron deficiency is by measuring differences in the size of the **Red Blood Cells**; normally, they are all about the same size. Called the red blood cell distribution width (RDW) test, it can be part of the routine red blood cell examination. Some doctors feel that variable-sized red blood cells are the very first sign of iron deficiency.

When performed: In searching for the specific cause of an anemia; when there is unexplained weakness and persistent tiredness; when the patient has a swollen, smooth, painful tongue; when monitoring patients on hemodialysis; when certain vitamin and other food deficiencies are suspected.

Normal values: Iron levels generally range from 75 to 175 mcg per 100 ml of serum. Normal values may vary depending on the laboratory's technique. The values may be slightly lower in women and children. Total iron-binding capacity ranges from 200 to 400 mcg per 100 ml. Serum ferritin ranges from 200 to 400 ng per 100 ml.

Abnormal values: Low blood values are found with anemia, infections, cancers, and pruritus (itching skin); after surgery; and in patients taking steroid drugs. Oral contraceptives, estrogens, or excessive dietary iron intake, especially from iron-fortified foods, may give elevated values. Extremely high levels of iron and iron-binding capacity are found with hemochromatosis, an inherited intestinal iron-absorption disease that can cause sufficient iron accumulation in the body so as to be fatal before the age of 30. Total iron-binding capacity is usually increased only with an iron-deficiency anemia; it is normal or decreased with other anemias. Total iron-binding capacity and transferrin may be artificially increased by birth control pills or other female hormones. Decreased ferritin is found with iron deficiency but not with anemia or infection; increased ferritin is found with excessive iron intake.

Risk factors: Negligible (see general risk factors for blood testing).

Pain/discomfort: Minimal (see general pain/discomfort factors for blood testing).

Cost: Total serum iron measurements are $5 to $10. Iron-binding capacity is $10 to $35; transferrin tests, $15 to $45. Iron testing is usually included in **Comprehensive Multiple Test Screening** panels, which range from $7 to $42; occasionally, iron-binding capacity and transferrin are also included in the panels. Ferritin tests are $15 to $20.

Accuracy and significance: Iron measurements alone are adequate for screening for anemia. In most instances, however, doctors make use of all the iron tests to reach a specific diagnosis, achieving a 90 percent accuracy rate.

IRON-BINDING CAPACITY, see *Iron*
ISHIHARA, see *Color Blindness*
ISOCITRIC DEHYDROGENASE

Testing for isocitric dehydrogenase (an enzyme found mostly in the liver) is particularly valuable in detecting and distinguishing liver disease. It can also reflect problems with the placenta during pregnancy. Most recently, it has been used to screen blood donors in order to eliminate the possibility of transmitting infectious hepatitis by blood transfusions. Blood is taken from a vein, and the serum is tested.

When performed: Primarily with suspected liver disease, especially to help differentiate disease that originates within the liver cells from disease that originates outside the liver (most commonly from the bile ducts) but that still reflects itself as liver pathology; when cancer of the liver, usually metastatic (migrated from another source), is suspected; during pregnancy as an indication of placenta problems.

Normal values: Normal levels range from 50 to 300 units per ml.

Abnormal values: Increased levels indicate liver disease, especially hepatitis or cancer. If a pregnant woman has no liver problem, an increase is a warning that something is wrong with the placenta.

Risk factors: Negligible (see general risk factors for blood testing).

Pain/discomfort: Minimal (see general pain/discomfort factors for blood testing).

Cost: From $15 to $25.

Accuracy and significance: With the advent of the newer **Hepatitis** tests and the greater use of **Amniocentesis,** this test is no longer widely used. However, it remains a significant measurement of liver disease when other liver function tests are equivocal. About 60 percent accurate.

ISOENZYMES, see *Aspartate Aminotransferase; Creatine Phosphokinase; Lactic Dehydrogenase*

ISOPROPYL ALCOHOL, see *Methanol*

ITAI-ITAI, see *Cadmium*

IVC, see *Radiography*

IVP, see *Radiography*

IVY BLEEDING TIME, see *Bleeding and Clotting Time*

J

JENKINS ACTIVITY SURVEY

Of the many factors being studied as potential indicators of increased risk of heart disease, especially heart attack, the psychological makeup of an individual is among those in the forefront. Studies of individual behavior patterns—particularly a person's competitiveness in activities such as employment, his ambitions, his attitudes toward time (sense of urgency), and even the way he speaks—have indicated two basic personality types in relation to heart disease risk. Type A is aggressive, highly competitive, always striving to get ahead, and extremely time-conscious. Type B is just the opposite: outwardly relaxed and seldom impatient. The Type B personality takes ample time for recreational activities and speaks more slowly and evenly than his Type A counterpart.

Doctors can sometimes determine a personality type by speaking with a patient over a perid of time and noting the nature of the patient's responses (especially the reaction to feigned hostility). The Jenkins Activity Survey provides a more standardized format for evaluating the coronary-prone personality. The test was first employed in 1965; since that time, nearly 100,000 people (primarily men) have taken it, demonstrating by the results that those who score as Type A have from five to eight times as many heart attacks as those who score as Type B.

The survey comprises 61 multiple-choice questions, which the patient completes in private. A sample question is: "Nowadays do you consider yourself to be (1) definitely hard-driving and competitive, (2) probably hard-driving and competitive, (3) probably relaxed and easygoing, or (4) definitely relaxed and easygoing?" The first answer indicates Type A; the second answer could be either Type A or Type B; the third answer is Type B; the fourth answer is rare.

There are now more than a dozen similar tests, including "structured" interviews as well as variations on the specific business and personal activities used to measure alleged coronary-prone behavior (socioeconomic status, social mobility, cultural background, and even smoking are predominant factors in some of the tests). Before the test is conducted, subjects should be told to view the questions as a measure of their attitudes and life ambitions rather than solely as a survey of heart disease potential.

A confirmatory test for the Type A personality is the Bortner test. Patients are asked to write a phrase, such as a familiar proverb, at their usual writing speed. They are then asked to write the same phrase slowly. Finally, they are asked to write it a third time as slowly as possible. Type A personalities seem unable to write very slowly; Type B perform the task with ease.

When performed: The survey is used primarily as a screening device to determine Type A or Type B personality traits, with particular association to heart disease. The test may be performed on healthy individuals and used as a future study or research index, or it may be performed on patients with known heart disease to help ascertain the test's validity. It may also be used to show a patient facets of his nature that he may be unaware of so he can better understand stress-inducing circumstances.

Normal values: While there are no normal values for such a test, obviously the more Type B answers, the less the individual reacts to stress in a supposedly unhealthy manner.

Abnormal values: Assuming the validity of the test in helping to detect coronary-prone individuals, the more Type A answers a person gives, the greater the risk of heart disease.

Risk factors: None.

Pain/discomfort: None.

Cost: Most doctors do not charge for this test when it is performed as part of an office visit.

Accuracy and significance: Although statistically, when Type A individuals are considered as a population, they seem to have a greater incidence of heart disease; when so-called Type A personalities are looked upon as individuals, there are many exceptions. Many Type A executives are not only content under pressure but show no signs of incipient heart disease. Conversely, those who are bored with their jobs and disappointed with their life achievements and do not fit in the Type A mold seem to have a high risk of heart disease. There are many people who do not fall into a Type A or Type B category, but unfortunately the Type A–Type B personality theory does not take these people into account. The test cannot be considered of great medical significance at this time and has no accuracy rating.

Note: Recently, the Jenkins Activity Survey has been applied to evaluate whether individuals with a Type A personality who had heart attacks had a better or worse prognosis (chance of, and degree of, recovery) than non–Type A's. The results showed no difference between Type A's and others when it came to how long both groups lived after the attack or how well the heart functioned after recovery took place.

JOINT ARTHROGRAPHY, see *Radiography*

JOINT FLUID, see *Synovial Fluid*

JOINT FLUID CULTURE, see *Culture*

JUGULAR VEIN PULSE, see *Pulse Analysis*

K

KAHN, see *Syphilis*

KALA-AZAR, see *Agglutination*

KAOLIN-CEPHALIN CLOTTING TIME, see *Partial Thromboplastin Time*

KARYOTYPING, see *Amniocentesis; Chromosome Analysis*

KATAYAMA, see *Hemoglobin*

KETONES (Ketone Bodies)

Ketones (two different acids and acetone) are produced in the body when glycogen (a form of carbohydrate) is not available to be utilized for energy. The body then draws upon its fat deposits, which are improperly oxidized and which then produce excessive amounts of ketones in both the blood and the urine. When insulin is absent or not immediately available to metabolize carbohydrates (as in diabetes), fats will be burned for body energy, creating more ketones than the body can utilize. Blood plasma from a vein is examined; urine is usually examined at the same time.

When performed: Especially when a patient is in a coma; to diagnose diabetic acidosis; when there is a question of toxemia in pregnancy; with hyperthyroidism and other metabolic abnormalities.

Since ketones are a "desirable" side effect of the no (or very low) carbohydrate, high protein and fat weight-loss diet, they are constantly tested for in the urine by the dieter as an indication that excess body fats are being metabolized.

Normal values: Ketones are not usually detected in the blood; however, up to 3 mg per 100 ml is considered within normal limits. There are very few ketones in the urine (125 mg per 24-hour sample, an amount that would not be detected by the usual urine acetone tests).

Abnormal values: More than 3 mg per 100 ml of serum is considered excessive. In diabetic acidosis, levels over 100 mg per 100 ml may be reached. Excessive ketones are found in the blood and urine in metabolic disorders, in starvation, and after a few days on a no-carbohydrate diet. They are also found in the urine with an inherited condition called maple syrup urine disease (the urine smells like fresh maple syrup) and with another inherited condition called renal glycosuria (the kidneys excrete sugar even though the blood sugar is normal). There may be a false elevation of ketones after administration of the **Bromsulphalein** test.

Risk factors: Negligible (see general risk factors for blood testing).

Pain/discomfort: Minimal (see general pain/discomfort factors for blood testing).

Cost: Blood tests for ketones average $9. Urine tests are usually performed with a paper dipstick; if performed in a doctor's office, there is usually no charge.

Accuracy and significance: Because ketones are found in so many abnormal conditions, they are significant only as a screening mechanism. They can be of value in following the progress of a diabetic who is unregulated; in this, they are 90 percent accurate.

KETOSTEROIDS, see *Cortisol*

KIDNEY SCAN, see *Nuclear Scanning*

KIDNEY STONE, see *Urinary Tract Calculus*

KINETOCARDIOGRAM, see *Apexcardiogram*

KISSING DISEASE, see *Mononucleosis*

KLINE, see *Syphilis*

KNEE ARTHROGRAPHY, see *Radiography*

KNEE ENDOSCOPY, see *Endoscopy*

KNEE JERK, see *Reflex*

KNEMOMETRY, see *Growth Hormone*

KOLMER, see *Syphilis*

KUHLMANN-ANDERSON, see *Intelligence Quotient*

KVEIM

The Kveim test is a special skin test to aid in diagnosing sarcoidosis (Boeck's sarcoid disease), a condition in which the lymph glands enlarge and fibrous nodules appear in the chest and other body areas. Sarcoidosis is often mistaken for tuberculosis; the Kveim test helps differentiate the two conditions.

The exact cause of sarcoidosis is not known, but it is believed to be a virus disease.

It is found mostly in young adults living in the south and in blacks far more than in whites. A tiny amount of known sarcoid tissue is injected into the skin; the injection site is watched for a reaction over the next six to eight weeks.

Another, more recent way of helping to diagnose sarcoidosis—or following the course of a patient with this disease—is by measuring the activity of serum angiotensin-converting enzyme, or SACE (see **Renin**). This test seems especially valuable when a patient shows very high **Calcium** levels in the blood.

When performed: When sarcoidosis or tuberculosis is suspected, usually after an abnormal chest X-ray; to prevent the need for a surgical procedure to enter the chest and obtain a nodule for **Biopsy**; with a chronic cough that cannot easily be diagnosed.

Normal values: There should be no reaction at the site of injection after eight weeks.

Abnormal values: In patients with sarcoidosis, a small growth appears at the injection site, usually within six weeks; when that growth is examined under the microscope, specific sarcoid granulomas are seen.

Risk factors: Negligible (see general risk factors for catheter and needle insertion).

Pain/discomfort: Minimal (see general pain/discomfort factors for catheter and needle insertion).

Cost: The cost for injecting the special tissue is approximately $10; the results are usually read during a routine office visit.

Accuracy and significance: From 80 to 90 percent of all patients with sarcoidosis have a positive reaction. However, the test can show a positive reaction to other conditions that cause lymph gland swelling. The test is significant in helping differentiate the causes of various diseases of the chest.

KYMOGRAPHY, see *Radiography*

L

LABILE FACTOR, see *Fibrinogen*

LACRIMAL, see *Schirmer's*

LACTASE DEFICIENCY, see *Lactose Tolerance*

LACTIC ACID

Lactic acid is an end product of sugar metabolism. When the body increases lactic acid production or fails to excrete lactic acid, the condition is called lactic acidosis (usually a complication of kidney, heart, or liver disease).

Lactic acidosis is characterized by a marked "anion gap." Normally, the amount of sodium plus the amount of potassium in the blood (anion group) equals the total amount of chloride and bicarbonate in the blood (cation group). When the difference between the two groups is greater than 30 (that is, when the cation group is decreased), an anion gap exists and is an ominous sign of lactic acidosis. Blood is taken from a vein, and the whole blood is tested.

When performed: When there is rapid, deep breathing, somnolence, stupor, or coma; when metabolic acidosis is suspected; when an anion gap exists.

Normal values: Lactic acid levels from 5 to 20 mg per 100 ml.

Abnormal values: Elevated blood lactic acid is indicative of lactic acidosis. It can also result from exercise, anemia, leukemias, diabetes mellitus, the taking of certain drugs such as epinephrine for asthma or phenformin for diabetes, and salicylate (aspirin) intoxication.

Risk factors: Negligible (see general risk factors for blood testing).

Pain/discomfort: Minimal (see general pain/discomfort factors for blood testing).

Cost: From $20 to $30.

Accuracy and significance: Although the test is 90 percent accurate in revealing excessive lactic acid in the blood, that is about all it does. It is used primarily in hospital and emergency situations on patients who are extremely ill. It is more a means of recording a patient's progress than an aid in diagnosing any specific disease.

LACTIC ACID DEHYDROGENASE, see *Lactic Dehydrogenase*

LACTIC DEHYDROGENASE (LDH)

Serum lactic dehydrogenase is an enzyme found in many body organs and in red blood cells, which when damaged or diseased, release the enzyme into the blood serum. LDH acts as a catalyst in carbohydrate metabolism. There are now at least six different forms (isoenzymes) of LDH, concentrated in varying amounts in such organs as the heart and liver and in the muscles; they are labeled LD1, LD2, etc.

Most commonly, the total LDH is measured; occasionally, the different forms of LDH are tested to help ascertain the location and sometimes the extent of body damage. Blood is taken from a vein, and the serum is examined. LDH is also measured in spinal fluid, in pleural (lung) fluid, and in the urine, where it is sometimes used as a screening test for kidney and bladder cancer.

When performed: When there is suspicion of a heart attack or cancer; to diagnose anemia; to aid in determining if a mother is carrying a child with an Rh problem; to distinguish hepatitis from other liver diseases; to aid in the diagnosis of pulmonary embolism.

Normal values: Normal LDH levels range from 200 to 600 units per ml of serum, or up to 250 IU. Because different laboratories use so many different methods for testing, normal values may vary greatly.

Abnormal values: Lower-than-normal values of LDH may be found after excessive X-ray exposure. Increased values are found after a heart attack. LDH levels do not become elevated as rapidly as certain other enzymes tested for when heart disease is suspected (see **Creatine Phosphokinase** and **Aspartate Aminotransferase**). When elevated, LDH levels persist much longer. Extremely high values of LDH are found with hepatitis, infectious mononucleosis, and anemias caused by deficiencies of vitamin B_{12} or folic acid. Elevated LDH levels are also seen with leukemia and other cancers, but the test is not specific enough to be the sole basis for diagnosis.

Elevated levels of certain isoenzymes of LDH indicate heart disease; others point to liver problems and are more disease-specific. When total LDH levels are elevated, an LDH heat fractionization test is sometimes performed. After LDH is subjected to high heat, only the heart-produced isoenzymes remain, helping to pinpoint the diagnosis.

LDH levels are increased in the spinal fluid following a stroke and with meningitis. In chest conditions that cause the surface of the lungs to give off fluid (pleurisy), the fluid has high LDH levels. With a urinary tract infection or a growth anywhere from the kidney to the bladder, urine LDH levels are elevated.

Risk factors: Negligible (see general risk factors for blood testing).

Pain/discomfort: Minimal (see general pain/discomfort factors for blood testing).

Cost: From $4 to $24 for total LDH. The test is usually included in **Comprehensive Multiple Test Screening** panels, which range from $7 to $42. When total LDH is analyzed for isoenzymes, the cost ranges from $20 to $78.

Accuracy and significance: Although blood levels of LDH increase with a variety of diseases, this test is most commonly used, together with other enzyme tests, to confirm the diagnosis of a heart attack. Its significance is really in helping to determine the cause of chest pain. Isoenzyme determinations are somewhat more specific but still cannot offer a definitive diagnosis. They are about 80 percent accurate.

LACTOGENIC HORMONE, see *Prolactin*

LACTOSE TOLERANCE (Intestinal Disaccharidase Deficiency)

Lactose is a type of sugar found in milk and milk products, including commercial yogurt, some soft (not hard) cheeses, and many different prepared foods such as bakery products that contain milk solids, baby foods, commercially prepared desserts, soft drinks, soups, and even frozen French-fried potatoes. Many drug preparations use lactose as a binder. Some people do not have sufficient lactase (an enzyme) to break down milk sugar; as a result, they have many different symptoms (mostly gastrointestinal cramps, bloating, and diarrhea) after drinking milk or eating milk products. Because lactose is broken down in the making of hard cheese, this food is usually tolerated by patients with milk intolerance. Intolerance to milk sugar is not an allergy, and the symptoms are not the same as an allergic reaction to milk protein. Usually, the symptoms result from ingesting an increased quantity of milk (people without lactase can usually drink a little milk or cream in coffee or on cereal). The condition is found most commonly in Orientals, Arabs, blacks, Italians, and Ashkenazi Jews.

In the lactose tolerance test, a patient is given a measured amount of a lactose solution to drink after a fasting blood sugar test (see **Glucose**) has been performed. An hour or two later, another blood sugar test is performed.

A newer and somewhat different way to diagnose lactose intolerance as well as related problems of carbohydrate malabsorption is through a breath-hydrogen analysis. This is of particular value when testing children, as it seems more of a game than a test. Instead of being stuck with a needle for blood measurements, the child blows into a balloon and the breath is then tested for its quantity of hydrogen gas. Breath is tested before and after the patient has had a drink of sugar water (sucrose). If the sugar is not absorbed normally, excessive hydrogen forms, indicating the enzyme deficiency as intestinal disaccharidase deficiency (disaccharides are forms of sugar).

There are other breath tests; one is called the triolein breath test, where radioactive triolein (a fat molecule) is given to see how much is absorbed by the intestines. Depending on absorption, the radioactivity is expelled by the breath attached to carbon dioxide and is measured by a scintillator (see **Nuclear Scanning**). This test approximates the measurement of fat in the feces to help diagnose malabsorption. Breath analysis is also used to help evaluate liver disease. When radioactive aminopyrine is ingested or injected, and the radioactive carbon monoxide in the breath is measured, it can help differentiate hepatitis from other forms of liver and bile problems. This test is called the aminopyrine breath test. The D-xylose breath test is a measure of bacteria in the intestines (see **Xylose Tolerance**); this is performed particularly after patients have had bowel surgery or when patients have stomach emptying problems and other delays in food transport within the bowel (see **Feces Examination**). Some patients complain of cramps and diarrhea after the tests, and there is the radioactivity factor to be considered when testing women and children.

When performed: When a patient complains of persistent abdominal or gas pains, especially if the patient's intake of milk has increased.

Normal values: Blood sugar, rather than lactose itself, is measured. Normally, after a patient drinks the lactose solution, the blood sugar will rise at least 40 mg per 100 ml within an hour or two.

Abnormal values: Failure of the blood sugar to rise more than 20 mg per 100 ml after drinking the lactose solution is indicative of lactose intolerance. Elderly patients with certain bone diseases may also show an abnormal result, as will some patients who have recently had gastrointestinal surgery or who have an "irritable" bowel.

Risk factors: Negligible (see general risk factors for blood testing).

Pain/discomfort: Minimal (see general pain/discomfort factors for blood testing).

Cost: The complete series of five or six blood glucose measurements ranges from $30 to $76. Some laboratories charge $1 for the bottle of lactose solution. Breath hydrogen gas measurements average $20. D-xylose testing averages $30.

Accuracy and significance: Although the measurement of blood sugar is the most common way to diagnose the inability to digest various forms of sugar, it is now considered an unreliable way of confirming the diagnosis; too many extraneous factors can cause a false-positive result. The breath hydrogen test, while 80 percent accurate, requires meticulous laboratory skills to obtain proper measurements. When an absolute diagnosis is required, a **Biopsy** of the small intestine is performed. Actually, an observed relationship between the consumption of foods containing lactose and the development of subsequent symptoms is usually sufficient; removal of lactose from the diet followed by relief of symptoms tends to confirm the diagnosis. And commercial lactase preparations (LactAid) are now available; when they relieve symptoms, they help substantiate the diagnosis.

LANGUAGE FUNCTION

Defects in language function (aphasia) may be of an expressive nature (difficulty in planning, coordinating, and using speech), a receptive nature (inability to understand what is said), or amnesic (inability to remember sounds). Testing for the type of aphasia helps locate the exact area of brain disease. The patient is asked to recite the alphabet, count forward and backward, spell words, and read a poem. Next, the patient is asked to repeat particular phrases such as *Methodist Episcopal* and the Peter Piper doggerel. Spoken and written commands such as "button your vest" or "hold out your hand and spread your fingers" are given and the response noted. Finally, the patient is asked to name familiar sounds such as the mewing of a cat, the ticking of a watch, and running water. There are many other tests for aphasia; the specific type depends on the physician's preference. All language function evaluations must take into account the patient's educational experience.

When testing children for language function, minor variations of the test are often used. Children are asked to repeat such familiar words as *cat, thumb,* and *running* to detect "baby talk." They are also asked to demonstrate voice tones; children with emotional problems appear limited in this respect.

Some doctors feel there is no such thing as "baby talk"; failure of an adult to use proper sounds (phonetics) is usually indicative of a disability such as minimal brain dysfunction. Persistent "baby talk" can also indicate abnormal anxiety and other mental health problems.

When performed: Whenever brain disease is suspected; in stroke; in certain infectious diseases that affect the brain such as syphilis.

Normal values: Normal patients have no difficulty speaking and understanding the language.

Abnormal values: Speech impairment almost always indicates disease of the left side of the brain. With receptive types of aphasia, the pathology is usually in the temporal (side) area; amnesic aphasia suggests frontal area brain disease; patients with expressive aphasia often accompanied by the inability to write out a word with eyes closed, signifies damage in the brain cortex (where motion and purposeful activity are controlled). Inability to know left from right, when accompanied by disturbed language function, may reflect brain disease.

Risk factors: None.

Pain/discomfort: None.

Cost: From $20 to $25 for the administration and interpretation of the test.

Accuracy and significance: Language function evaluations are not specific and have no accuracy ratings, but they can help detect brain damage, and when properly interpreted, they can help pinpoint the area of the brain involved. Some doctors believe the tests are equally significant in helping uncover emotional problems, especially in children.

LAP, see *Leucine Aminopeptidase*

LAPAROSCOPY, see *Endoscopy*

LATEX AGGLUTINATION, see *Agglutination*

LATEX FIXATION, see *Agglutination*

LATS, see *Thyroid Function*

LAV, see *Acquired Immunodeficiency Syndrome*

LDH, see *Lactic Dehydrogenase*

LEAD

Lead is a trace element (only a trace is normally found in the body) that can produce a toxic reaction (plumbism) when sufficient amounts enter the body. At one time, most paint had a lead base. Infants who chewed on toys or cribs painted with lead-based paint were apt to suffer lead poisoning. Today, most paints are lead-free; however, old walls, furniture, and toys that have been painted over may still have lead paint underneath, posing a hazard if the paint chips or peels. Lead poisoning can also occur in people whose occupation puts them in contact with lead and people who are exposed to heavy vehicular traffic (policemen).

Whole blood, urine, and body tissues such as liver, bone, and hair (see **Hair Analysis**) may be examined. The urine may also be examined for delta aminolevulinic acid (ALA) and coproporphyrin as a screening test for those whose jobs involve contact with lead.

When performed: To aid in the diagnosis of lead poisoning; in children with pica (the regular eating of dirt and other foreign material); during pregnancy.

Normal values: Normally, traces of lead up to 35 mcg per 100 ml may be found in the blood; once, this was universally considered the upper limit of normal. Today, most doctors feel that if a child shows screening lead levels greater than 25 mcg per 100 ml it is considered sufficiently elevated to warrant close investigation.

Abnormal values: Levels over 35 mcg per 100 ml of whole blood or over 100 mcg in a 24-hour urine specimen are indicative of lead intoxication. More than 50 mcg per gram of hair reveals plumbism.

Risk factors: Negligible (see general risk factors for blood testing).

Pain/discomfort: Minimal (see general pain/discomfort factors for blood testing).

Cost: From $15 to $45 when blood and urine are examined. When body tissues are examined, there is often an additional charge for obtaining the specimen; its amount depends on the specimen's location and operative procedures.

Accuracy and significance: All tests for lead poisoning are 95 percent accurate; lead is either present in excessive amounts or it is not. Lead testing is assuming even greater significance in the evaluation of children with learning disabilities.

LEARNING ABILITY NECK REFLEX, see *Reflex*

LEARNING DISABILITY

Until recently, a child's ability to learn, especially as observed in the school environment, was considered a nonmedical condition. It is now known that an inability to perform equally to one's peers at the normal grade level can result from an inherited condition causing mental retardation; a developmental defect; a physical handicap such as impaired hearing, vision, or muscle incoordination; an allergy causing hyperactivity; or even a reaction to medications taken to control hyperactivity. While there are numerous tests to help diagnose a learning disability (see **Aminoaciduria, Amniocentesis, Chromosome Analysis, Electroencephalogram, Electromyography, Hearing Function, Intelligence Quotient, Language Function, Phenylketonuria, RAST, Sweat, Thyroid Function, Visual Acuity,** to name but a few), learning problems are first identified through achievement tests that measure reading, writing, and arithmetic performance correlated to the child's age, experience, and family background.

For example, dyslexia (difficulty in understanding the written word; mentally reversing printed letters—hence, not comprehending or distorting the meaning of a sentence or paragraph) is probably the most common learning disability. Its cause can lie in the brain, the eyes, or another part of the body. Writing disabilities frequently come from a lack of coordination between the brain and the muscles. A mathematics disability seems to reflect problems of memory and can exist with or without a reading problem.

The basic screening test for most of these conditions is the achievement test, a measure of a child's performance compared to the child's peers and expected ability. Achievement tests are the key to isolating the problem area. While they were once used almost exclusively in schools, many pediatricians now use them as part of an overall examination and evaluation. The tests are published under a variety of names: the Metropolitan Achievement Test, the Stanford Achievement Test, Sequential Tests of Educational Progress (STEP), Tests of Academic Progress and the Iowa Tests of Educational Development are only a few. Many states prepare and publish their own tests; most proficiency tests for specific subjects are a form of achievement test. The readiness tests given children prior to entering kindergarten also serve as excellent screening tests for learning disabilities.

When performed: Primarily to pinpoint the specific learning disability and to help account for the physical problems relating to the disability; to track the progress of therapy of a learning-disabled patient; to screen family members when a learning disability has been uncovered; to ascertain the presence or absence of certain skills in children.

Normal values: Although each test has its own scoring system, the majority are based on what a child should have learned, or the performance skills a child should have achieved, at the time of testing.

Abnormal values: Inability to read, write, or do arithmetic at a level equal to the majority of one's peers (age, sex, school grade).

Risk factors: None.

Pain/discomfort: None other than possible embarrassment at failure before the causes are known.

Cost: Approximately $25 when performed in a doctor's office, hospital, or by a professional tester. Many of these tests can be purchased by parents at school supply stores at a cost of $1 to $5.

Accuracy and significance: When the tests are properly administered, they are about 70 percent accurate as an aid in the diagnosis of learning disabilities. It is equally important that a child's background be considered. A child brought up in a sophisticated urban environment, for instance, might call a milking pail a champagne bucket and be quite correct.

LE CELL, see *Antinuclear Antibodies*

LECITHIN/SPHINGOMYELIN RATIO, see *Pregnancy*

LEE-WHITE COAGULATION, see *Bleeding and Clotting Time*

LEFT VENTRICULAR EJECTION TIME, see *Systolic Time Intervals*

LEGIONNAIRES' DISEASE, see *Agglutination*

LEISHMANIASIS, see *Agglutination*

LEPTOSPIROSIS, see *Agglutination*

LES, see *Gastroesophageal Reflux*

LEUCINE AMINOPEPTIDASE (LAP)

Leucine aminopeptidase is an enzyme produced by the liver, the pancreas, and the small intestine. LAP tests are performed when various other enzyme tests seem to conflict, especially in diagnosing liver disease and in determining whether elevated levels of **Alkaline Phosphatase** are caused by liver problems as opposed to bone disease. Blood is taken from a vein, and the serum is tested.

When performed: Primarily to distinguish bile duct obstruction from liver cell disease.

Normal values: Depending on the method used by various laboratories, normal values can differ; one measure is from 5 to 25 standard units per ml.

Abnormal values: LAP is increased when the bile ducts are obstructed (causing liver disease); it is normal or lower than normal when liver pathology comes from within the liver cells.

Risk factors: Negligible (see general risk factors for blood testing).

Pain/discomfort: Minimal (see general pain/discomfort factors for blood testing).

Cost: From $10 to $25.

Some doctors consider this test outmoded, and it is possible that a health insurance company or government-sponsored medical program will not reimburse the doctor or patient for the cost of the test.

Accuracy and significance: Although the test is not commonly used, occasionally it is employed to substantiate a diagnosis. It is about 50 percent accurate.

LEUKOCYTE, see *White Blood Cell*

LEUKOCYTE ADHERENCE INHIBITION, see *White Blood Cell*

LEUKOCYTE ANTIBODY, see *HLA*

LEUKOCYTE DIFFERENTIAL, see *Blood Cell Differential*

LEUKOCYTE ESTERASE, see *Urine Examination*

LEUKOCYTE SCANNING, see *Nuclear Scanning*

LEWIS, see *Cystometry*

LIMULUS AMEBOCYTE LYSATE, see *Gonorrhea; Synovial Fluid*

LIMULUS ASSAY see *Synovial Fluid*

LIPASE

Lipase, an enzyme secreted by the pancreas, helps to break down triglyceride fats (see **Lipids**) so they can be utilized by the body. In the blood, lipase levels usually parallel those of **Amylase** (another fat-splitting enzyme produced by the pancreas), and the two are generally tested together. Blood is drawn from a vein, and the serum is examined.

When performed: When disease of the pancreas is suspected and a definite diagnosis is not certain.

Normal values: Normal levels of lipase range from 0.2 unit to 1.5 units per ml.

Abnormal values: Serum lipase levels are elevated in pancreatitis (but not as much as amylase levels), in cancer of the pancreas and certain intestinal ulcers, and in patients using opiate drugs (morphine, codeine).

Risk factors: Negligible (see general risk factors for blood testing).

Pain/discomfort: Minimal (see general pain/discomfort factors for blood testing).

Cost: From $10 to $40.

Accuracy and significance: The test is merely a confirmation of the diagnosis of pancreatic disease. At times, it is employed because lipase levels remain elevated far longer than amylase levels. It is about 70 percent accurate. (Also see **Pancreas Function**.)

LIPIDS

The total lipids test includes the measurement of the three major lipids (fats) in blood serum: cholesterol (an alcohol, not a true fat, yet still so categorized medically), triglycerides, and phospholipids. The test also includes the free fatty acids and other fats, but at present, these have no diagnostic significance. Phospholipids (e.g., lecithin) also offer little diagnostic information, but a few physicians employ the phospholipid/cholesterol ratio as an experimental indication of atherosclerosis (see **Cholesterol**).

Triglycerides comprise the greatest amount (by weight) of lipids in the blood as well as in the foods we eat and are considered true fats (olive oil is made up in large part of triglycerides). While triglycerides come primarily from fats in the diet, like cholesterol they can also be manufactured by the liver. Triglycerides are the blood fats that reflect light; thus, in samples taken after a fatty meal or when there is some metabolic defect, they may be seen as a turbid layer in a test tube of serum that has been left standing. Alcohol and carbohydrates, more than fatty foods, cause a great increase in blood triglyceride levels.

The triglyceride test may be performed independently, but it is commonly measured along with cholesterol. The two tests, coupled with observation of the serum after refrigeration overnight in a test tube, are considered together to arrive at a classification of hyperlipidemia when an excess of serum lipids exists. Lipidemia (the normal amounts of fat in the blood) is often confused with lipoproteinemia, which is another classification of the various densities of the protein molecules that attach themselves to and carry the lipids in the blood (see **Lipoproteins**).

Blood is taken from a vein, and the serum or plasma is tested. For triglycerides, the patient should follow a normal diet for at least two weeks before the test and should then eat nothing for 14 hours before the blood is taken. Certain drugs such as hormones, steroids, birth control pills, and diuretics must not be taken for a month before the tests.

When performed: Blood lipids are measured to reflect familial (inherited) disorders of fat metabolism (not necessarily disease-producing); they can point to possible liver, kidney, and thyroid diseases and at times signify bile tract obstruction; today, however, they are tested mostly as an experimental indication of atherosclerosis.

Normal values: Total lipids usually range from 400 to 1,000 mg per 100 ml (they are normally increased after a meal containing fat). Triglycerides range from 30 to 145 mg per 100 ml; phospholipids, from 125 to 350 mg per 100 ml; the phospholipid/cholesterol ratio, from 0.7 to 1.8.

Abnormal values: There is as yet no scientific agreement on the relative merits of serum lipid measurements for the prognosis of heart and artery disease. Thus, while six varieties of hyperlipidemia (elevated serum lipid levels) have been postulated as a guide to the degree of risk for atherosclerosis, these hypothetical abnormalities are just that—hypothetical. The types are classified according to whether triglycerides, cholesterol, or both are elevated (along with the appearance of the plasma and the patient's symptoms, if any).

Type I, while very rare, shows only high triglycerides. Patients may suffer abdominal pain, but the risk of heart disease is thought to be low.

There are two kinds of type II: the most common, IIa, shows only an increased cholesterol level; IIb shows elevated cholesterol and triglycerides. Both are alleged to be indications of heart disease.

Type III, extremely rare, shows high cholesterol and triglyceride levels but also shows elevated glucose (sugar) levels. It, too, is alleged to be a warning sign of heart disease.

Type IV, similar to but more common than type III, shows only a marked triglyceride elevation.

Type V, rare, also shows only a triglyceride elevation and is believed to be a combination of types I and IV.

It has been postulated that the lower the phospholipid/cholesterol ratio (decreased phospholipids), the greater the possibility of atherosclerosis. Again, the reasoning behind the classification of lipids is to discover if there is a way to utilize such typing as a means of identifying those at risk for atherosclerosis.

Falsely elevated triglyceride levels are commonly found in patients taking thiazide diuretics, steroid hormones, and birth control pills.

Risk factors: Negligible (see general risk factors for blood testing).

Pain/discomfort: Minimal (see general pain/discomfort factors for blood testing).

Cost: Triglyceride and total lipid measurements are $5 to $22. They are usually included in **Comprehensive Multiple Test Screening** panels, ranging from $7 to $42. Phospholipid measurements are $8 to $18. When all lipid tests are performed concurrently, the fee is $20 to $25.

Accuracy and significance: Most lipid tests are still for purposes of research, as no absolute evidence of a direct relation with heart disease has yet been scientifically proved. While the significance of the various lipid measurements is still under study, it should be remembered that wide fluctuations of the various lipid levels also occur with a number of other diseases. However, for the detection of an inherited problem of cholesterol metabolism, the tests are considered 90 percent accurate. Whether treatment of these metabolic disabilities will be of value has yet to be determined.

LIPOPROTEINS

When **Lipids** (fat molecules) combine in the blood with protein molecules, they are called lipoproteins. Lipoproteins are classified according to their density: those with more fat and less protein have the least density (lightest weight); those with the least fat and the most protein have the highest density. Classifying the different lipoproteins is called phenotyping.

The lipoprotein containing the least amount of protein (1 percent), consists largely of triglycerides and is called a chylomicron. The very-low-density lipoproteins (VLDL), sometimes called prebeta, contain more than half triglycerides as well as almost equal amounts of cholesterol and phospholipids and up to 10 percent proteins. The low-density lipoproteins (LDL), sometimes called beta, are nearly half cholesterol, with almost equal amounts of triglycerides and phospholipids along with 20 percent proteins. LDLs have been reported to be coated with a particular protein called apoprotein B, or apo B; if, genetically, one inherits a mutation of a normal apo B gene, it seems to be the cause of abnormal amounts of LDLs that are related to atherosclerosis. Normally, apo B helps transfer cholesterol-containing LDLs from the blood into the cells; a defective apo B gene cannot perform this task, and the LDLs remain in the blood.

In 1985, physicians began testing for the apoproteins (also called apolipoproteins). Some believe that levels of apo A-I are, at this time, the best indicators of heart disease, but this test's value is only limited to a highly select group of patients. Testing for apo B (also called apo B-100) to compare it as a ratio to apo A-I, and also to total cholesterol, is also being evaluated as a coronary disease marker. Apo E is yet another lipoprotein under study. The value of all apoprotein readings as heart disease risk factors has yet to be proved.

The high-density lipoproteins (HDL), sometimes called alpha, are composed mostly of proteins and phospholipids. The presence of increased amounts of high-density lipoproteins in the blood has been associated with a noticeable lack of heart and artery disease. There are two known subfractions of HDL at present: HDL_2 and HDL_3. It is thought that only HDL_2 is related to heart disease. Of interest, women prior to the menopause—with large amounts of estrogens—have the greatest amounts of HDL_2 (it has been thought that estrogens may be protective factors against heart disease). Thus, in tests for **Cholesterol,** the amount of high-density lipoproteins is more important than simply total cholesterol alone. HDL levels are rarely influenced by the type of fat (saturated or polyunsaturated) a person eats; they are increased by exercise, weight loss, niacin (vitamin B_3), and moderate amounts of alcohol and they are decreased on a high-carbohydrate diet.

The four different lipoproteins are also utilized in ascertaining the six types of hyperlipidemia (see **Lipids**). Type I shows almost all chylomicrons. Type II has two variations: IIa is mostly very-low-density lipoproteins; IIb is mostly both very-low-density lipoproteins and low-density lipoproteins. Type III shows abnormal low-density and very-low-density lipoproteins. Types IV and V show increased very-low-density lipoproteins. Type V also shows an increased amount of chylomicrons. The classifications are primarily measurements to see if predisposition to atherosclerosis (heart and artery disease) can someday be predicted. Blood is taken from a vein for testing.

When performed: To study and classify people with elevated lipids (cholesterol or triglycerides) as a possible aid in detecting patients with greater-than-average risk of heart and artery disease.

Normal values: Standards have now been proposed for some of the lipoproteins. The average LDL cholesterol level is considered to be 150 mg per 100 ml, the assumed "normal" range being between 100 and 200 mg per 100 ml. HDLs average 55 mg per 100 ml, with the "normal" range said to be between 30 and 80 mg per 100 ml. There are some doctors who feel that when all the subfractions of HDLs are taken into account, the upper limits of normal could go as high as 300 mg per 100 ml. Normal values for chylomicrons and VLDLs are still under study. There are several apolipoproteins that can be measured (apo A-I, apo A-II, etc.), but normal blood levels of these have not, as yet, been definitely related to atherosclerosis.

Abnormal values: The presence of excessive amounts of very-low-density lipoproteins is tentatively assumed to be a prognostic sign of atherosclerosis. In contrast, large amounts of high-density lipoproteins are believed to be a prognostic sign of some built-in protection against atherosclerosis.

Risk factors: Negligible (see general risk factors for blood testing).

Pain/discomfort: Minimal (see general pain/discomfort factors for blood testing).

Cost: HDL testing ranges from $10 to $20. It is commonly included in **Comprehensive Multiple Test Screening** panels, which are $7 to $42. LDL testing is $10 to $30; VLDL testing averages $20. When the various lipoproteins are measured at one time (this usually includes lipid measurements), the charge is $30 to $40.

Accuracy and significance: As with lipid testing, lipoprotein measurements are primarily in the nature of research. The medical significance of all of these tests is still under study, especially their significance in relation to diet, stress, smoking, and ordinary daily activities. It is known, for example, that misleading apoprotein values can occur after trauma.

LIQUID CRYSTAL THERMOGRAPHY, see *Thermography*

LISTERIOSIS, see *Agglutination*

LITHIUM

Lithium salts have been found to be effective in the treatment of manic-depressive illness—primarily to prevent and treat the mania, but occasionally to lessen the depression. Because of the toxic effects of lithium, patients who are on maintenance treatment must be monitored closely so that they can benefit from the drug with as few adverse effects as possible.

The blood level of lithium is tested the day after treatment starts. It is then tested three times a week until the proper maintenance level is established. Afterward, it is tested monthly (sooner if symptoms appear). The patient must not take lithium for eight hours prior to the test. Blood is drawn from a vein, and serum is examined.

When performed: To follow patients with manic-depressive disease who are being treated with lithium; to adjust the dosage of the drug as necessary.

Normal values: Normally, there is no lithium in blood serum. A therapeutic blood level of lithium is considered to range from 0.5 to 1.5 mEq per liter. But even at the therapeutic level, the patient may have side effects, such as excessive thirst and urination, upset stomach, diarrhea, slight tremor, and increased white blood cell count.

Abnormal values: Blood levels of lithium over 1.5 mEq per liter are considered toxic. When there is a toxic amount of lithium in the blood, the patient may suffer from vomiting, muscle weakness, convulsions, leukocytosis, coma, and death (at 4 mEq per liter). Diuretics or a low-salt diet can cause an increased serum level of lithium.

Risk factors: Negligible (see general risk factors for blood testing).
Pain/discomfort: Minimal (see general pain/discomfort factors for blood testing).
Cost: From $10 to $28.
Accuracy and significance: The test is considered 90 percent accurate as a measure of lithium in the blood. At times, **Sodium** measurements must be made in order to assure the doctor of true lithium levels. The test is a very important tool with which to monitor patients taking the drug; indeed, it can be lifesaving.

LIVER ENZYME, see *Isocitric Dehydrogenase*

LIVER SCAN, see *Nuclear Scanning*

LOMBARD, see *Hearing Function*

LONG-ACTING THYROID STIMULATOR, see *Thyroid Function*

LOWER-BOWEL X-RAY, see *Radiography*

LOWER ESOPHAGEAL SPHINCTER, see *Gastroesophageal Reflux*

LOWER GI SERIES, see *Radiography*

LUMBAR PUNCTURE, see *Cerebrospinal Fluid*

LUMBAR THERMOGRAPHY, see *Thermography*

LUNDH, see *Pancreas Function*

LUNG, see *Pulmonary Function*

LUNG FLUID, see *Thoracentesis*

LUNG SCAN, see *Nuclear Scanning*

LUNG SECRETION, see *Sputum*

LUPUS ERYTHEMATOSUS (LE) CELL, see *Antinuclear Antibodies*

LUTEINIZING HORMONE, see *Estrogen; Testis Function*

LYME DISEASE, see *Agglutination*

LYMPHADENOPATHY-ASSOCIATED VIRUS, see *Acquired Immunodeficiency Syndrome*

LYMPHANGIOGRAPHY, see *Radiography*

LYMPHOCYTE TYPING (B and T Cells)

One particular white blood cell (see **Blood Cell Differential**), the lymphocyte, is now classified into two distinct types of cells: the B cell (it is thought that this form originates in the bone—hence, the letter *B*—and in various bursa or body cavities containing lymph tissue) and the T cell (it is thought that the thymus gland—hence, the letter T—controls the production and maturation of this form, even though T cells are also formed in the bone). Each of the two cell types seems to have a distinct purpose. The B cells make antibodies (see **Agglutination**) found in the blood, tears, and other body fluids that fight the antigens of specific diseases and are sometimes called "helper" cells. T cells seem to be more generalized in their control of immunity to certain diseases as well as in attacking viruses. They are sometimes called "killer" cells. T cell reactions also are believed to be the way that the skin reacts to injections of disease material by showing redness and swelling (see **Skin Reaction**). Although the two lymphocytes look the same under the ordinary light microscope, they can be distinguished through an electron microscope or by mixing them with sheep red blood cells (only the T cells will cling to the sheep cells and produce a distinctive rosette pattern).

By determining the quantity of the two lymphocytes in the blood (taken from a vein), in the lymph nodes, or in **Bone Marrow** (taken by aspiration, or **Biopsy**), it is possible to diagnose the specific type of leukemia and assess the possible response to treatment. It is also possible to determine whether certain conditions are cancerous; the state of a patient's immunity; and the activity of some autoimmune conditions such as systemic lupus erythematosus.

When performed: To detect and differentiate between certain cancers such as the leukemias; to help detect and evaluate conditions of immunodeficiency; to help diagnose various skin diseases, particularly when cancer might be the cause of a psoriasislike rash and other common rashes; to help diagnose Hodgkin's disease (enlargement of the lymph glands and spleen); to test the possible effect of certain drugs on a patient prior to organ transplant or skin grafting; to assist in the prognosis of certain cancerous conditions.

Normal values: From 5 to 25 percent B cells and 45 to 85 percent T cells (while the range seems wide, most people average 10 percent B cells and 65 percent T cells). It is also considered normal to have approximately 20 percent null cells, or cells that appear to be either B or T.

Abnormal values: Lower-than-normal amounts of B cells suggest decreased immunity (a patient may have one of several serious infections such as pneumonia); an increased amount of B cells is present in certain leukemias. Decreased T cells indicate an extreme susceptibility to virus, parasitic, and certain fungus diseases and an unusual sensitivity to certain drugs that can cause decreased immunity. Patients with T-cell deficiency may not react to diagnostic skin tests. An increase in T cells points to leukemia and other cancers. (Also see **Acquired Immunodeficiency Syndrome**.)

Risk factors: Negligible (see general risk factors for blood testing; for bone marrow aspiration or lymph node biopsy, see general risk factors for catheter or needle insertion).

Pain/discomfort: Negligible (see general pain/discomfort factors for blood testing). The needle used to obtain a biopsy or bone marrow specimen may cause some discomfort (see general pain/discomfort factors for catheter and needle insertion).

Cost: From $90 to $150.

Accuracy and significance: While the test is considered 90 percent accurate when used in lymph cell diseases, it is of less value in helping to distinguish other conditions. However, when other diagnostic tests are equivocal, lymphocyte typing may offer an answer. As B- and T-cell numbers can vary from day to day, some doctors believe each patient's normal limits must be determined before an accurate evaluation can be made and appropriate drugs administered.

Note: By using the flow microfluorometry test, where lymphocyte-type blood cells are labeled and identified, it is possible to select the best treatment for patients with aplastic anemia (a form of anemia where the **Bone Marrow** is destroyed by chemicals, drugs, radiation, or infection).

LYMPHOCYTIC CHOREOMENINGITIS, see *Virus Disease*

LYMPHOGRANULOMA VENEREUM, see *Frei*

LYSOZYME

Lysozyme (or muramidase) is an enzyme that destroys certain bacteria, thus causing certain disease symptoms to subside. Lysozyme occurs naturally in some body fluids such as tears, saliva, serum, and breast milk; it is also found in some plants and in egg whites. The natural occurrence of lysozyme in mother's milk and saliva may account for the traditional beliefs that mother's milk helps protect babies from certain diseases and that licking a wound is beneficial. Lysozyme is also found in large amounts in monocytes (large **White Blood Cells**). Blood serum and/or urine is examined.

When performed: Lysozyme values are studied in patients with myelomonocytic and lymphocytic leukemia.

Normal values: In serum, 7 to 14 mcg per ml is a normal finding; in urine, 2 mcg per ml.

Abnormal values: Patients with myelomonocytic leukemia have elevated levels of lysozyme (as high as 230 mcg per ml). Patients with lymphocytic leukemia have decreased values (3 to 12 mcg per ml).

Risk factors: Negligible (see general risk factors for blood testing).

Pain/discomfort: Minimal (see general pain/discomfort factors for blood testing).

Cost: From $20 to $40 on blood or urine.

Accuracy and significance: A very specific test to differentiate between two types of leukemia; about 90 percent accurate.

M

MACROGLOBULIN (Sia)

Macroglobulins are serum globulins (see **Albumin/Globulin** and **Immunoglobulin**) that are up to 10 times heavier than the usual globulins. They are usually measured as an entity, but they can be broken down into separate parts; the largest portion (usually about two-thirds) is known as alpha-2. Macroglobulins comprise only about 5 percent of all globulins. In the Sia test, blood is taken from a vein for examination. The serum is diluted with water so that total macroglobulins are precipitated out of the solution.

When performed: Primarily when Waldenstrom's macroglobulinemia (a rare disease found most often in older men and characterized by anemia, enlarged liver and spleen, and hemorrhage) is suspected; when leukemia, certain cancers, and prolonged infections cannot be specifically diagnosed.

Normal values: Total macroglobulins average 0.4 g per 100 ml of serum (slightly higher in women). The alpha-2 portion ranges from 0.1 to 0.4 g per 100 ml.

Abnormal values: Increases of up to three times normal values (especially of alpha-2 macroglobulins) are found in Waldenstrom's macroglobulinemia. Total macroglobulins are increased in leukemia, multiple myeloma, certain cancers, and chronic infections. Increased macroglobulins can falsely increase the erythrocyte sedimentation rate. (See **Sedimentation Rate**.)

Risk factors: Negligible (see general risk factors for blood testing).

Pain/discomfort: Minimal (see general pain/discomfort factors for blood testing).

Cost: The Sia test for generalized total macroglobulins is $8 to $15. Special tests to isolate alpha-2 macroglobulin are $20 to $25. When all macroglobulin components are measured, the fee is $90 to $100.

Accuracy and significance: Most often, the tests are used to help support the diagnosis of Waldenstrom's macroglobulinemia; it is not an absolute diagnostic criterion. Since they are primarily screening tests, they have no relative accuracy value.

Note: With the use of a special instrument called a viscometer, the ability of blood to flow easily (as does water) or with difficulty (as does molasses) can be measured. Increased viscosity (molasseslike) is an indication of Waldenstrom's macroglobulinemia, polycythemia, and several other diseases, especially of the liver. High frequency hearing loss is also found associated with increased blood viscosity.

MADDOX ROD, see *Strabismus*

MAGNESIUM

One of the most abundant minerals in the body, magnesium is found in all cells and is active in many biochemical processes, particularly in enzyme reactions. Magnesium is important to the regulation of the body's calcium supply and usage. A normal diet (particularly nuts and vegetables) affords the body about 0.5 g of magnesium every day. Blood is collected from a vein, and serum is examined.

When performed: The test is performed whenever patients exhibit symptoms such as twitching and quivering muscles, irritability, and weakness. It is also used to determine whether these symptoms are caused by lowered **Calcium** levels rather than by lowered magnesium levels. Low magnesium levels seem to prevent effective potassium therapy, so the test is especially important when a patient has a low serum potassium level but shows no positive response to administration of potassium and when a heart attack is suspected but is not easily confirmed; and to confirm **Malnutrition.**

Normal values: Serum magnesium levels range from 1.5 to 2.5 mEq per liter (2 mg per 100 ml). Values vary with different laboratory techniques.

Abnormal values: Lower-than-normal values are found with parathyroid, thyroid, and adrenal gland hyperactivity and with malnutrition, chronic alcoholism, pancreatitis, and diuretic therapy. Higher-than-normal values are found with dehydration and with inactive adrenal glands as well as after a heart attack.

Risk factors: Negligible (see general risk factors for blood testing).

Pain/discomfort: Minimal (see general pain/discomfort factors for blood testing).

Cost: From $6 to $36. The test is usually included in **Comprehensive Multiple Test Screening** panels, which range from $7 to $42.

Accuracy and significance: Although magnesium abnormalities are reflected in a wide variety of diseases and nutritional conditions, the test is also considered to have some significance in helping diagnose muscle irritability. It is usually performed with a **Calcium** test. Some doctors think the serum magnesium level is a more accurate measurement of heart muscle damage, especially if that damage is very small, than cardiac enzyme tests **(Creatine Phosphokinase, Lactic Dehydrogenase).** It is considered to be about 80 percent accurate.

MAGNETIC RESONANCE IMAGING (MRI)

This diagnostic test, originally called nuclear magnetic resonance (the name was changed at the request of radiologists so that patients would not think it was part of **Nuclear Scanning,** a different medical specialty), is somewhat similar to **Computerized Tomography** (CT), in that it produces three-dimensional-appearing images of various organs and structures within the body. And as with positron emission transaxial tomography (PETT), it also offers images that indicate how certain organs and tissues are functioning. The difference between magnetic resonance imaging and CT or PETT is that this machine does not use X-rays or any form of ionizing radiation that can be harmful to the body; to date, MRI has not been shown to cause any adverse biological effect. Instead of X-rays (see **Radiography**), MRI uses principles of magnetism; the magnetic field that it generates around the body causes certain atoms in the nucleus of body cells to "line up," and then by sending and receiving radio signals, which are fed into a computer, the position of those atoms is recorded, and a distinct picture of that part of the body being investigated can be studied at length. The magnets used in MRI are quite powerful; they range from 1,500 gauss to 20,000 gauss (a *gauss,* or G, is the term used to indicate a magnet's strength; the effect of the earth's magnetic field on a compass needle is 1 G, while that of a toy magnet such as is used to hold papers on metal is about 10 G). The patient lies inside a large, tunnel-like tube in a specially protected room to prevent the magnetic attraction of susceptible substances; any metallic object, such as a fountain pen or keys, will be quite forcibly hurled toward the magnet, and patients with a metal prosthesis or pacemaker cannot be placed inside the magnet. Because this device has only been in extensive clinical use since 1981, its true value has not yet been determined. It has, however, been shown to be particularly valuable—in some instances offering more and better information than CTs or **Ultrasound**—in heart and blood vessel diseases (the use of potentially dangerous contrast dyes is not necessary), brain lesions, chest and spine disorders, and especially in helping diagnose pelvic problems in women. It is said to be able to detect breast lesions that other techniques may miss and can differentiate between cysts and growths. It has shown considerable promise in helping diagnose congenital heart disease and pericardial pathology (the latter can be particularly difficult to diagnose), and it is now being used to evaluate blood-flow abnormalities in the arteries as well as the heart. More recently, MRI has been able to locate the exact area of a myocardial infarction (the dead heart muscle tissue that comes from a heart attack). On the negative side of the picture, at the present time, a patient is required to lie very still for much longer periods of time than with CTs, and MRI does not seem to be as effective as other devices in diagnosing certain bone disorders. The newest application of MRI is to help differentiate the various types of dementia due to Alzheimer's disease and Huntington's chorea (an inherited brain condition that causes dementia and involuntary movements) from dementia due to blood vessel problems.

New as MRI is, it has already led to even more sophisticated developments; magnetic resonance spectroscopy (MR spectroscopy) allows almost immediate measurements of the heart muscle's metabolism—particularly valuable to know immediately after a heart attack. This test can also show how the heart will respond to various forms of therapy. And it is expected that this test will also be applied to other body organs and to indicating the response of a cancer to treatment.

When performed: When brain disease is suspected and CT is not helpful; when searching for growths within the chest or abdomen; when knowledge of the pattern of blood flow is needed to aid in diagnosis of blocked heart arteries (it is said to show atherosclerotic lesions); when heart defects, especially of the valves, are suspected; and with infertility problems in women. It is sometimes used to avoid the dangers of angiography (see **Radiography**).

Normal values: As with X-rays and CTs, MRI should show no abnormalities in size, position, and function of body organs and should show no new growths within the body.

Abnormal values: As with X-rays and CTs, much depends on the experience of the doctor who must interpret the images. As those who work with this diagnostic device become more familiar with its potential, more and more abnormal conditions will be able to be detected.

Risk factors: As noted, anyone with an implanted metal device such as a heart pacemaker or some surgical clips—especially those used to close blood vessels—should not enter (or even come near) a magnetic resonance imaging device. The magnetic force could cause a clip to come loose and result in hemorrhage. Warnings have also been issued that women in the early stage of pregnancy should not be exposed to the magnetic field; there have been reports that these women have suffered headaches, swelling of the hands, and peeling of the skin. Animals exposed to MRI have shown abnormal **White Blood Cell** changes.

Pain/discomfort: The primary discomfort seems to be the claustrophobic feeling many patients suffer while lying inside the narrow, closed-in tunnel. And some patients find it extremely uncomfortable to have to lie quite still for up to 15 minutes at a time; at present, even breathing can blur the image, but this drawback is expected to be corrected in the very near future.

Cost: Due to the price of the machine (twice that of a CT scanner), the average MRI test runs around $600 to $900. If performed in a hospital, the room and other related charges must be added. There are, however, mobile MRIs that can travel to doctors' offices to lessen the expense. As of December 1985, some insurance plans will only pay for certain MRI testing (e.g., brain, spinal cord); other uses may not be reimbursable. Medicare payments for MRI testing are limited to brain, nervous system (including multiple sclerosis), adrenal gland, and genitourinary system problems; heart, lung, and some functional tests are excluded from payment.

Accuracy and significance: At present, MRI can be more accurate than CT is assisting in the diagnosis of some conditions while not as accurate in others. Most doctors believe it to be the state of the art, or the best diagnostic tool yet, for uncovering the most difficult diagnoses, but specific accuracy rates are as yet unknown.

MAGNETIC RESONANCE SPECTROSCOPY, see *Magnetic Resonance Imaging*

MAKE-A-PICTURE STORY, see *Thematic Apperception*

MALABSORPTION, see *Xylose Tolerance*

MALARIA

Cases of malaria have increased in recent years as more and more people travel to areas of the world where the disease is endemic. There are four different types of parasites that cause the disease in humans: Plasmodium falciparum (the most serious), Plasmodium vivax, Plasmodium ovale, and Plasmodium malariae. The anopheles mosquito is a carrier of the parasite, and its bite when infected spreads the disease. Blood is taken from a vein or fingertip and stained (with Wright's stain, Field's stain, or Giemsa's stain). The sample is then examined under the microscope for direct identification of malarial organisms. **Agglutination**-type tests are also used to measure the incidence of malaria in population groups (especially when the disease might be spread through needles used by drug addicts), to evaluate treatment, and to help determine the type of parasite.

When performed: When symptoms such as recurring fever, chills, anemia, and paroxysms suggest malaria; when a patient has recently returned from traveling in areas where the disease exists (such as West Africa).

Normal values: Normally, there are no malarial organisms in the blood.

Abnormal values: Identification of any one of the various species of malarial parasites in a blood sample is indicative of infection.

Risk factors: Negligible (see general risk factors for blood testing).

Pain/discomfort: Minimal (see general pain/discomfort factors for blood testing).

Cost: From $15 to $30. This usually includes two to three separate microscopic examinations of the blood.

Accuracy and significance: The test is very specific (98 percent accurate) when malarial parasites are present. The inability to find malarial parasites in the blood, however, does not mean a person is without the disease. To assume significance, the test might have to be repeated several times, particularly during or immediately after an attack of chills and fever.

MALATHION INSECTICIDE POISONING, see *Cholinesterase*

MALE-FEMALE IDENTITY, see *Chromosome Analysis*

MALE SEX ORGAN FUNCTION, see *Testis Function*

MALNUTRITION

Malnutrition is different from malabsorption (see **Xylose Tolerance**), although the latter can cause the former. In essence, *malnutrition* is a generalized term that denotes one or more nutritional deficiencies (e.g., vitamins, proteins, minerals); it can come about as much from an excess of a food or foods (causing a loss of some other nutrient) as from a lack of an essential food substance. It is especially common in hospitalized patients where the diet may not compensate for the nutritional needs brought about by treatments (e.g., surgery, X-ray therapy, drugs). Other causes of malnutrition include: economic factors, cultural food habits, psychological problems, alcohol and drugs, infections, cancer, thyroid disease, and several inherited disorders—to mention but a few.

There are many tests to help detect malnutrition, sometimes called nutrition status testing; most are described under their own headings: **Albumin/Globulin** (decreased albumin), **Iron, Schilling, Folates, Magnesium, Blood Cell Differential,** and all the various vitamin and mineral measurements. In addition, there are, of course, weight observations (loss of weight being an obvious reason to search for a possible cause of malnutrition) and **Anthropometric Measurements**—primarily skinfold thickness measurements, usually of the middle part of the upper arm, using skinfold calipers. The goal is to determine the fat content under the skin; when it is less than normal (based on a table that takes age and sex into account), it can be the first sign of malnutrition, particularly of a protein deficiency. These tests are also performed on patients whose drugs do not seem to be working as expected. Anthropometrics are considered accurate enough to assist in a diagnosis, and they are quite inexpensive; in most instances, doctors do not charge for these measurements. (Also see **Skin Reaction.**)

MAMMOGRAPHY, see *Radiography*

MANGANESE

Research has suggested that people with epilepsy have lower-than-normal blood levels of the mineral manganese. It is not known whether decreased manganese in the blood is the cause of epilepsy or a result of the disease. Close relatives of patients with epilepsy also seem to have low blood manganese levels, although they may exhibit no symptoms of epilepsy. Because manganese is found in virtually all foods, it was once assumed that there could be no manganese deficiency. Adding extra manganese to the diet of a patient with epilepsy has, in a few cases, improved the patient's condition. Blood is taken from a vein, and the whole blood is tested.

The accidental ingestion or inhalation of manganese (prevalent among those who work with paints, fertilizers, and in the manufacture of drugs and glass) can cause edema, apathy, lung infection, liver disease, and symptoms similar to parkinsonism.

When performed: It may well become routine to test all patients with epilepsy for blood manganese levels; the test is also performed when manganese poisoning, usually from industrial sources, is suspected.

Normal values: Normal manganese levels range from 15 to 50 mcg per liter.

Abnormal values: Patients with epilepsy, and their immediate relatives, average 5 to 10 mcg per liter; increased values are found with manganese poisoning.

Risk factors: Negligible (see general risk factors for blood testing).

Pain/discomfort: Minimal (see general pain/discomfort factors for blood testing).

Cost: From $40 to $60.

Accuracy and significance: Testing for manganese in patients with epilepsy and their families is still considered in the investigational stage. When the test is used to help diagnose the cause of industrial toxicology, it can be of major significance; here it is considered to be 80 percent accurate.

MANOMETRY (ESOPHAGEAL), see *Gastroesophageal Reflux*

MANTOUX, see *Skin Reaction*

MAPLE SYRUP URINE DISEASE, see *Aminoaciduria*

MARIJUANA, see *Drug Abuse*

MASTER TWO-STEP, see *Electrocardiogram*

MATERNITY, see *Parentage; Pregnancy*

MAUZERALL-GRALNICK, see *Porphyrins*

MAXIMUM BREATHING CAPACITY, see *Pulmonary Function*

MAXIMUM EXPIRATORY FLOW RATE, see *Pulmonary Function*

MAXIMUM MIDEXPIRATORY FLOW RATE, see *Pulmonary Function*

MAXIMUM VOLUNTARY VENTILATION, see *Pulmonary Function*

MAZZINI, see *Syphilis*

MCH, see *Red Blood Cell Indices*

MCHC, see *Red Blood Cell Indices*

MCV, see *Red Blood Cell Indices*

MEAN CORPUSCULAR HEMOGLOBIN, see *Red Blood Cell Indices*

MEAN CORPUSCULAR HEMOGLOBIN CONCENTRATION, see *Red Blood Cell Indices*

MEAN CORPUSCULAR VOLUME, see *Red Blood Cell Indices*

MEASLES, see *Virus Disease*

MEDITERRANEAN ANEMIA, see *Hemoglobin*

MELANOGEN-MELANIN

Malignant melanoma is a skin condition consisting of black spots that are believed to start from an inherited nevus (mole); it is the most dangerous of all skin cancers. Many patients with melanomas secrete colorless melanogen in the urine, which then turns to dark brown or black melanin after several hours' exposure to air. The addition of ferric chloride hastens the reaction. A single urine sample is used for testing.

When performed: When a patient has blue-black, brown-black, or jet black moles or pigmentation on the skin, or when a light brown mole turns darker.

Normal values: No melanogen (turning to melanin) should be detected in urine.

Abnormal values: The presence of melanin in any quantity usually confirms the diagnosis of malignant melanoma. At times, a black-colored urine must be distinguished from alkaptonuria (see **Aminoaciduria**).

Risk factors: None.

Pain/discomfort: None.

Cost: From $10 to $20.

Accuracy and significance: The test is significant if melanin is found in the urine. The absence of melanin, however, does not guarantee the absence of melanoma. It is considered to be about 70 percent accurate.

MELENA, see *Occult Blood*

MELIOIDOSIS, see *Agglutination*

MENOPAUSE, see *Estrogen*

MENTAL DEPRESSION, see *Depression*

MENTAL STATUS, see *Cognitive Capacity Screening; Facial Recognition*

MERCURY

Mercury is a metallic element that can be toxic when taken into the body in sufficient amounts. Mercury can enter the body by inhalation if it is in the air; by contact with the skin (many skin ointments used to include mercury); by injection, as when it is used as a diuretic drug; and mostly by ingestion, as when eating fish containing even a trace of the metal. There are two different forms of mercury: the inorganic form (such as that used in thermometers), which causes vomiting, diarrhea, and kidney failure (most mercury is ultimately stored in the kidneys); and the organic form (such as that used in drugs), which causes weakness, brain damage, loss of balance, mental illness, and muscle pains.

When small amounts of mercury are taken into the body over long periods of time (years), no symptoms may appear until they build up to a toxic level. Urine is most frequently examined for mercury; blood from a vein may also be tested, as well as hair, nails, and other tissues. (See **Hair Analysis.**)

Other tests for suspected environmental-related poisoning include a test for fluoride (from ant or roach poisons) and what is called heavy metal screening (e.g., antimony, arsenic, chromium, **Phosphorus,** and **Cadmium**), which may be performed on blood or urine; these are usually employed when there is some related occupational exposure and bizarre symptoms cannot be explained. For example, chromium poisoning may be associated with photography and exposure to paints and dyes; it can cause an extensive dermatitis with ulcers and has also been blamed for lung cancer. Arsenic poisoning is usually reflected by abdominal pains—anywhere from 2 to 12 hours after ingestion. If the exposure is to very small amounts, there may be no symptoms at all for weeks, or there may be vague muscle pains and a difficulty in urination. While blood is usually tested for evidence of the heavy metal, it is also common to test the hair and the nails, especially for chronic exposure. Antimony causes bleeding in the bowels and the kidneys as well as liver damage. Barium, also used in insecticides, can cause muscle twitchings and rigidity (resembling tetanus, or "lockjaw"), as well as heartbeat irregularities and anemia. There is virtually no end to the metals and chemicals that can be tested for to ascertain the cause of some puzzling disease; the secret of successful diagnosing of heavy metal and other poisoning is to think of the probable cause. (Also see **Toxic Chemical Exposure.**)

When performed: On people who work with mercury (dental assistants, mirror makers, people who manufacture or use certain insecticides); with patients who seem to have mental illness, especially irritability or depression, when there is no known cause or provocation and when no psychiatric diagnosis can be made; when there is weakness, muscle tremors or cramps, brain damage, or kidney damage that cannot be diagnosed.

Normal values: There should be less than 10 mcg of mercury per 100 ml of urine and less than 2 mcg per 100 ml of blood. Hair and nails normally show a slight trace of the metal, usually less than 10 mcg per gram.

Abnormal values: While the amount of mercury varies tremendously in different individuals before it causes symptoms, in most instances a urine level greater than 20 mcg per 100 ml, a blood level greater than 20 mcg per 100 ml, or tissue amounts greater than 100 mcg per gram are indicative of mercury intoxication.

Risk factors: Negligible (see general risk factors for blood testing).

Pain/discomfort: Minimal (see general pain/discomfort factors for blood testing).

Cost: From $11 to $35 for most metals; $20 to $40 for screening.

Accuracy and significance: The test is quite specific for mercury toxicity when large abnormal values are found. It is especially significant in explaining psychiatric symptoms that can come from mercury poisoning. Metal testing is considered to be 90 percent accurate.

METANEPHRINS, see *Catecholamines*

METHACHOLINE INHALATION CHALLENGE, see *Pulmonary Function*

METHADONE, see *Drug Abuse*

METHANOL

Methanol (sometimes called methyl alcohol or wood alcohol) is occasionally ingested accidentally in place of ethanol (ethyl alcohol), the basis for liquors. One ounce of ethanol is usually metabolized and excreted by the body in three hours (depending on the quantity taken in). In contrast, it takes the body more than 24 hours to eliminate each ounce of methanol. More than an ounce of methanol can cause blindness and even death. Sterno is a solid form of methanol. Related products, used as sweetening agents, have recently been found in imported wines from several countries.

Isopropyl alcohol (regular rubbing alcohol) and ethylene glycol (the primary ingredient of automobile antifreeze) are also poisonous, but to a somewhat lesser degree than methanol. (Ethylene glycol causes oxalate crystals in the urine; see **Urinary Tract Calculus**.) Blood from a vein or urine may be tested.

When performed: When a patient has a combination of breathing and vision difficulties or is in a coma and no diagnosis can be made; when the ethyl **Alcohol** test is positive, but there are no signs of drunkenness.

Normal values: There should be no trace of methanol, isopropyl alcohol, or ethylene glycol in the blood or urine.

Abnormal values: Any amount found in the blood or urine is abnormal; values greater than 50 mg per 100 ml of blood can be fatal.

Risk factors: Negligible (see general risk factors for blood testing).

Pain/discomfort: Minimal (see general pain/discomfort factors for blood testing).

Cost: From $15 to $30 when performed alone. From $40 to $50 when tested together with isopropyl alcohol and ethylene glycol.

Accuracy and significance: The test can be very significant, even lifesaving, when performed on a patient who appears drunk but whose breath has no alcohol odor. It is considered to be 90 percent accurate.

METHEMOGLOBIN, see *Hemoglobin*

METROPOLITAN ACHIEVEMENT, see *Learning Disability*

METYRAPONE, see *Cortisol*

MHPG, see *Catecholamines*

MICROBIAL CULTURE, see *Culture*

MIDDLE-EAR INFECTION, see *Tympanometry*

MIELKE TEMPLATE, see *Bleeding and Clotting Time*

MILK ALLERGY, see *Agglutination*

MILK INTOLERANCE, see *Lactose Tolerance*

MINI-OBJECT, see *Cognitive Capacity Screening*

MINNESOTA MULTIPHASIC PERSONALITY INVENTORY (MMPI)

The MMPI is perhaps the most widely used test in clinical psychology; it is employed to assess ostensibly normal subjects as well as those with alleged disabling personality traits. The test consists of 550 statements printed on separate cards (for example, "I wish I could be as happy as others seem to be," "I am sure I am being talked about," "Someone has been trying to influence my mind"). The subject sorts the cards into piles indicating whether he agrees, disagrees, or "cannot say."

Essentially, the test covers nine traditional psychiatric diagnostic categories: hypochondria, depression, hysteria, psychopathic deviate, masculine-feminine interest (homosexuality), paranoia, psychasthenia, schizophrenia, and hypomania. It has since been extended to cover many new diagnostic interpretations. The responses are assessed to provide a coded profile. For example, an affirmative answer to the statement "I think I would like the work of a librarian" is supposed to indicate feminine occupational identification. Certain statements are used to determine whether the subject is lying. For example, an affirmative response to the statement "My sex life is satisfactory" (a statement that is a component of the lie-scale section of the test) is considered an indication that all the patient's responses are questionable. One criticism of the original form of this test is that its standards are based on a sample of the city of Minneapolis rather than on a broader, more representative population. The test is particularly open to censure when it is employed on individuals of diverse ethnic backgrounds.

When performed: The MMPI is used to uncover pathological tendencies as well as to reveal a profile of a individual's personality. It is also used for student counseling and screening of potential employees. Some clinics, usually those treating orthopedic problems such as bad back, perform the MMPI on all patients to help evaluate the psychological component of pain complaints.

Normal values: Similar patterns of responses in thousands of cases form the basis for coding individual profiles. The response profiles are used for differential diagnosis as well as for personality description.

Abnormal values: Certain response profiles are supposed to differentiate normal from pathological personalities (indicating paranoia, schizophrenia, depression, hypochondria, and other psychiatric conditions).

Risk factors: None.

Pain/discomfort: None.

Cost: From $50 to $100.

Accuracy and significance: Much of the significance of this test depends on the circumstances under which it is administered and the interpretation of the tester. There is no consensus among medical professionals as to its accuracy or value.

MIOSIS, see *Pupillary Reflex*

MITE INFESTATION, see *Scabies Infestation*

MMPI, see *Minnesota Multiphasic Personality Inventory*

MONOCLONAL ANTIBODIES, see *Agglutination*

MONONUCLEOSIS

The many and varied complaints of patients with infectious mononucleosis—including sore throat, headache, swollen glands (enlarged lymph nodes), abdominal pain, bleeding, and neurological problems—make diagnosis difficult. The specific cause of the disease is the Epstein-Barr virus, a member of the **Herpes** family of viruses. The disease was once thought to be spread by kissing and thus was called the "kissing disease." In infectious mononucleosis, the patient's antibody level reaction to sheep red blood cells rises. The heterophile antibody (an immunoglobulin) test is the primary aid for diagnosis. Blood is taken from a vein and the serum tested as in the

Agglutination test. The Forssman antibody test is even more specific. There are several other "spot" tests to detect mononucleosis antibodies; most require only one drop of fingertip blood placed on a chemically treated spot on a slide (Mono-Diff, Mono-Test, Mono-Spot). A marked increase in atypical lymphocytes in a **Blood Cell Differential** also points to infectious mononucleosis. Other tests for infectious mononucleosis, all based on the same principle, include the Paul-Bunnell (named after the two doctors who introduced it) and the Davidson differential; some doctors feel the latter test is a bit more specific.

When performed: When there is suspicion of infectious mononucleosis; to differentiate infectious mononucleosis from other diseases.

Normal values: Normally, there may be very small amounts of antibody to sheep red blood cells (below a dilution of 1:112).

Abnormal values: Antibody levels are elevated to a dilution of 1:224 or more in approximately 70 percent of patients with mononucleosis; elevated levels may persist for weeks.

Risk factors: Negligible (see general risk factors for blood testing).

Pain/discomfort: Minimal (see general pain/discomfort factors for blood testing).

Cost: There is usually no charge for the "spot" test when performed in a doctor's office. When performed in a laboratory, the charge is $6 to $10. Virus testing is $90.

Accuracy and significance: The various "spot" and biochemical tests for mononucleosis are considered to be 85 percent accurate. The test is significant in helping the doctor differentiate mononucleosis from other diseases with similar symptoms.

MORO RESPONSE, see *Hearing Function*

MORPHINE, see *Drug Abuse*

MOSENTHAL

The specific gravity of urine is usually a routine measurement; normally, it should be high when the urine is concentrated (contains more solid matter), most frequently on awakening, and lower after a large amount of fluid is ingested. At times, however, more precise tests of specific gravity are required to pinpoint the location of a kidney problem; they are called urine concentration tests.

For the Mosenthal test, the patient cannot drink any liquids (the usual food diet is allowed) for 24 hours prior to testing. The first specimen of urine is voided on awakening and measured for specific gravity. The patient stays in bed for an additional hour and then voids again for another specific gravity measurement. The patient gets up and is active for one more hour, after which a third and final urine specimen is taken. Some doctors test only for specific gravity; others also perform a **Chloride** test on the urine.

The Fishberg test is a shortened version of the Mosenthal. Very little liquid is taken with dinner the night before the test, and no food or liquids are taken during the night. When the patient awakens, a urine sample is collected; two additional samples are taken an hour apart. The patient stays in bed the entire time. The test cannot be performed when a patient is taking diuretic drugs or certain hormones or is eating an unusual diet (especially one low in protein).

When performed: Whenever kidney disease is suspected; when adrenal or pituitary hormone problems, liver disease, or unexplained edema (water retention) exists.

Normal values: No matter what version of the test is used, at least one urine sample should show a specific gravity of 1.025 or greater, indicating the kidney's ability to concentrate urine when liquids are withheld.

Abnormal values: A specific gravity value of less than 1.020 indicates kidney problems. As the specific gravity decreases in value, greater kidney pathology is indicated. On occasion, a low specific gravity will result from pituitary problems or the failure of the hypothalamus to produce antidiuretic hormone (**Vasopressin,** ADH), but this can be distinguished from kidney disease by administering vasopressin and noting the patient's response.

Risk factors: None.

Pain/discomfort: None.

Cost: There is usually no charge for measuring the specific gravity of the urine samples brought to the doctor's office. A hospital may charge $12 a test.

Accuracy and significance: The test is considered a useful screening procedure for suspected kidney disease. It is not sufficiently significant to provide a particular diagnosis, despite its accuracy rate of 98 percent as a measurement.

MOTOR DEVELOPMENT

There are several measurements of infant motor development (how early in life and how well a child learns to use his muscles and coordinate his activities). The most popular is the Gesell Developmental Schedule, in which a child's physical activities are compared against a set of norms or standards determined by studying thousands of children during different stages of development. For example, at 4 weeks old, a child should be able to rotate his head and clench his fists. At 5 months, he should be able to grasp a rattle; at 1 year, he should be able to throw a ball; at 4 years, he should be able to walk up and down stairs properly and hop on one foot. There are "schedules" for ages up to 6 years.

Observations are also made of the child's language ability, drawing ability, and certain social activities such as personal grooming. The primary purpose of observation is to detect neurological (nervous system or muscle) pathology as early as possible. The Bayley Scale is another motor development measurement.

When performed: The Gesell test has become almost routine in pediatric examinations to aid in diagnosing developmental problems. It is also performed when a child appears to be slow in acquiring the usual developmental traits for his age (for example, not walking when expected to; not responding to stimuli).

Normal values: There are schedules (or expected standards) of physical activity for various ages, a few examples of which are described above (the schedules run into hundreds of observations).

Abnormal values: Failure to perform several activities expected at a given age; when a child appears to have multiple developmental problems, neurological or other pathology must be considered.

Risk factors: None.

Pain/discomfort: None.

Cost: From $25 to $50, depending on the time required and the number of comparisons made; the older the child, the greater the number of observations.

Accuracy and significance: When properly performed and carefully interpreted, the tests are considered to be 90 percent accurate in noting developmental disability, but they do not pinpoint the cause.

MRI, see *Magnetic Resonance Imaging*

MUCIN CLOT, see *Synovial Fluid*

MULTIPLE MYELOMA, see *Bence-Jones Protein*

MULTIPLE SCLEROSIS, see *Hot Bath; Immunoglobulin*

MULTIPLE TEST PANEL, see *Comprehensive Multiple Test Screening*

MUMPS, see *Agglutination; Skin Reaction; Virus Disease*

MURAMIDASE, see *Lysozyme*

MUSCLE ENZYME, see *Aldolase*

MUSCLE REFLEX, see *Reflex*

MUSCLE STIMULATION, see *Electromyography*

MUSCLE TENSION, see *Electromyography*

MUSCULAR DYSTROPHY ENZYME, see *Creatine Phosphokinase*

MYASTHENIA GRAVIS, see *Edrophonium*

MYCOSIS, see *Fungus*

MYELOGRAPHY (MYELOGRAM), see *Radiography*

MYELOMATOSIS, see *Bence-Jones Protein*

MYOGLOBIN, see *Hemoglobin*

MYOGRAPHY, see *Electromyography*

MYOPIA, see *Visual Acuity*

N

NAIL BIOPSY, see *Biopsy*

NARCOTICS, see *Drug Abuse*

NASAL AIRWAY RESISTANCE, see *Smell Function*

NEARSIGHTEDNESS, see *Visual Acuity*

NEOCEPT, see *Pregnancy*

NEONATAL HYPOTHYROID, see *Thyroid Function*

NEPHROCALCINOSIS, see *Urinary Tract Calculus*

NEPHROLITHIASIS, see *Urinary Tract Calculus*

NERVE CONDUCTION, see *Electromyography*

NERVE THERMOGRAPHY, see *Thermography*

NERVOUS STRESS, see *Electromyography*

NEUROBLASTOMA, see *Catecholamines*

NEUROGRAPHY, see *Electromyography*

NEWBORN DEFECT SCREENING, see *Genetic Disorder Screening*

NEWBORN SCREENING, see *Aminoaciduria; Galactosemia; Hemoglobin; Phenylketonuria; Red Blood Cell; Thyroid Function*

NIACIN (Vitamin B$_3$)

Skin rashes, headache, nervousness, diarrhea, loss of appetite, insomnia, and inflammation of the tongue are all symptoms of niacin (vitamin B$_3$) deficiency. Nicotinic acid and niacinamide are forms of this vitamin. Niacinamide is sometimes used in therapy because it causes fewer side effects. Niacin is found mostly in yeast, meats, fish, poultry, and eggs and in small amounts in vegetables. Pellagra is the specific disease that may result from lack of sufficient niacin and is known in medicine as the 3-D disease: characterized by diarrhea, dermatitis, and dementia (mental depression). Niacin is measured by testing for its metabolic end products in the urine.

When performed: In mental illness, especially schizophrenia, mania, depression, and paranoia; when skin diseases cannot be easily diagnosed; in patients on vegetarian diets; with alcoholism.

Normal values: The metabolic end products of niacin should range from at least 0.6 to 1.59 mg in a six-hour urine specimen.

Abnormal values: Less than 0.6 mg for a six-hour urine specimen indicates a vitamin B$_3$ deficiency sufficient to cause disease (pellagra).

Risk factors: None.

Pain/discomfort: None.

Cost: From $5 to $10.

Accuracy and significance: The test is considered to be 70 percent accurate and is performed to confirm the diagnosis of pellagra, but the symptoms and signs of the disease, plus a successful therapeutic trial of vitamin B$_3$, allow a diagnosis long before the test is needed.

NICOTINIC ACID, see *Niacin*

NILE BLUE FAT STAIN, see *Pregnancy*

NITRITE, see *Urine Examination*

NITROBLUE TETRAZOLIUM (NBT), see *Blood Cell Differential*

NONGONOCOCCAL URETHRITIS, see *Chlamydia Identification; Complement Fixation*

NONISOTOPIC IMMUNOASSAY, see *Agglutination*

NONMATERNITY, see *Parentage*

NONPATERNITY, see *Parentage*

NONPROTEIN NITROGEN (NPN), see *Urea Nitrogen*

NONSPECIFIC URETHRITIS, see *Chlamydia Identification*

NONSTRESS FETAL ASSESSMENT (NST)

The nonstress test for fetal assessment, sometimes called the fetal heart rate acceleration test (FHRAT), helps to evaluate potential problems of pregnancy. It is used almost routinely for those pregnant women for whom the doctor feels there is a greater-than-average risk of problems such as high blood pressure, diabetes, or previous pregnancy problems (see **Fetal Monitoring**).

In the past, when a difficult pregnancy was suspected, a small amount of the hormone oxytocin was administered to increase contractions of the uterus. The procedure is known as the oxytocin challenge test (OCT) or the contraction stress test (CST). No matter what the impetus, the purpose is to stimulate fetal activity (induce the baby to kick or move in the womb) and then to note if the baby's heart rate increases as it should. Usually, the mother lies in a bed which elevates her head and knees. When the baby kicks or moves, the mother presses a button that records the baby's heartbeat.

The breast stimulation stress test (BSST) is a new version of fetal assessment tests. While it is less a measure of the response of the fetal heart, it is considered a reasonable monitor of fetal well-being, especially in cases of high-risk pregnancies. The patient, with breasts covered, is asked to stroke and squeeze the breast and then to roll the bare nipple between the fingers followed by gentle tugging on the nipple until a uterine contraction is felt. A nurse monitors the contractions, and stimulation is stopped when the contraction starts. One protocol has the process performed three times until three contractions are felt within a 10-minute period of time. If the three contractions are not recorded, the test is repeated over a 20-minute period. Usually, 90 percent of patients have sufficient contractions to allow an interpretation of the fetus's condition. BSST is considered more convenient and more practical than the OCT because it does not require the injection of a drug.

When performed: On pregnant women, primarily those who are known to have, or are suspected of having, pregnancy problems; when there is doubt as to the position or exact location of the placenta; when there is a question about the baby's position and condition (such as the possibility that the umbilical cord is wrapped around the baby's neck or the possibility that the baby's size is not in accord with the duration of the pregnancy); when a pregnancy exceeds the estimated delivery date; when the mother stops feeling normal movements in the womb. BSST may be performed weekly or even twice a week once the fetus is sufficiently mature to react.

Normal values: The baby's recorded heartbeat should increase at least 15 beats per minute within 20 minutes following kicking or movement. This is called reactive, or positive.

Abnormal values: Failure of any acceleration of the baby's heartbeat during fetal movement. This is called nonreactive. Most often, if there is a nonreactive response to the nonstress test, a stress test using oxytocin is administered before considering the response abnormal. Certain drugs, such as beta blockers used to treat high blood pressure, can cause a false positive result.

Risk factors: None with the use of the nonstress fetal assessment test; there is always a minor risk when the hormone is used.

Pain/discomfort: None, although some pregnant women find the test anxiety-provoking.

Cost: From $40 to $80, depending on the time required.

Accuracy and significance: The procedure is 80 percent accurate in helping to observe and predict the condition of the fetus and the course of some but not all pregnancy problems. The test can be lifesaving for the infant.

Recent evidence has revealed that if there is excessive stimulation of the uterus, a false-positive test may result. Therefore, a positive test should be confirmed by a different corroborative test before any action is taken. Both drugs and nipple stimulation can cause false-positive uterine contractions.

NORADRENALIN, see *Catecholamines*

NOREPINEPHRINE, see *Catecholamines*

NORTHERN BLOT, see *Chromosome Analysis*

NPN, see *Urea Nitrogen*

NST, see *Nonstress Fetal Assessment*

NUCLEAR MAGNETIC RESONANCE, see *Magnetic Resonance Imaging*

NUCLEAR SCANNING (Radioactive Uptake, Scintillation, Radioisotope)

Nuclear scanning, or radionuclide organ imaging, may be performed on many parts of the body to aid in diagnosing and treating disease. Its primary function is to outline the size, shape, and exact location of an organ (liver, kidney, vein, etc.) or a chamber or duct within an organ. Nuclear scanning tests are also fairly precise in measuring organ function.

A radioactive material (radioisotope or radionuclide) is injected or ingested into the body; depending on the organ to be studied, it may be inserted into an arm vein or administered through a catheter (thin, hollow tube) that starts in an arm or leg vein or artery and is pushed through the blood vessels to the specific organ being tested. In a heart scan, for example, the catheter may start in the arm or the neck and end directly inside the heart chamber being studied. To test the thyroid, a patient drinks radioactive iodine. Various chemicals are known to select certain body organs, and after being made radioactive, they can be detected within the organ by rectilinear scanners or gamma cameras, both of which work on the same principle as the Geiger counter in detecting uranium. A faster modification of the process is called scintography.

The amount of radioactivity in the injected chemicals is so small as to cause no known harmful effects to the body. Virtually all radioactivity is gone within a day or so. The scanning machines that detect the radioactivity do not give off any radiation.

In many instances, the radioactivity is visualized on a photographic plate or an X-ray plate. Sometimes, a computer printout is made on paper outlining the organ being studied. The results show the size and shape of the organ as well as any part of the organ that failed to pick up radioactive material—usually indicating a defect (disease, tumor). Any excess of radioactivity in an area usually means the organ is enlarged or hyperactive. Through measurement of the flow of radioactive material through an organ, the function of that organ can be determined. When the kidneys are tested, measurement of blood flowing into and out of the kidney is called a renogram; measurement of the size, shape, and position of the kidney is called a renal scan. Usually, both kidneys are measured at the same time to better detect which kidney, if only one, is affected.

In some cases, instead of a diagram or illustration of the radioactivity, a counter is placed over the organ and the amount of radioactivity is "counted" and recorded as to its intensity. This technique is often used in testing organ function, since it is easier and continuous.

Most often, the nuclear scanning test is referred to by the name of the organ or area being studied; examples are discussed below.

Abdominal scan: One of the most difficult diagnoses of all is to locate the source of suspected abdominal bleeding. This is because patients with this problem do not bleed all the time; a test such as **Endoscopy** or **Radiography** could show a normal result if performed at the moment bleeding had temporarily stopped. However, by injecting a radioactive chemical into the bloodstream and monitoring it with scintography, it is possible to detect intermittent bleeding from the gastrointestinal tract—especially when the test is carried out over a 30-minute period of time. (Also see **Fluorescein Eye Stain**.)

Bile acid breath scan: After the patient eats a special meal containing a radioactive substance, the radioactivity of the **Carbon Dioxide** (CO_2) in the exhaled breath is measured. With intestinal dysfunction—such as malabsorption, delayed transit of food, and bacterial overgrowth in the bowel (see **Xylose Tolerance**)—the radioactive CO_2 is increased. At times, the radioactivity of the feces is also measured to help distinguish malabsorption from bacterial overgrowth (see **Feces Examination**).

Biliary (gallbladder) scan: Because of the poor accuracy rate of cholangiography (see **Radiography**) testing, scintography of the gallbladder and its ducts to and from the liver has been employed, especially to ascertain whether or not the bile ducts are open and functioning. Although **Ultrasound** testing of the gallbladder is considered to be most accurate when searching for gallstones, biliary scanning can help detect infections of the bile ducts and gallbladder; these conditions can cause pain and discomfort similar to gallstones. Biliary scanning also has the advantage of following the actions, or nonactions, of the gallbladder over a period of several hours. The test is helpful, too, in detecting "leaks" in the bile duct system and relating the pancreas to the patient's symptoms.

Bone scan: Usually, radioactive strontium is used (since it replaces calcium), and a uniform uptake (or concentration) throughout all the bones is normal. An increased concentration in a specific area is abnormal and usually represents cancer, but arthritis and fractures can sometimes give a similar picture. Radioactive gallium is used in testing for hidden bone infections, since gallium seems to seek out inflammatory tissue. Usually, a bone scan is performed a few hours after injection of the material.

Brain scan: Radioactive chemicals (mostly technetium) are used for brain imaging; normal brain tissue will not pick up most of the tracer material. A concentration of radioactive material usually indicates an increased number of blood vessels and a disease process. The scanning is performed twice, immediately after the injection of radioactive material and then 24 hours later.

Esophagus and stomach scan: When patients have difficulty in swallowing (dysphagia), they are sometimes given a syrupy radioactive solution to swallow. This is also called a radionuclide transit (RT) test, during which the path of the radioactive material is followed by a gamma camera. Many doctors prefer this test to the barium swallow (see **Radiography**), as the barium swallow can be performed only once, and interpretation of the barium's path is highly subjective. An esophageal scan can be performed several times without risk of excessive radiation exposure. **Gastroesophageal Reflux** is also evaluated in a reverse form of esophageal scan; radioactive measurements follow the reverse flow to see if the stomach's contents go back into the esophagus.

Heart, or cardiac, scan: Radioactive thallium is injected into a vein and is absorbed by heart tissue, allowing visualization of the size and shape of the heart. This test is particularly valuable when pericarditis (excessive fluid around the heart) is suspected. Scanning takes place immediately after injection of the chemical. Other radioactive chemicals are used to outline the inside chambers of the heart. A blood pool scan shows heart contractions clearly and can help indicate the amount of damage after a heart attack.

In perfusion imaging, radioactive chemicals can be directed into the coronary arteries supplying oxygen to the heart muscle to reveal blocked or narrowed arteries. This procedure is also used while a patient is exercising to detect heart muscle that has inadequate circulation only when under physical stress. *Cold spot* imaging is another term for visualizing the heart with radioactive chemicals. *Cardiac catheterization* is yet another term used; however, it is also applied to angiology or angiography (see **Radiography**) when dye, rather than radioactive chemicals, is utilized.

Kidney and bladder scan: At times, radioactive chemicals are injected into the bloodstream just before the blood reaches the kidney. The rate of kidney filtration (renogram scanning) and the rate of bladder filling and emptying (cystogram scanning) are measured as a means of testing the function of these organs.

Leukocyte scan: When leukocytes **(White Blood Cells)** are attached to radioactive indium 111, they concentrate in areas of abscess and inflammation and can help locate a suspected but hidden abscess. This can be valuable in patients with unexplained bowel disease and especially after surgery when a patient has an unexplained fever. If the test is negative, it is considered strong evidence against there being a hidden, serious infection.

Liver scan: Nuclear scanning is probably the best way to study the liver without surgery. Radioactive gold or rose bengal (a dye) is injected into a vein. Normally, the chemical is absorbed by the liver within 20 minutes and shows a uniform appearance when viewed by the scanner. If, however, there is pathology (growth, cirrhosis, or abscess), that area will not take up the chemical, and the absence of radioactivity indicates disease.

Lung scan: There are two kinds of lung scanning: a perfusion scan and a ventilation scan. They may be performed separately or together to aid in diagnosis. The perfusion scan is more common. Radioactive albumin is injected into a vein, and the scanning is performed immediately. The primary purpose of a perfusion scan is to diagnose pulmonary embolism. When the two different lung scans are performed together, it is also possible to evaluate pulmonary function in emphysema and other lung obstructions, to locate a growth and follow the course of that growth before and after treatment, to measure the size of the heart, and to discern areas of infection and lung collapse. The ventilation scan is performed by having the patient breathe in radioactive xenon gas and then passing the scanner over the lungs. Inhaled radioactive xenon can show normal or abnormal bronchial passageways and areas of the lung that do not receive air.

Pancreas scan: A radioactive selenium–amino acid compound is injected in a vein. The pancreas normally takes up this amino acid immediately, and the radioactive element allows imaging of the organ in about 10 minutes. Pancreatic disease is difficult to diagnose, and this test helps detect cancer, cysts, and infection by the organ's failure to show absorption of the radioactive material. At times Triolein is injected as a means of diagnosing malabsorption or fat-absorption problems.

Placental scan: When there is doubt about the exact position of the fetus during pregnancy, the injection of an extremely tiny dose of radioactive albumin will help show the location of the placenta so as to place the fetus. When there is suspicion of intrauterine bleeding, usually due to a damaged placenta, this test will help diagnose the condition and can be lifesaving to the patient.

Radiation poisoning: After exposure to radiation, various organs of the body may be scanned (most commonly, it is the thyroid gland) as a means of detecting radioactivity. This is similar to deliberately placing nuclear material in the gland, but here the test is used to detect unwanted radiation such as might occur in the air after a nuclear power plant accident or after atomic testing.

Red blood cell survival scan: To reach a precise evaluation of hemolytic anemia and other causes of red blood cell destruction or loss, some of the patient's blood is withdrawn and radioisotopes are attached to the red blood cells. The blood is then scanned weekly for a month; the loss of radioactive-tagged cells indicates the rate of hemolytic anemia.

Salivary gland scan: When there is a suspected blockage of the ducts that empty the salivary glands into the mouth, usually due to a stone or infection, radioisotopes can be injected into the glands to locate the blocked area. This test can also help predict how a patient with Bell's palsy (a paralysis of the main facial nerve on one side) will respond to treatment. If the unaffected side of the face shows a response to salivary stimulus similar to the affected side, it is considered a good sign for recovery.

Spinal fluid scan: Radioactive albumin is injected into the lower-back spinal fluid space (see **Cerebrospinal Fluid**) and observed as it passes around the cord into the brain spaces. The chemical takes about 24 hours to reach the brain area and remains there for two to three days. This test is especially valuable in diagnosing hydrocephalus (abnormally large head); it is also indicated when there is suspicion of a spinal fluid leak. The test is sometimes called cisternography, spinal cord scan, or intrathecal scan.

Spleen scan: The same chemicals used for a liver scan are often employed to visualize the spleen; however, radioactive red blood cells (erythrocytes) give an even better image (since the spleen's function is to remove ineffective erythrocytes from the blood). The test is used to help diagnose an unknown mass in the upper left portion of the abdomen, to evaluate the size and functioning of the spleen, and to diagnose spleen injury. Spleen scanning takes place about four hours after red blood cell injection.

Testicular or scrotal scanning: Sometimes called an orchiogram, this consists of an injection of radioactive material into the testicular artery and is used to diagnose pain and/or swelling in one or both testicles. It is particularly useful in diagnosing epididymitis (an infection of the cordlike duct next to the testicle) and when an undiagnosable tumor is felt.

Thyroid scan: See **Thyroid Function.**

Vein scan: Various radioactive chemicals injected into a vein will be absorbed in blood clots if a thrombus or phlebitis is present. The clot is easily visualized. The test may also predict patients who are prone to thromboembolism.

Note: Radioimmunoassay is a technique (not a specific test) that uses radionuclides (as employed in scanning) for measuring minute quantities of hormones, certain drugs, and antigens that can cause disease (see **Agglutination; RAST**). It is another method to verify hormone deficiency or excess, drug toxicity, allergy, and infections.

When performed: In general, scanning is performed when it is necessary to visualize an organ and to follow the progress of certain diseases. More specific indications for nuclear scanning are noted in the descriptions of the scanning procedures above.

Normal values: Normal values are noted in the specific scanning descriptions above.

Abnormal values: Whether an organ should or should not pick up and reflect radioactivity is discussed under each organ-scanning procedure. The normality, abnormality, and degree of abnormality are determined by a physician with extensive experience in the field.

Risk factors: Depending on the organ being scanned and the particular technical process, the risk ranges from negligible (see general risk factors for blood testing) to slight when there is a single injection of radioactive material (see general risk factors for X-ray and radioactive substance application). The increase of risk parallels the number of instruments used and the complexity of the procedure (see general risk factors for catheter and needle insertion and for contrast substance use). Whenever catheters are inserted and directed to a sensitive area of the body (heart, brain, and other internal body organs), the risk increases in proportion to the distance the catheter must travel. Catheters within the heart and major arteries, particularly those to the lungs, can cause fluctuations in heart rhythm and have been known to stop the heart's beating completely (cardiac arrest). Catheters have also been known to damage the heart's valves. In summary, the more complicated a procedure, the longer it takes, or the larger the body area being scanned, the greater risks associated with nuclear scanning become.

Yet another risk, albeit an indirect one, from employing radioactive substances used in nuclear scanning, and in other nuclear medicine investigations, is that when a nursing mother has such a test, she may pass on radioactive milk to her child. It has been suggested that breast feeding be stopped for a period of time should a nursing mother require a medical test using a radioactive substance.

Pain/discomfort: Pain and discomfort are minimal when the test involves only the injection of a radioactive substance (see general pain/discomfort factors for blood testing). When the test necessitates the insertion of a catheter (see general pain/discomfort factors for catheter and needle insertion), many patients complain of the manipulation of their bodies for prolonged periods of time. Unless the procedures are explained in detail before the test, patients tend to be quite apprehensive, especially when a catheter is directed to the heart. Some patients undergoing a lung scan complain of a sense of suffocation.

Cost: There is a wide range of fees for nuclear scanning. Much depends on the organ being evaluated, the time needed for study, and the difficulty in directing the radioactive chemical to the particular organ. For example, thyroid nuclear scanning ranges from $50 to $120. A simple kidney scan is $50 to $200. Liver, spleen, pancreas, esophagus, and stomach scans are $100 to $300. Lung scans run $200 to $300. Bone or cardiac scans are $300 to $500. If the procedure is performed in a hospital, there is usually an additional charge, depending on the services employed and the length of time a patient remains hospitalized after completion of the tests. If a special computer is used to enhance the observed image, there may be an additional charge of $100.

Accuracy and significance: In general, nuclear scanning is considered reasonably accurate, but much depends on the organ or area of the body being scanned. For example, heart scans can be extremely significant in differentiating the causes of chest pain. A number of doctors believe thallium scanning (without catheterization) is quite precise in locating damage to heart muscle and indicating its scope. When a thallium scan is performed while a patient is exercising, and the test appears normal, angiography (see **Radiography**), with its use of catheters, is not necessary. Lung scanning is not absolutely precise unless large defects exist. The majority of doctors think only incontestably normal scans are diagnostic, while abnormal scans are not always especially specific. Overall, nuclear scanning is considered to have an accuracy rate of from 50 to 80 percent.

NUMBER CONNECTION

A patient with the disease known as portal system encephalopathy (PSE; the word *portal* refers to the liver) shows a variety of abnormal mental symptoms. The patient's behavior can appear psychotic, and the thought process can be confused. At times, the patient's symptoms can imitate delirium tremens (DTs). The disease is caused by the liver's inability to function properly, which leads to an excessive accumulation of **Ammonia** in the blood, particularly in and around the brain. While it can result from alcoholism, it also results from other liver diseases and has been known to be an adverse consequence of abdominal surgery. It was once called hepatic coma, but this referred to the condition when it was irreversible and ultimately fatal. Today, PSE can be treated if discovered early. One way to recognize some of the disease's first symptoms is by a change in the patient's handwriting, but this is not something usually seen by a doctor. Should there be the suspicion of PSE, a number connection test can be ordered. This test uses numbers scattered all over a sheet of paper. The patient is asked to connect the numbers in correct order with a pencil line. It resembles the child's game where a picture was formed when consecutive numbers were connected. There are several different versions of the test, so it may be repeated at regular intervals to note the progression or regression of the disease. Although there are various chemical tests to aid in the diagnosis of liver disease, many doctors consider the number connection test one of the best indications of the amount of liver damage.

When performed: When liver disease is suspected; to help diagnose personality changes; as a confirmation of alcoholism; to help uncover the cause of coma once the patient is conscious.

Normal values: The ability to put numbers in sequence, neatly and rapidly.

Abnormal values: The inability to put numbers in sequence, even with help; the need to take increasing lengths of time to connect the numbers as the test is repeated.

Risk factors: None.

Pain/discomfort: None.

Cost: Usually administered by a nurse or doctor's assistant in the doctor's office; there can be a $10 charge.

Accuracy and significance: Considered a 70 percent accurate measure of the extent of liver damage. It is usually performed with **Albumin/Globulin, Bilirubin, Ammonia,** and other liver-function tests.

NUTRITION STATUS, see *Malnutrition*

NYSTAGMUS, see *Caloric*

O

OCCULT BLOOD

In medicine, the word *occult* means "present but invisible." Thus, occult blood procedures test for blood that can be seen only through microscopic or chemical examination. Virtually all body fluids, excretions, and secretions can be tested for occult blood; most often, the test is performed on feces and urine (see **Feces Examination** and **Urine Examination**). It has been proposed that if everyone's feces were properly tested for occult blood twice a year, almost all deaths from bowel cancer could be eliminated.

A person can lose about an ounce of blood a day from the bowel (amounting to a pint in two weeks) without noticing any bleeding. In contrast, visible bleeding occurs when more than 2 ounces of blood enter the bowel (from a bleeding ulcer, from a growth in the colon or large intestine, or from hemorrhoids). When that blood mixes with the stomach acid in the bowel, it turns black and is termed melena. Thus, a general assumption is that black, tarry bowel movements indicate bleeding somewhere in the upper intestinal tract, while bright red blood indicates lower-bowel and rectal bleeding.

There are many different tests for occult blood; the most common are the guaiac (Hema-Chek, Hemoccult), orthotoluidine, and benzidine. The orthotoluidine test is the most sensitive but will give a false-positive result when the patient's diet includes meat. The guaiac test usually does not react to dietary meat but is the least sensitive. In most instances, a patient is told not to eat any meat or even to brush his teeth for at least three days before the test, since the slightest trace of blood from meat or from irritation of the gums can give a false-positive result. Some of the newer tests are esthetically easier to perform; they eliminate the need to take a sample of the feces (Cs-T, or Coloscreen Self-Test; Early Detector; EZ-Detect). One test, called HemoQuant, indicates the quantity of blood coming from the gastrointestinal tract; it is also claimed not to give false-positive results due to ingestion of certain vegetables, medications, and vitamin C, but red meat must still be avoided.

When performed: Whenever gastrointestinal or kidney disease is suspected; whenever a patient has an anemia that cannot be diagnosed.

Normal values: Urine, feces, and other body secretions should show no occult blood.

Abnormal values: A positive occult blood test, after eliminating all extraneous causes (brushing the teeth, irritating the throat, blowing the nose too hard, meat in the diet, taking an excessive amount of iron pills), is considered abnormal. Occult blood can be found in the bowel with patients taking aspirin or other drugs that irritate the stomach. Alcoholic gastritis may also cause a positive test. False-positive results can be caused by eating turnips, horseradish, and other foods; false-negative results can come from taking large doses of vitamin C just prior to being tested. A positive test does not automatically indicate colon cancer; it simply means there is some bleeding source in the bowel. As a matter of fact, in patients younger than 50, no more than 3 percent of all positive tests turned out to involve cancer. Between the ages of 50 and 70, the positive test indicated cancer in 12 percent, and after age 70, it indicated cancer in only 23 percent of all patients.

Eating beets will color the feces red but will not cause a positive test. A positive urine occult blood test usually indicates pathology somewhere in the urinary tract, from the kidneys to the bladder to the ducts that carry the urine.

Risk factors: None.

Pain/discomfort: None.

Cost: Usually, there is no charge for an occult blood test performed in the doctor's office (Hema-Chek, Hemoccult); the patient brings the test paper, provided by the doctor, from home to the office. When more specific tests are performed in a laboratory, the charge is $4 to $17. Most often, doctors suggest that patients purchase their own do-it-yourself medical test kit for home use for $3 to $6; repeated positive test results are then investigated more thoroughly. Hospitals may charge up to $20 for the test.

Accuracy and significance: Although the test is valuable, unfortunately it can show 30 to 60 percent false-positive results when applied to feces. And there have been instances where the test failed to detect blood known to be present, although most often, this was due to improper technique. When applied to urine, the test is considered to be 90 percent accurate. If the test is positive more than once, and all the extraneous factors that could cause a false-positive result have been considered, the finding is significant enough to warrant an extensive search for the cause of hidden bleeding.

(A feces specimen should not be taken from a toilet bowl in which any of the automatic cleaning compounds or devices are used.)

OCT, see *Nonstress Fetal Assessment*

OCULAR HYPERTENSION, see *Tonometry*

OCULAR MUSCLE, see *Strabismus*

OCULAR PLETHYSMOGRAPHY, see *Plethysmography*

OLFACTORY PERCEPTION, see *Smell Function*

OPG, see *Plethysmography*

OPHTHALMODYNAMOMETRY, see *Tonometry*

OPHTHALMOSCOPY, see *Fundoscopy*

OPTOKINETIC, see *Caloric*

ORCHIOGRAM, see *Nuclear Scanning*

ORGANIC PHOSPHATE POISONING, see *Cholinesterase*

ORGAN IMAGING, see *Computerized Tomography; Nuclear Scanning; Radiography; Ultrasound*

ORGAN TRANSPLANT, see *HLA*

ORIENTAL SORE, see *Agglutination*

ORTHOTOLUIDINE, see *Occult Blood*

OSMOLALITY

Osmolality is a measure of the osmotic pressure of a liquid. In medicine, osmotic pressure indicates the amount of dissolved material (minerals, hormones, etc.) in a body fluid, most commonly blood or urine. Large amounts of sodium, sugars, fats, and other substances increase the blood's osmolality; in fact, the amount of sodium alone in the blood can sometimes be used as a reasonable measure of serum osmolality. Bold osmolality regulates body water (the feeling of thirst, when water is needed, and the control of urine output), and it depends primarily on blood electrolytes (see

Chloride; Potassium; Sodium). Blood is taken from a vein, and the serum is tested. Urine is also tested for osmolality.

The osmolality test is considered more accurate than the urine specific gravity test (see **Mosenthal**), which offers somewhat similar measurements (specific gravity measures the presence and quantity of all the particles of varying sizes that are contained in the liquid). A common method of testing for osmolality is to measure the exact degree at which the liquid freezes, since soluble particles in a liquid affect the freezing point.

When performed: When dehydration is suspected; in alcoholism; when excessive amounts of fats are in the blood (hyperlipidemia); in uncontrolled diabetes and in unexplained instances of edema (water retention); to measure the effects of intravenous therapy.

Normal values: Normally, osmolality should range from 280 to 295 mOsm per liter (about the same as normal plasma) in blood and 300 to 1,200 mOsm per liter of urine.

Abnormal values: Levels are increased (hyperosmolality) with water loss (vomiting, diarrhea, excess sweating) or inadequate water intake (300 mOsm per liter is considered moderate to severe dehydration), with brain or kidney damage, and with diabetes insipidus. Decreased levels occur when excess water is taken in or administered (such as with intravenous therapy) and when diuretic drugs are used (which cause excretion of a great deal of sodium ions, lessening the amount of blood electrolytes). Markedly decreased levels in the urine indicate failure of the kidney's concentrating ability.

Risk factors: Negligible (see general risk factors for blood testing).
Pain/discomfort: Minimal (see general pain/discomfort factors for blood testing).
Cost: From $18 to $38.

Accuracy and significance: The test is considered to be about 80 percent accurate and is most often performed in a hospital, where the effects of intravenous solutions can be monitored. Osmotic pressure is considered a reasonable measurement of the body's state of hydration or dehydration. When blood and urine osmolality are measured together, they help to confirm the diagnosis of diabetes insipidus (a hormone imbalance causing a patient to drink unusually large quantities of fluid and to urinate excessively; see **Vasopressin**).

OSMOTIC FRAGILITY, see *Red Blood Cell*

OSTEOPOROSIS TESTING, see *Bone Mineral Density Analysis*

OTIS, see *Intelligence Quotient*

OTOTOXICITY, see *Hearing Function*

O₂, see *Oxygen*

OVA AND PARASITE, see *Feces Examination; Parasite*

OVULATION, see *Body Temperature*

OVULATION PREDICTOR, see *Body Temperature*

OVULATION TIME, see *Body Temperature; Tackmeter*

OvuSTICK, see *Body Temperature*

OXALATE

Eating many foods that naturally contain the chemical oxalate (sorrel, spinach, cabbage, tomatoes, rhubarb, and even chocolate) usually has no adverse effect; in some people, however, it can cause hyperoxaluria (an abnormally excessive amount of oxalate in the urine). If it then combines with calcium, oxalate can on occasion cause kidney stones. A rare inherited condition known as primary hyperoxaluria, or oxalosis, (as distinguished from secondary, or ordinary, hyperoxaluria), causes kidney infections and high blood pressure. Oxalate is measured in urine. Since oxalate levels can be lowered by altering the diet, the test aids not only in diagnosis but also in following the progress of treatment. Kidney stones of oxalate can also form when a patient has a bowel infection such as colitis or diverticulitis. Patients seem even more susceptible to oxalate stones after surgery for intestinal disease; they also occur following intestinal bypass surgery performed to help patients lose weight.

When performed: The test is used whenever a patient has symptoms of kidney or bladder stones. It is also performed when there are certain intestinal inflammation problems that do not respond to therapy; when the intestine has been operated on for cancer or ulcers; or when, in rare instances, an intestinal bypass procedure is performed to promote weight loss. (It is believed that the presence of excessive oxalates after surgery represents a vitamin B_6 deficiency from poor intestinal absorption.) Oxalate levels are measured when there is suspicion of ethylene glycol (automobile antifreeze) or oxalic acid (bleach) poisoning.

Normal values: Oxalate levels normally range from 0 to 40 mg per 24-hour specimen of urine.

Abnormal values: Levels greater than 50 mg per 24-hour sample of urine are considered abnormal. With hyperoxaluria, the urine usually shows white, cloudy formations.

Risk factors: None.
Pain/discomfort: None.
Cost: From $13 to $30.

Accuracy and significance: The test is 80 percent accurate and indicates excessive oxalate levels in the urine. The significance of the test is such that when increasing oxalate levels are found, a diet can be prescribed to reduce the oxalates and help prevent the formation of kidney stones.

OXYGEN

Oxygen in the blood is measured in a variety of ways. The *oxygen content* is the amount of the gas actually present in the blood. The *oxygen capacity* is the amount of oxygen that would be found in the blood if all it could hold were present. Both measures indicate just how much oxygen is available to support life, or the percentage of oxygen saturation of the blood. And blood oxygen is measured as the *partial pressure of oxygen* (P_{O_2}), sometimes called *oxygen tension*.

Oxygen is rarely tested alone; it is almost always measured along with the blood's

Carbon Dioxide (CO_2) and **pH** (hydrogen ions that indicate the acidity of the blood; although the blood is in fact alkaline, "acid" is used to differentiate between the increase and decrease in the pH). Once the Po_2 and the pH are known, the amount of oxygen attached to hemoglobin (hemoglobin saturation) can be determined. These three different tests are known as the blood gas group.

Whole blood is taken from an artery for most oxygen testing; in an emergency, it can be taken from a vein to measure content or saturation. The sample must be collected in a syringe that is coated inside with oil to prevent any air from reaching the blood; the needle tip must be sealed immediately and the syringe packed in ice. A new device now measures Po_2 simply by touching the skin. Elderly patients should be reclining when the blood is taken, since blood oxygen is lowest in that position and yields a truer value.

When performed: Primarily in respiratory diseases and in conditions that affect the lungs and interfere with transfer of oxygen to the blood; to determine if oxygen therapy will be effective; when there is heart failure; when there is suspected hypnotic or narcotic drug overdose; as a means of better evaluating kidney problems.

Normal values: Normal values for the different measures of oxygen are as follows:

Oxygen tension (Po_2): 85 to 105 mm Hg (after 40 years of age, it may be lower).

Oxygen content: 15 to 23 volumes percent for arterial blood and 10 to 16 volumes percent for venous blood.

Oxygen capacity: 16 to 24 volumes percent (levels depend on how much hemoglobin is present, since each gram of hemoglobin holds 1.39 ml of oxygen).

Oxygen saturation: from 94 percent to 100 percent of capacity for arterial blood and from 60 percent to 85 percent of capacity for venous blood.

Abnormal values: Oxygen values are decreased (hypoxemia) with any chronic obstructive lung disease (such as emphysema) or during an asthmatic attack. Almost any respiratory complication of disease can reduce oxygen utilization as reflected by lowered oxygen values for all the tests. Polycythemia (too many red blood cells) will also lower oxygen values. Exercise can decrease the amount of oxygen in the blood.

Risk factors: Negligible (see general risk factors for blood testing).

Pain/discomfort: Minimal (see general pain/discomfort factors for blood testing).

Cost: All forms of oxygen are usually measured at the same time along with other blood gases (carbon dioxide and pH); the fee is $30 to $140 for oxygen testing and $40 to $50 for a test of other blood gases. Eight-hour monitoring costs up to $300.

Accuracy and significance: Although oxygen measurements are usually performed on extremely ill and hospitalized patients, the primary purpose of the tests is to confirm the physician's judgment as to the level of blood oxygenation. Oxygen tests are 80 percent accurate and can provide an early warning of hypoxemia. The significance of this test lies in the constant monitoring of the patient's blood for its oxygen content and the ability to prevent damage to tissues such as the brain from the loss of oxygen.

OXYTOCIN CHALLENGE, see *Nonstress Fetal Assessment*

P

PACING, see *Radiography*

PACKED BLOOD CELL VOLUME, see *Hematocrit*

PAH CLEARANCE (SODIUM P-AMINOHIPPURIC), see *Creatinine*

PAIN, see *Thermography*

PALMER, see *Gastroesophageal Reflux*

PANCREAS ENZYME, see *Amylase*

PANCREAS FUNCTION

The pancreas is a 7-inch, 3-ounce, elongated gland that lies just behind the stomach. In addition to **Insulin,** a hormone necessary for blood sugar and carbohydrate metabolism, it also secretes **Glucagon,** another hormone that helps control the amount of insulin in the body. These hormone secretions are called *endo*crines because they leave the gland directly without the need for ducts as with other glands, such as the salivary glands. The pancreas also makes and gives off other products, primarily enzymes, that aid in food digestion—**Amylase** being the primary one; trypsin, chymotrypsin, and **Lipase** being others. The gland even secretes bicarbonate to neutralize stomach acid, which could destroy the enzymes. These *exo*crine substances (*exocrine* meaning they leave the gland by way of a duct) empty into the duodenum (that first part of the small intestine that begins where the stomach ends) at the same place the gallbladder empties bile into the intestine.

Pancreatic disorders, in addition to diabetes, include acute and chronic pancreatitis, an infectious condition that causes extremely severe abdominal pains. The infection can also cause hemorrhage and shock. Stones may form in the gland's ducts that block passage of the enzymes (the stones can also block passage of bile at the same time). And the pancreas is more than usually subject to a form of cancer that is rapidly fatal. Three of the most common causes of pancreatic problems are alcohol ingestion (usually from excessive alcohol use, but even a small amount can precipitate pain in some people), drug addiction, and gallstones.

Yet another pancreatic dysfunction is pancreatic insufficiency; many doctors feel this is really a form of chronic pancreatitis with relapses in between attacks. Primarily, it is evidenced by steatorrhea, or an excess of fat in the feces (see **Feces Examination**), and it is considered one of the main causes of malabsorption (see **Xylose Tolerance**). Suspicion of this condition, as well as other pancreatic disorders, should also make the doctor think of cystic fibrosis (see **Sweat**).

Some other causes of pancreatic dysfunction are excessive exposure to X-rays in the abdominal area, various drugs used to suppress inflammation and immunity, **Malnutrition** (especially insufficiency of protein), and following stomach or bowel surgery. Some signs of a pancreas problem, other than pain, include weight loss, loss of appetite, and abdominal distention.

Although this gland is extremely important for the absorption of nutrients, disease and dysfunction of the pancreas are difficult to diagnose. Measuring blood levels of amylase and lipase have been the most common, but not-too-accurate tests, and pancreas scanning (see **Nuclear Scanning**) can sometimes be of help. Other pancreas function tests (usually, endocrine secretion of hormones is not included in this evaluation) include: the bentiromide test, in which a chemical compound (the chemical is part para-aminobenzoic acid, or PABA, the same effective ingredient as in suntan and sunscreen products) is swallowed, absorbed by the intestine, and then excreted in the urine, where it can be measured as an indication of the adequacy of pancreatic enzyme secretion. At present, this is considered the simplest test, although it, too, is not very accurate; many other intestinal conditions can cause a false-positive result, and false-negative results have occurred even when pancreatic disease was present. One major advantage is that the patient is not required to swallow a long tube, which can be quite uncomfortable. And there are some dietary restrictions that must be followed to help increase this test's accuracy: prunes, cranberries, and certain vitamin products must not be eaten for several days prior to testing, nor can some enzyme food supplements or sunscreen products be used.

The secretin stimulation test requires that a tube be passed from the mouth or nose through the stomach into the intestine, where the pancreatic products empty. This is usually performed under the fluoroscope to assure the tube's proper location. Then, after injecting certain pancreas-specific hormone drugs (such as secretin) into the body to cause the gland to give off enzymes, the secretions are withdrawn through the tube and evaluated. With the Lundh test, the pancreas is stimulated by the patient's drinking a special liquid meal—as opposed to being injected with drugs—and the secretions are removed through the tube and tested. The pancreatic Schilling test is somewhat similar to the **Schilling** test for anemia; it is, however, an indirect test and requires the use of radioactive substances. A recent test measures the amount of trypsin in the blood; this test seems particularly valuable when pancreatic disease is assumed to come from alcoholism or cystic fibrosis (see **Sodium** and **Sweat**). At times, trypsinogen—the precursor of trypsin—is measured in the blood; while somewhat technically easier to determine, its levels, too, are reduced with pancreatic disease. Another pancreatic hormone, called pancreatic polypeptide (PP), will, at times, fail to increase after being stimulated by secretin (as in the secretin stimulation test), as it should if the pancreas is normal. Secretin and cholecystokinin are both hormones normally given off by the walls of the duodenum after eating.

Another test is called the fluorescein dilaurate tubeless indicator (the word *tubeless* is self-explanatory). The dye fluorescein (see **Fluorescein Eye Stain**) is swallowed, and the amount that shows up in the urine indicates pancreatic function. **Endoscopy, Ultrasound,** and **Computerized Tomography** are three other means of evaluating the pancreas, especially when searching for cancer of the pancreas (the fourth leading cause of cancer deaths in the United States). Monoclonal antibody measurements (see **Agglutination**) and leukocyte adherence inhibition assays (see **White Blood Cell**) are now being used as pancreas tests. The most accurate test for cancer of the pancreas is endoscopic retrograde pancreatography (see **Radiography** and **Glucagon**).

When performed: Primarily when a patient has unexplained abdominal pain. These tests are also utilized when malabsorption seems evident (poor growth, weight loss), when diarrhea persists, when cystic fibrosis is suspected, and when apparent liver problems cannot be explained by liver-function testing. If cancer is suspected, or if it is found in some other part of the body, pancreatic-function tests may be used to locate the primary cancer site.

Normal values: With the bentiromide test, at least 50 percent of the drug should be found in the urine after six hours. After the secretin test to stimulate the pancreas is performed, the bicarbonate removed by the tube should be greater than 80 mEq per L. After the patient drinks the special meal that is part of the Lundh test, the intestinal juices are again analyzed for bicarbonates and, at times, for one or more of the enzymes. In the Schilling test, the urine is analyzed for radioactive cyanocobalamin. This chemical, as with the others, should show a relatively normal or usual amount based on the laboratory's previous testing; normal and abnormal results are, in a sense, relative and based on past experience. Serum trypsinlike immunoreactivity, as with trypsin testing alone, can show normal amounts unless a patient has chronic pancreatitis with steatorrhea. Normal fluorescein excretion should be at least 30 percent of that swallowed.

Abnormal values: In general, a decreased amount of bicarbonate, drug, chemical, or enzyme indicates decreased pancreatic function.

Risk factors: Negligible when blood or urine is tested (see general risk factors for blood testing). When the tube is swallowed, there can be irritation and possibly bleeding where the tube makes contact. An allergic response to some of the drugs has been reported.

Pain/discomfort: Swallowing the tube is considered quite uncomfortable by most patients; once swallowed, it can become even more irritating as it remains inside— sometimes for hours. For blood testing, there is minimal discomfort (see general pain/discomfort factors for blood testing).

Cost: The bentiromide test runs from $40 to $50. Secretin and other tests requiring use of the swallowed tube and X-rays can cost from $150 to $300. The other tests can cost from $25 to $100, depending on the chemical or drug used, the time required, and the number of enzymes measured.

Accuracy and significance: In general, tests for pancreatic function are only from 50 to 80 percent accurate. While most doctors consider the secretin test the most accurate, the discomfort it causes tends to limit its use. The indirect, or chemical, tests are reasonably accurate for diagnosis when used in conjunction with the patient's history and the physical findings. It is rare for any one of the tests to have an accuracy rate of 80 percent or better, but they are all that can be offered at the present time. Much depends on the specific condition being searched for when it comes to choosing the test or tests to be undertaken. The only foolproof way of diagnosing pancreatic dysfunction is by direct inspection (surgery).

PANCREAS SCAN, see *Nuclear Scanning*

PANCREATIC SCHILLING, see *Pancreas Function*

PANCREATOGRAPHY, see *Radiography*

PAPANICOLAOU (PAP), see *Cytology*

PARACENTESIS, see *Thoracentesis*

PARAHORMONE, see *Parathyroid*

PARAINFLUENZA, see *Virus Disease*

PARASITE

Although the word *parasite* literally refers to a plant or animal form that attaches itself to and exists on another living organism, in medicine the term usually refers to an infestation by some form of wormlike organism that causes disease. When doctors suspect that a patient is suffering from a parasitological invasion, they usually order an "ova and parasite" test—most often as part of a **Feces Examination**. *Ova* refers to the egg stage of a parasite's development; it is sometimes easier to detect egg forms than it is to see actual adult parasites. Not all parasites assume the familiar wormlike shape. Some are single cells that slither around (the amoeba that causes diarrhea, abdominal cramps, and abscesses); some move quite actively and have tiny hairs called flagella protruding from their single-celled bodies (the giardia that is becoming the most common cause of gastrointestinal illness, which is usually acquired during foreign travel, and the trichomonas that cause vaginitis); and some combine both attributes (the trypanosomes that cause sleeping sickness, muscle and heart infections, and many different types of difficult-to-diagnose fevers.

In actuality, **Malaria** is really a parasitic disease, as are trichinosis (in which worms, most often acquired from eating inadequately cooked pork, lodge in muscles, causing severe pain), schistosomiasis (swimmer's itch), **Toxocariasis**, and all the many different tapeworm illnesses, which are becoming much more common thanks to the public's growing taste for raw or undercooked meat and fish. Pneumocystis carinii (P. carinii) is the parasite that causes the most common type of pneumonia found in AIDS (see **Acquired Immunodeficiency Syndrome**) and there is a new blood test that can distinguish this infection; in the past, it was necessary to diagnose this disease surgically with an open-lung **Biopsy**.

There are many other different, and usually rare, parasitic infestations. Doctors are aided in arriving at a diagnosis through various tests such as **Complement Fixation, Agglutination, Counterimmunoelectrophoresis, Skin Reaction**, and **String**, as well as direct examination of the blood, urine, feces, and other body tissues and secretions. The most important step in discovering that a parasite has caused a disease is to consider its possibility, something that is not always an obvious choice in today's practice of medicine. When an illness is difficult to diagnose, and especially if the patient's eating habits have recently changed, or if he or she has recently traveled to areas where these parasites are common (particularly the tropics), tests for parasites whose effects relate to one's symptoms should be carried out.

PARATHYRIN, see *Parathyroid*

PARATHYROID (Parahormone, Parathyrin, PTH)

Until recently, **Calcium** testing was the principal way to diagnose parathyroid disease. The parathyroid glands (usually four tiny, isolated glands buried within the thyroid gland substance but distinctly different from the thyroid) help control the body's need for and use of calcium. Calcium is necessary for muscle contraction—especially heart muscle—nerve transmission, blood clotting, and to keep the body's myriad cells alive. With hyperparathyroidism, or an excess of parathyroid hormone, calcium increases in the blood (**Phosphorus** usually decreases); when parathyroid hormone production diminishes, calcium does also. Hyperparathyroidism usually results from a parathyroid gland tumor, but it is also found with rickets (vitamin D deficiency) and abnormalities of other endocrine glands. When hyperparathyroidism is present, it is often accompanied by a stomach ulcer, kidney stones, high blood pressure, heart rhythm abnormalities, bone pain, or even psychosis. For testing, blood is taken from a vein; when a more precise diagnosis is needed the hormone is also tested for its two components, C-terminal and N-terminal. Decreased parathyroid hormone (hypoparathyroidism) commonly occurs following the surgical removal of the thyroid gland as a treatment of thyroid disease. It can also occur after X-ray treatments to the neck for thyroid disease and after treatment for parathyroid tumors. And for some as yet unknown reason, it has been found in patients suffering from candidiasis (a fungus infection of the mouth called "thrush"; the fungus can also infect the lungs and vagina).

With hypoparathyroidism, there is often an extreme sensitivity of the muscles, which can tighten and twitch involuntarily. There can be muscle pains, particularly in the abdomen, frequent urination, and abnormal mental manifestations such as depression and delirium. With severe cases, there is hair loss, as well as loose teeth, brittle nails, and eye cataracts.

There is also an inherited condition known as pseudohypoparathyroidism, in which parathyroid hormone may be present but does not act on the kidneys as it should. Last, there is pseudo-pseudohypoparathyroidism, a condition that imitates pseudoparathyroidism but one in which the blood's calcium remains normal (unlike the other hypoparathyroid disorders).

Occasionally, the Ellsworth-Howard test is used to help eliminate pseudohypoparathyroidism; by injecting the patient with parathyroid hormone, its effect on the kidney's ability to handle calcium and phosphorus can be observed.

A more recent test for hyperparathyroidism is the measurement of cyclic adenosine monophosphate (cAMP) in the patient's urine; elevated amounts usually corroborate the suspected diagnosis, although normal values have been found even when the disease was known to exist. At times, parathyroid hormone may be injected into the patient to measure the cAMP response.

When performed: Primarily when blood calcium tests are abnormal; when there are repeated episodes of muscle pains and tetany (muscle twitching); when there are repeated episodes of kidney stones; when abnormal bone X-rays cannot be explained; when personality changes cannot be diagnosed.

Normal values: Total parathyroid hormone should be from 100 to 600 pg per ml; however, as laboratory procedures differ, each laboratory may have its own standard. C-terminal and N-terminal measurements also vary but range between 200 to 1,200 pg per ml. Calcium measurements must be made simultaneously with and correlated with parathyroid hormone values.

Abnormal values: With hypoparathyroidism, parathyroid hormone levels are generally lower than normal; with pseudohypoparathyroidism and hyperparathyroidism, the levels are elevated. They are normal with pseudo-pseudohypoparathyroidism. Hormone levels must always be evaluated together with blood calcium values to help arrive at a specific diagnosis.

Risk factors: Negligible (see general risk factors for blood testing).

Pain/discomfort: Minimal (see general pain/discomfort factors for blood testing).

Cost: From $50 to $100 for total parathyroid hormone; if C-terminal and N-terminal measurements are made, the fee is approximately $200. All costs also include calcium measurements.

Accuracy and significance: Parathyroid hormone measurements are only about 70 percent accurate, as all of the hormone is not always detected. The significance of the test is in its differentiation among the many causes of calcium disorders and the various parathyroid syndromes.

PARENTAGE

In the United States, approximately one out of every three births is considered to be illegitimate—in the strict legal sense of the word; in some urban areas, more than 50 percent of all newborn children are alleged to be illegitimate. In light of recent court decisions giving the same legal rights to illegitimate children that legitimate children have (support, inheritance, and many other benefits), knowledge of parenthood has become important for legal as well as social reasons. There is also the need to protect men who are falsely accused of fatherhood and to assure mothers that the children they bring home from the hospital are really theirs.

The term *paternity test* is a misnomer. Disputed parentage tests do not prove whether a man or woman is really the biological parent of a child; rather, they can only help prove that the man or woman *could not possibly be* the biological parent. At this time, nearly 100 different tests can be performed, all of which point out that certain of the mother's or father's biological traits were or were not inherited by the child. Some are based on blood types (such as the O, A, B, AB, Rh, and hemoglobin groups); some are based on immunological characteristics that are transmitted from parent to child (such as enzyme defects, various globulin levels, and cell compatibility). See **HLA.**

Sometimes only one test is needed to show that a child could not possibly be the issue of an alleged parent (for example, if an accused father has type AB blood and the child has type O blood). More often than not, however, seven basic tests are performed; it is claimed that these tests offer a probability of exclusion of 93 percent. After 62 different tests are performed, the probability of exclusion reaches 98 percent.

When such tests are performed today, an individual must have an instant-development photograph taken of his face and then affix his signature to the back of the photograph along with his thumbprint. This identifying material is attached to the report to show the specific individual on whom the tests were made. (In the past, it was not unusual for a man to go to a laboratory, give the name of the accused father, and offer his blood for testing after earlier, private tests confirmed that the substitute man's blood would exclude him from parentage.) With children, photographs and footprints are used for identification. In addition, the tests are performed in two separate laboratories at the same time . Saliva may also be tested as a confirmatory measure, comparing inherited characteristics of the enzymes.

A recent addition to parentage testing is plasminogen (PLG) exclusion (see **Fibrinogen**). This is yet another genetic marker that can be isolated from blood plasma or serum. While this test is said to be as accurate as many other non-parent-designating "markers"—especially in initial or routine testing—it takes far less time (only a few hours) and is far less costly.

When performed: The test is used most often in legal disputes concerning births out of wedlock. The most common dispute involves a man accused of being the father of a child. In quite a few instances, however, a mother will claim that the child brought home from the hospital is not hers because of alleged child substitution.

Normal values: There are no normal values in disputed parentage tests, since, even if all known tests show that a person could be the parent of a child, there is always a small margin of doubt. If, however, the tests show that parentage would be impossible, they are considered completely accurate. (For example, a woman with type A_2 blood could not possibly be the mother of a child whose blood type was A_1B, no matter who the father was.)

Abnormal values: The only possibility of error occurs when the laboratory's testing serum contains traces of other typing factors not noted on the label (this is not a rare occurrence).

Risk factors: Negligible (see general risk factors for blood testing).

Pain/discomfort: Minimal (see general pain/discomfort factors for blood testing).

Cost: The fee for determining the blood type is approximately $5 for each individual involved. Should this test be all that is needed, the only other charges are those related to medical/legal certification. However, should additional blood type or group tests be required, the cost can range from $100 to $600, depending on the number of different tests needed.

Accuracy and significance: When the test shows that either the alleged mother or the alleged father could not be the biological parent, it is close to 95 percent accurate. When tests show only the probability of parenthood, the degree of accuracy depends on the number of different tests performed—the maximum accuracy that can be achieved is 98 percent. In actual practice, absolute exclusion is revealed only about 30 percent of the time.

In 1985, The American Association of Blood Banks, the American Medical Association, and the American Bar Association published a set of "Guidelines for Reporting Estimates of Probability of Paternity." Among these are: the use of genetic markers (see **Genetic Disorder Screening**) and observed phenotypes (physical characteristics), as well as the application of mathematical expressions and probability estimates—including a "paternity index." Its purpose is to standardize reporting and improve communications between all those involved in parentage disputes.

PARENTHOOD EXCLUSION, see *Parentage*

PAROTITIS, see *Virus Disease*

PAROXYSMAL NOCTURNAL HEMOGLOBINURIA, see *HAM*

PARTIAL PRESSURE OF CARBON DIOXIDE, see *Carbon Dioxide*

PARTIAL PRESSURE OF OXYGEN, see *Oxygen*

PARTIAL THROMBOPLASTIN TIME (PTT)

This test, sometimes called activated clotting time, measures the time for a clot to form after related clotting chemicals (such as calcium) are added to the blood. The word *activated* simply means an activator is added to shorten the time it takes to perform the test; the activator also makes the test more accurate, and when used, this test is called the activated partial thromboplastin time. Thromboplastin is one of the 12 factors in the body that cause blood to clot. The partial thromboplastin time test measures the efficacy of 8 of those factors, primarily Factors VIII and IX (the antihemophilia factors). It is gradually replacing the older **Bleeding and Clotting Time** tests. Blood is drawn from a vein, and plasma is examined. The test serves the same function as the blood clotting time, which must be measured immediately after the blood is taken; the advantage of the PTT is that the blood sample may be measured later in a laboratory.

When performed: As a general screening test to help detect clotting disorders; as an aid to diagnosing hemophilia and monitoring therapy for that disease; whenever heparin is prescribed to prevent blood clots as a means of controlling the dosage of that drug.

Normal values: Normal partial thromboplastin time averages 35 to 50 seconds, depending on the laboratory.

Abnormal values: Elevated PTT levels (more than 50 seconds) occur with hemophilia and with patients taking heparin.

Risk factors: Negligible (see general risk factors for blood testing).

Pain/discomfort: Minimal (see general pain/discomfort factors for blood testing).

Cost: From $6 to $32.

Accuracy and significance: The test is 80 to 90 percent accurate and is better than the routine bleeding and clotting time tests; it is particularly significant when following the progress of a patient receiving heparin. To ensure the efficacy of partial thromboplastin time measurements, the test must be performed before heparin is administered to establish a baseline measurement.

Note: Although the PTT is the most commonly performed test for clotting disorders, many new, related tests are being used to help uncover the specific cause of bleeding problems. The reptilase time test (it gets its name because the test reagent comes from snake venom) is also used when a patient is being given heparin to prevent clotting; reptilase will not be affected by the heparin. The thrombin time helps determine the role of fibrinogen in the clotting process (see **Fibrin Degradation Products**). And in fact, there are now separate tests for all the blood coagulation (clotting) factors, and some subfactors, that are used to relate bleeding problems to other disease conditions as well as to inherited causes. Usually, these tests are reserved for patients already diagnosed as having a coagulation disturbance. They cost from $35 to $100 each.

In 1985, a test was introduced that can be performed during the 18th week of pregnancy to determine whether or not the fetus could have hemophilia. It uses a DNA probe, or **Chromosome Analysis**, as a means of identifying those males at risk by detecting the genes corresponding to the disease. At present, the test is performed on a sample of the mother's blood, but it is also expected to be used with **Chorionic Villi Sampling**.

PAST-POINTING, see *Caloric*

PATCH, see *Skin Reaction*

PATERNITY, see *Parentage*

PAUL-BUNNELL, see *Mononucleosis*

PBI, see *Thyroid Function*

PCG, see *Phonocardiogram*

PCO$_2$, see *Carbon Dioxide*

PEAK EXPIRATORY FLOW RATE, see *Pulmonary Function*

PEAK FLOW MONITORING, see *Pulmonary Function*

PEG, see *Immunology; Radiography*

PELLAGRA, see *Niacin*

PENICILLINASE, see *Culture*

PENILE PLETHYSMOGRAPHY, see *Plethysmography*

PENILE TEMPERATURE, see *Body Temperature*

PENILE TUMESCENCE MONITOR, see *Impotence*

PENILE XENON WASHOUT, see *Impotence*

PEP, see *Systolic Time Intervals*

PEPSINOGEN

Pepsinogen is a substance secreted by certain stomach cells and converted by stomach acid to the digestive enzyme pepsin. Normally, it is present in blood serum. Recent research studies of men with stomach cancer, who had blood samples collected for other reasons years before they showed any evidence of cancer, revealed that a great many of these men had lower-than-normal pepsinogen levels prior to the onset of their cancer. It has since been observed that changes in the stomach lining cells, which may or may not be precancerous, decrease the blood's pepsinogen levels. Yet long-time smokers, many with symptoms of gastritis (an inflammation of the stomach wall) and a tendency to ulcers rather than cancer, have higher blood levels of pepsinogen. The blood for testing is usually taken from an arm vein.

When performed: As a screening test to evaluate the risk of stomach cancer; as a confirmatory test in the diagnosis of stomach cancer; to help differentiate among the causes of stomach pain and bleeding.

Normal values: For men, 30 to 45 ng per ml; for women, 20 to 40 ng per ml. If reported by mcg, both sexes average 45 to 150 mcg per ml for a 24-hour period.

Abnormal values: Less than 40 ng per ml is reason to suspect the presence of stomach cancer; greater than 60 ng per ml is reason to suspect the presence of gastritis. Smokers have higher-than-normal levels (greater than 75 ng per ml) without signs or symptoms of gastritis.

Risk factors: Negligible (see general risk factors for blood testing).
Pain/discomfort: Minimal (see general pain/discomfort factors for blood testing).
Cost: From $25 to $35.

Accuracy and significance: it has been postulated that men with a low pepsinogen level have seven times the risk of having stomach cancer than do men with normal or elevated pepsinogen levels. Whether women show the same risk factor has not been determined as yet. The test is considered 35 to 50 percent accurate in helping to diagnose stomach cancer, gastritis, and ulcers.

PERFUSION IMAGING, see *Nuclear Scanning*

PERFUSION SCAN, see *Nuclear Scanning*

PERICARDIAL pH, see *pH*

PERICARDIOCENTESIS, see *Thoracentesis*

PERIMETRY, see *Visual Field*

PERIODIC ACID SCHIFF SMEAR, see *Fungus*

PERIPHERAL COLD STIMULATION, see *Cold Pressor*

PERIPHERAL VISION, see *Visual Field*

PERITONEOSCOPY, see *Endoscopy*

PEROXIDE HEMOLYSIS, see *Tocopherols*

PERSONALITY, see *Depression, Minnesota Multiphasic Personality Inventory; Rorschach; Thematic Apperception*

PERTHES, see *Tourniquet Test for Varicose Veins*

PERTUSSIS, see *Agglutination*

PET, see *Computerized Tomography*

PETECHIAE, see *Capillary Fragility*

PETECHIOMETER, see *Capillary Fragility*

PETT, see *Computerized Tomography*

pH

The pH is a measure of how much hydrogen gas is in the blood; it reflects the number of hydrogen ions that are present per liter. A pH of 7, which is neutral (neither acid nor alkaline), means there are 100 nanoequivalents of hydrogen ions per liter of blood. The body functions best when the blood pH is 7.40—that is, when it contains about 40 nanoequivalents of hydrogen ions per liter. Therefore, the blood is normally very slightly alkaline (on the base side when considered on an acid-base relationship).

The balance is so delicate that when the pH goes below 7.38 (a difference of only 2 nanoequivalents of hydrogen—far less than a billionth of a gram), normal body functions are disrupted and the pathological condition of acidemia (acidosis) exists.

The body immediately struggles to correct the condition, which can be fatal if allowed to persist. A drop in pH also causes severe constriction of arteries and a lack of oxygen to tissues. Should hydrogen ions be lost from the body (or neutralized) and the blood pH rise above 7.44, the opposite pathology occurs—a condition known as alkalemia (alkalosis). If the alteration is caused primarily by bicarbonate, it is called metabolic; if the change is caused by carbon dioxide, it is called respiratory. Either condition reflects an acid-base balance disturbance.

Since most normal metabolic reactions in the body tend to create acids, the blood is always slightly alkaline (to neutralize the acids). Breathing out carbon dioxide (which is acid) also helps keep the pH properly balanced. Preferably, blood from an artery is tested; properly collected venous blood can be measured in emergency situations. The blood must not be exposed to air. The pH is also measured in urine, spinal fluid, lung fluid, semen, and many other body secretions. Vaginal pH measurements have been shown to help uncover the specific cause of an abnormal vaginal discharge; normally, vaginal secretions are very acid—around 4.0—but when the pH rises, or becomes less acid, it usually signifies an infection. Measuring the pH from the pericardium (the sac that surrounds the heart) when it fills with fluid (fluid is not normally present) can reveal whether the problem is from an infection or from some other, noninfection cause (hypothyroidism, cancer, kidney disease). And pH measurements inside the esophagus (see **Gastroesophageal Reflex**) help determine the cause of heartburn.

When performed: Almost always in conjunction with **Carbon Dioxide** and **Bicarbonate** tests and frequently with **Oxygen** testing; whenever there are respiratory or kidney problems that cannot be positively diagnosed; when a patient is in a coma or very confused; following vomiting or diarrhea; with severe muscle cramps; when certain drug poisoning is suspected.

Normal values: Normal pH in the blood ranges from 7.38 to 7.44. The body will not survive a pH lower than 6.8 or higher than 7.8.

Abnormal values: Levels below 7.35 indicate acidosis: either respiratory (from a lung condition that prevents the normal exchange of oxygen and carbon dioxide from the blood to the air, such as asthma, emphysema, an injury that causes a blood clot in the lung, or fractured ribs) or metabolic (from poisoning by drugs such as aspirin or from diabetes, diarrhea, or kidney disease). A pH above 7.45 indicates alkalosis: either respiratory (from deliberate fast breathing, certain drugs, or liver disease) or metabolic (from taking diuretics, steroids, or alkaline antacids for ulcers or burning stomach, or from vomiting or adrenal disease).

Urine pH is normally acid, especially on arising, but it becomes more acid (sometimes abnormally so) with kidney disease or lung disease and after taking certain drugs or eating a great deal of meat. Urine becomes less acid (and sometimes alkaline) with various drugs and when the diet is high in vegetables and fruits. Spinal fluid is normally alkaline but becomes acid when excessive drugs are administered and in certain lung diseases. Most other body fluids are alkaline; when they become acid, pathology is usually indicated (an acid semen means decreased fertility).

Risk factors: Negligible (see general risk factors for blood testing).

Pain/discomfort: Minimal (see general pain/discomfort factors for blood testing).

Cost: Although pH is usually measured as part of testing blood gases at a fee of $40 to $50, at times it is measured separately at a fee of $15 to $20. There is seldom a charge for urine survey testing; if performed in a laboratory, the fee is from $12 to $30.

Accuracy and significance: When pH is measured with carbon dioxide and bicarbonates, it can help differentiate between the various causes of acidosis and alkalosis. Knowledge of serial pH measurements can lead to the precise treatment of acidosis and alkalosis conditions, which can be lifesaving. In contrast, pH measurements in the urine are not critical; simple paper dipstick tests are usually sufficient. About 90 percent accurate.

PHB, see *Porphyrins*

PHENOLSULFONPHTHALEIN (PSP)

Kidney function is often tested by injecting phenolsulfonphthalein dye into the bloodstream and measuring the amount of the dye excreted in the urine after specific time intervals (15 minutes, 30 minutes, one hour, and two hours). The test does not depend on the amount of urine produced. Six milligrams (1 ml) of the dye is injected intravenously half an hour after the patient has drunk two glasses of water.

When performed: The test is used whenever kidney disease or urinary tract obstruction is suspected and with edema (water retention) or hypertension. It may also be performed with catheters inserted in each ureter (the tube that carries urine from each kidney to the bladder) to discover if only one kidney is damaged.

Normal values: Normally, about 25 percent of the dye is excreted in the urine in the first 15 minutes, 50 percent in the first 30 minutes, 65 percent after the first hour, and 75 percent by the second hour.

Abnormal values: Excretion of PSP may be reduced in kidney disease and urinary tract obstruction. Excretion of PSP may be increased in liver disease and high blood pressure. Many drugs (diuretics, aspirin, penicillin, certain vitamins) can cause abnormal PSP results.

Risk factors: Negligible (see general risk factors for blood testing).

Pain/discomfort: Minimal (see general pain/discomfort factors for blood testing).

Cost: From $6 to $22 for dye evaluation only. The doctor usually injects the dye in the office; rarely is there a charge for the procedure.

Accuracy and significance: Although the test is still performed, it is gradually being replaced by more sensitive kidney-function tests. The ease with which the test is performed makes it a useful screening test for kidney disease, but it is not a specific test; it is considered to be about 50 percent accurate.

PHENOTYPING, see *Lipoproteins*

PHENOXY ACID SCREENING, see *Toxic Chemical Exposure*

PHENYLALANINE, see *Phenylketonuria*

PHENYLEPHRINE, see *Finger Wrinkle*

PHENYLKETONURIA (PKU)

Phenylketonuria is an inherited amino acid enzyme deficiency that can cause mental retardation because of the body's inability to metabolize a protein amino acid, phenylalanine, which is then abnormally found in the urine. It occurs once in every 10,000 births and is most common among people from northern Ireland and western Scotland. Early treatment of this metabolic disorder—by a diet low in phenylalanine (using synthetic proteins in place of plant and animal proteins)—can prevent mental retardation; thus, the testing of newborn infants is essential to early diagnosis and treatment. A very small amount of phenylalanine is necessary for normal growth, and children differ markedly in how much they can eat without showing symptoms.

The primary test for phenylketonuria is the blood Guthrie bacterial inhibition assay (GBIA). A small amount of blood is usually drawn from the infant's heel for testing. The test cannot be performed until at least 24 hours after the infant has had his first milk meal. (Breast-fed infants must be tested again after one month.) Urine can also be tested for PKU, but blood will show a positive reaction much sooner than urine. If the Guthrie test is positive, a blood phenylalanine analysis is performed to confirm the diagnosis.

The dinitrophenylhydrazine (DNPH) test and ferric chloride urine test help detect PKU as well as other inherited metabolic defects. There are also special plastic strips coated with chemicals that turn color when dipped into the urine (or even placed on a wet diaper) of a child with phenylketonuria, but occasionally they give a false-positive reaction.

When performed: Testing of newborn infants for PKU is now mandatory throughout the United States, although some states will not test children when the parents object. In other situations, the test is utilized when mental retardation is suspected.

Normal values: Normally, there are less than 4 mg per 100 ml of demonstrable phenylalanine in the blood.

Abnormal values: When a child has PKU, the blood concentration of phenylalanine is kept between 3 and 7 mg per 100 ml. A concentration greater than 20 mg per 100 ml indicates a metabolic disorder. The urine will show 100 mcg per ml or more with PKU.

Risk factors: Negligible (see general risk factors for blood testing).

Pain/discomfort: Minimal (see general pain/discomfort factors for blood testing).

Cost: From $8 to $10 for blood screening. When performed with the routine infant screening tests to detect **Thyroid Function** and other inborn errors of metabolism, the charge ranges from $20 to $25. When chemical spot tests are used, such as paper dipsticks in the infant's urine or a drop of chemical on the infant's diaper, the fee is $3 to $5.

Accuracy and significance: Although this test has, in the past, been considered to be 98 percent accurate, in 1984 a study reported on 357 babies who were first reported to have a positive test result; follow-up testing revealed only two actually had PKU. Thus, the possibility of false positives must be kept in mind; a single positive test should not be accepted at face value. It is also known that chemicals used in the manufacture of some disposable diapers can cause both false-positive and -negative reactions; they should not be used for this test. The significance of the test is in terms of the mental retardation it has already prevented.

PHEOCHROMOCYTOMA, see *Catecholamines*

PHLEBOGRAPHY, see *Radiography*

PHLEBORHEOGRAPHY, see *Plethysmography*

PHLEGM, see *Sputum*

PHONOCARDIOGRAM (PCG)

The phonocardiogram is similar to the **Apexcardiogram** (ACG), in that it uses a measuring apparatus called a transducer, which records on paper a representation of the heart sounds—especially those made by the heart valves when closing. The major difference between the PCG and the ACG is the graphic tracing of the heart sounds. The PCG is illustrated by a continuous series of short, wavy lines (which actually look like vibrations); the stronger the sound, the greater and larger the line vibration recording from the baseline. The ACG is illustrated by a continuous rising and falling line (more like a series of large waves). The PCG is always recorded along with an ACG and a standard **Electrocardiogram** (ECG) or **Echocardiogram** in order to identify the exact position of the heart (contraction, relaxation) at the time of the sound.

When performed: When abnormal heart sounds and their timing need to be recorded for permanent records; to confirm or differentiate the sounds heard through the stethoscope; after surgical replacement of heart valves to determine success and performance.

Normal values: The PCG (especially in conjunction with the ECG) shows a standard vibration pattern for heart sounds when the heart valves are normal in size and length.

Abnormal values: Heart valve disease (aortic stenosis, mitral stenosis, etc.) shows a unique change from the normal pattern. There is also a specific pattern when the heart is enlarged—to the point where the two normal heart sounds are recorded as one.

Risk factors: None.

Pain/discomfort: None.

Cost: When performed with a standard electrocardiogram, the fee ranges from $80 to $100.

Some doctors consider this test inadequate when used alone, and it is possible that a health insurance company or government-sponsored medical program will not reimburse the doctor or patient for the cost of the test.

Accuracy and significance: The primary purpose of the phonocardiogram is to offer the doctor a more precise reading of a patient's heart action. The test provides a graphic record of heart sounds and heart valve disturbances. As such, it can be a valuable adjunct to the diagnosis of unusual heart and valve disease, although only about 70 percent accurate; much depends on the expertise of the technician and physician.

PHOSPHATASE, see *Acid Phosphatase; Alkaline Phosphatase*

PHOSPHATES, see *Phosphorus*

PHOSPHATIDYL GLYCEROL, see *Pregnancy*

PHOSPHOLIPIDS, see *Lipids*

PHOSPHORUS

Phosphorus metabolism is directly related to calcium metabolism and is associated with many body functions, most controlled by the parathyroid glands. Ninety percent of the phosphorus in the body is stored in the skeleton. Approximately 1 g of phosphorus is ingested daily by the average adult, primarily from dairy foods, meat, nuts, and vegetables. Although the test is reported as phosphorus, usually phosphate ions (phosphorus combined with something else such as oxygen phosphates) are measured. It is possible to be poisoned by inorganic phosphorus as opposed to organic phosphorus (see **Cholinesterase**). Matches, fireworks, and some rodent poisons contain phosphorus, which may cause symptoms imitating liver disease. Blood is collected from an arm vein, and the serum is examined. Phosphorus is also tested in urine and feces.

When performed: In kidney disease, hypoparathyroidism, suspected vitamin D deficiency (rickets), and undiagnosed nerve and muscle disease when phosphorus poisoning is suspected.

Normal values: Normal phosphorus levels range from 2.5 to 4.5 mg per 100 ml of serum (higher in children).

Abnormal values: Phosphorus levels may be increased in kidney disease, hypoparathyroidism, conditions of bone destruction and repair (healing fractures, certain bone diseases), hypervitaminosis D (excess vitamin D), and sometimes in patients taking Dilantin, pituitrin, or heparin. Phosphorus levels may be decreased in certain rare diseases of the kidney tubules, alcoholism, hyperparathyroidism, and vitamin deficiency. Increased urine and feces phosphorus usually reflects a decrease in the serum.

Risk factors: Negligible (see general pain/discomfort factors for blood testing).

Pain/discomfort: Minimal (see general pain/discomfort factors for blood testing).

Cost: From $4 to $27. Usually included in **Comprehensive Multiple Test Screening** panels, which range from $7 to $42.

Accuracy and significance: Although the test is a 90 percent accurate measure of phosphorus levels in the blood, abnormal values exist in so many conditions that the test is not useful for a specific diagnosis unless it is utilized in conjunction with other tests. To avoid false results, the glassware employed in the test must be kept free of cleaning solutions containing phosphorus. Patients who suddenly stop using alcohol a day or two before the test, or who are surreptitiously taking diuretic drugs, can also cause the test to yield abnormal values.

PHOTODENSITOMETRY, see *Bone Mineral Density Analysis*

PHOTOMOTOGRAPHY, see *Thyroid Function*

PHOTON ABSORPTIOMETRY, see *Bone Mineral Density Analysis*

PHYTOHEMAGGLUTIN, see *Acquired Immunodeficiency Syndrome*

PILOCARPINE STIMULATION, see *Sweat*

PINHOLE, see *Visual Acuity*

PINPRICK, see *Sensory*

PINWORM, see *Feces Examination*

PIRQUET, see *Skin Reaction*

PITUITARY FUNCTION

Although there are a few tests that directly measure the hormones given off by the pituitary gland, most pituitary-function tests are reflections of other gland and organ functions that are either activated or controlled by pituitary hormones. They include: **Vasopressin, Growth Hormone, Thyroid Function, Cortisol, Prolactin, Estrogen, Testis Function,** and **Pregnancy.** At times, most often as a consequence of brain surgery or after a patient has received a great many X-ray treatments to or near the pituitary area, hormones given off by the pituitary gland, called releasing factors or stimulating factors (they cause other glands to give off their particular hormones), are injected and the effect of these "activating" hormones is observed. Usually, these tests are performed in a hospital over a period of several days, at a cost of from $1,500 to $2,000, depending mostly on the price of hospitalization. Recently, some of these tests have been performed quite successfully in doctors' offices for less than $500. At other times, various drugs (e.g., chlorpromazine, better known as Thorazine) are used because they can block the release of certain pituitary hormones, and their effect may reveal a pituitary dysfunction. Testing for related hormones is the way pituitary function is most often measured—with measurements of the growth hormone, and that hormone's response to provocation, being the primary test. The latest way to assess pituitary function is to combine at least four different hypothalamic releasing factors such as growth, thyroid, etc. with **Vasopressin** injections at the same time; the combination seems to increase abnormal hormone values in a much shorter period of time (within an hour).

PITUITARY GONADOTROPIN, see *Testis Function*

PIXEL SCALE, see *Computerized Tomography*

PKU, see *Phenylketonuria*

PLACENTAL LACTOGEN

Human placental lactogen (HPL), also known as human chorionic somatomammotrophin (HCS), is a hormone produced by the placenta (the blood supply around the fetus during pregnancy). It first appears in the blood after about the fifth week of pregnancy and gradually increases in amount until the baby is born, after which it disappears. Its appearance and gradual increase are an indication of normal pregnancy. Blood is taken from a vein, and the serum is tested.

When performed: The HPL test is used whenever there is suspicion of trouble during pregnancy, especially if the patient has a sudden onset of vaginal bleeding. It has been suggested that the test be routinely performed during all pregnancies as a means of detecting potential miscarriage.

Normal values: No HPL is usually found until after the fifth week of pregnancy. At that time, about 0.5 mcg per ml can be detected. The level then rises to between 7 and 10 mcg per ml just before delivery.

Abnormal values: Slightly increased values may be found with a large placenta (multiple births), but the test is not a positive indicator. A sudden decrease in HPL during pregnancy is considered a warning sign that a miscarriage is about to occur, usually because the fetus either is abnormal or is having some difficulty (such as insufficient oxygen or separation of the placenta from the uterus). Certain rare tumors may cause an increased amount of HPL in the blood.

Risk factors: Negligible (see general risk factors for blood testing).
Pain/discomfort: Minimal (see general pain/discomfort factors for blood testing).
Cost: From $25 to $45.
Accuracy and significance: Although the test may have to be performed several days in succession, it is a particularly significant guide for an obstetrician managing a high-risk pregnancy. Many obstetricians consider it an 80 percent accurate forecast of complications in the placenta and an abnormal pregnancy.

PLACENTAL PROTEIN, see *Estrogen Receptor*

PLACENTAL SCAN, see *Nuclear Scanning; Ultrasound*

PLASMA PROTEINS, see *Albumin/Globulin*

PLASMA RENIN ACTIVITY, see *Renin*

PLASMA THROMBOPLASTIN ANTECEDENT, see *Fibrinogen*

PLASMINOGEN, see *Fibrinogen; Parentage*

PLATELET COUNT

Platelets, or thrombocytes, are minuscule bodies (less than half the size of red blood cells) that are essential to the blood-clotting process. They are manufactured in bone marrow at the rate of about 100,000 each day. When bleeding occurs, platelets group or clump together (aggregate), swell up, stick to the injured area, and attempt to act as plugs to stop the bleeding. The normal life span of platelets is about eight days. Only one drop of blood is necessary for examination and may be taken from the fingertip, heel, or earlobe or from a tube of blood drawn for other tests. Platelets are usually counted manually under the microscope; electronic counting is also performed. Platelets are examined, too, for size (young, larger platelets are more effective for clotting).

Note: The newly developed platelet aggregation tests (aggregometer, Profiler) help distinguish between inherited (hemophilia, Von Willebrand's disease) and acquired bleeding problems. Drugs such as aspirin and aspirinlike products used for arthritis and generalized pain can keep platelets from aggregating and thus cause bleeding. This new test is also used as an indication of susceptibility to stroke in older people.

When performed: When there are obvious bleeding tendencies; before surgical procedures or tooth extractions; with fractures; to check liver function; when polycythemia or certain kinds of anemia are suspected; when leukemia is being treated.

Normal values: There should be between 150,000 and 500,000 platelets per cu mm (lower for children). Normal values vary with different laboratory methods.

Abnormal values: Platelets are usually increased (more than 500,000 per cu mm) in rheumatoid arthritis, most cancers, trauma (hemorrhage), polycythemia, and some anemias (iron deficiency). They are decreased in bleeding tendencies (usually less than

20,000 per cu mm before bleeding occurs), purpura (a condition in which even the slightest bruise causes a black-and-blue mark from bleeding under the skin), some anemias, certain leukemias, and infectious mononucleosis.

Risk factors: Negligible (see general risk factors for blood testing).

Pain/discomfort: Minimal (see general pain/discomfort factors for blood testing).

Cost: From $5 to $24. Platelet aggregation can cost from $100 to $240.

Accuracy and significance: Platelet counts are 90 percent accurate and very significant in reaching a diagnosis of bleeding tendencies. They are especially important when following patients receiving chemical treatment for leukemia, which tends to destroy body platelets. Platelet aggregation is about 60 percent accurate.

PLETHYSMOGRAPHY

Venous thrombosis (a clot attached to the wall of a vein), usually in a deep vein of the leg (and far more common in the left leg than in the right, for reasons as yet unknown), is becoming a common illness. Deep-vein thrombosis (and its potential consequence, pulmonary embolism or lung clot) frequently follows surgical procedures when patients must lie quietly for long periods after the operation. Phlebography (see **Radiography**) is the best way to diagnose deep-vein thrombosis (thrombophlebitis); however, when X-ray is difficult or when it is impossible to locate a vein in the foot for injection of a radiopaque dye (because of excessive swelling, low pain threshold, etc.), venous impedance plethysmography is used. This is a noninvasive technique (the skin is not broken with injections) and is a safe, fairly reliable way to test for thrombosis.

In venous impedance plethysmography, a standard blood pressure cuff with measuring wires is connected to an impedance analyzer, which records the blood flow through the vein around the area of the leg where the clot is suspected. The blood pressure cuff is inflated to create pressure around the upper leg and thus slow or stop the flow of blood in the veins below the cuff. The pressure is released suddenly and the rate of venous blood flow is recorded. The test can be performed at home, in a doctor's office, or at the bedside of a hospitalized patient.

Ocular plethysmography is a test to detect and evaluate blood flow through the carotid arteries to the brain. With the patient sitting in a chair, special cups are placed over the eyes while the pulsations behind the eyes are recorded. The eyes are tested simultaneously to determine if one carotid artery pulse is slower than the other, which indicates blockage.

Penile plethysmography, using similar equipment, is used to differentiate psychological from physical **Impotence.**

When performed: Whenever there is swelling of the leg (usually but not always painful) that cannot be specifically diagnosed; prior to and following extensive surgical procedures, especially when the patient has been forced to lie on the operating table for a long period of time; whenever patients are bedridden for more than several days at a time; as a screening test for the prevention of thrombosis and pulmonary embolism and occasionally to follow the progress of the treatment of a clot; in cases of impotence.

Normal values: After the pressure in the blood pressure cuff is applied, the impedance analyzer should show a slow steady rise as the lower veins fill up but are unable to empty; as soon as the pressure is released, a sudden surge of blood into all the leg veins should be recorded.

Abnormal values: When a thrombus (clot) is present, a vein will show very slow filling, and when the pressure above the vein is released, the sudden surge of blood will not be recorded. Abnormal values for other uses of plethysmography depend on the physician's experience and interpretation.

Risk factors: None.

Pain/discomfort: There may be some embarrassment when penile plethysmography is performed. When ocular plethysmography is performed, a few patients find the eye cups uncomfortable but not painful.

Cost: Venous impedance plethysmography, usually applied to the legs, is $50 to $110. Penile plethysmography averages $100. Ocular plethysmography is $75 to $130.

Accuracy and significance: Plethysmography is considered to be about 80 percent accurate. While a number of doctors believe venous impedance plethysmography is probably the most significant way to identify thrombosis, other doctors will not accept a diagnosis of a leg vein clot unless it can be seen on an X-ray. Today, penile plethysmography is being replaced by the penile tumescence monitor. Ocular plethysmography is a significant noninvasive way to measure blood flow to the brain without risk to the patient. If contact lenses are left in place while ocular plethysmography is performed, inaccurate values can result.

PLEURAL FLUID, see *Thoracentesis*

PLUMBISM, see *Lead*

PNEUMOCYTIS, see *Parasite*

PNEUMOENCEPHALOGRAPHY, see *Radiography*

PNEUMONIA, see *Complement Fixation*

PNEUMOTACHOMETER, see *Smell Function*

POLIOMYELITIS, see *Complement Fixation*

POLYDIPSIA, see *Vasopressin*

POLYETHYLENE GLYCOL ASSAY, see *Immunology*

POLYSOMNOGRAPHY, see *Sleep Monitoring*

POLYURIA, see *Vasopressin*

PORPHYRINS

Porphyrins are pigments that come from red blood cells and from the liver; when present in the urine, they indicate disease (porphyria). Erythropoietic (red blood cell) porphyria is a rare, inherited condition characterized by the excretion of red-tinted urine shortly after birth. Hepatic (liver) porphyria may be inherited or acquired after birth as a consequence of drug use, alcoholism, or exposure to certain chemicals such as lead and fungicides. Virtually all people who have excessive porphyrins in their system are hypersensitive to sunlight. Exposure to sun results in edema, blisters, and other skin lesions, mostly ulcers and scarring. Other symptoms that occur with porphyria include generalized body pains (most commonly in the stomach), confusion, and convulsions. During an acute attack, a patient may have high blood pressure, an extremely rapid pulse, and fever.

The porphyrin test measures a number of different types of porphyrins (such as coproporphyrins, protoporphyrins, and uroporphyrins); it is usually not necessary to distinguish the type of porphyrin to establish a diagnosis. Two specific products that immediately precede the formation of porphyrins are porphobilinogen (PHB) and delta aminolevulinic acid, called ALA (see **Lead**). Determination of these specific products helps pinpoint the diagnosis by showing whether the porphyria is erythropoietic or hepatic, inherited or acquired. A 24-hour sample of urine is the most common test. Porphyrins may also be measured in the feces, in the blood serum taken from a vein, and in red blood cells alone.

When performed: Primarily when a patient complains of reddish or reddish purple urine; when there is photosensitivity, hyperpigmentation, ulceration of the skin, excessive hair growth, undiagnosed stomach pains, unexplained convulsions, and other nervous disease manifestations that cannot be otherwise diagnosed; as an indication of a possible acute attack of porphyria and as a measure of progress while treating the disease; as an aid in testing for lead poisoning.

Normal values: Normally, there are no porphyrins in the urine and no more than 1,000 mcg in a 24-hour feces specimen. There may be up to 100 mcg per 100 ml in red blood cells and up to 60 mcg per 100 ml of blood serum.

Abnormal values: Porphyrins are increased in the urine in porphyria, liver disease, certain cancers, and lead poisoning. They may also be increased with alcoholism, the use of estrogens (including birth control pills), psychic trauma, menstruation, and pregnancy. Eating beets or blackberries or taking certain laxatives containing phenolsulfonphthalein (Ex-Lax), danthron, or cascara may give a false porphyrinlike color to the urine, as will certain azo-dye urinary anesthetics (Pyridium) and rifampin, an antibiotic. Patients who are malingering have been known to add ketchup or tomato juice to their urine in order to simulate illness.

Risk factors: Negligible (see general risk factors for blood testing).

Pain/discomfort: Minimal (see general pain/discomfort factors for blood testing).

Cost: Urine porphyrin measurements are $12 to $30; feces porphyrin measurements, $50 to $70. Fees for blood porphyrin measurements depend on the particular laboratory procedure and range from $20 to $100.

Accuracy and significance: Porphyrin measurements are 90 percent accurate and are very significant in helping to diagnose and differentiate between the various types of porphyrias. They are of significant aid in determining why some patients cannot tolerate sunlight and whether hyperpigmentation of the skin is present, and are helpful to women who have excessive hair on the face, the cause of which has not been diagnosed.

Recently, the American Porphyria Foundation has said that the Watson-Schwartz urine test for PHB may not be reliable, since its results can be normal between porphyric attacks and may be normal in relatives with acute intermittent porphyria, and it is often performed improperly and even misinterpreted by laboratories. They recommend the Mauzerall-Gralnick method as being more precise and without false-positive results.

PORTAL SYSTEM ENCEPHALOPATHY, see *Number Connection*

POSITRON EMISSION TRANSAXIAL TOMOGRAPHY, see *Computerized Tomography*

POSTAGE STAMP, see *Impotence*

POTASSIUM

Potassium is a blood electrolyte (see **Sodium**) that is essential to maintaining the proper balance of fluids within body cells. (Sodium acts in the same manner but is responsible for the water *surrounding* the body cells.) Potassium is particularly important to help carry out enzyme reactions throughout the body and to regulate heart muscle action. The typical daily diet contains about 3 g of potassium (less than half as much as sodium), but the body excretes almost all of it. Foods richest in potassium include dates, apricots, bananas, oranges, and tomatoes. Most problems come from too little potassium in the body, a condition caused more by reactions to drugs than by disease or lack of the mineral in the diet. Very little potassium is lost in sweat (which contains large amounts of sodium).

Blood is taken from a vein, and the serum is examined. In this test particularly, but also in many others, the common practice of asking the patient to clench and open the fist (to help find a vein in the arm) or leaving the tourniquet on too long can cause great errors in measurement. Potassium is also measured in the urine, the spinal fluid, sweat, and saliva.

The most accurate measurement of potassium is total body potassium. The patient lies inside a steel-walled room; a special radioactive form of potassium is injected and then a nuclear counter is passed over the entire body for 30 minutes to detect the amount of radioactive potassium present (see **Nuclear Scanning**) which in turn reveals total body potassium.

Once serum or total body potassium has been determined, a physician can reasonably estimate potassium changes by alterations in the **Electrocardiogram**.

When performed: When there are symptoms of muscle weakness, lethargy, heart rhythm abnormalities, or hormone problems; when patients are taking diuretic drugs; to help determine the source of acidosis, which can cause coma.

Normal values: Potassium levels should range from 4 to 5.5 mEq per liter in serum and 25 to 100 mEq per liter in a 24-hour urine sample.

Abnormal values: Elevated amounts of potassium (hyperkalemia) are found with kidney failure, liver disease, and adrenal cortical hormone deficiency. A large amount of potassium in the blood, usually secondary to kidney failure, can cause the heart to stop beating. Urine levels are most often the opposite of serum levels (high blood potassium with low urine amounts). A few exceptions, however, exist with malabsorption (the potassium is not taken into the bloodstream through the intestines) and with diarrhea.

Serum potassium levels may be decreased in diabetes, vomiting, and diarrhea; from taking laxatives, diuretic drugs, and certain forms of penicillin; with heart rhythm irregularities; and when there is a magnesium deficiency.

Salivary changes in potassium occur with adrenal disease, and sweat changes occur with certain inherited conditions.

Risk factors: Negligible (see general risk factors for blood testing).

Pain/discomfort: Minimal (see general pain/discomfort factors for blood testing).

Cost: From $4 to $25. Usually included in **Comprehensive Multiple Test Screening** panels, which range from $7 to $42.

Accuracy and significance: The test is 90 percent accurate, but it is important that the collection of blood for testing be precise. Should a quantity of red or white blood cells and platelets be present and break down during the collection process, abnormally false elevation will result. The test is significant as a confirmation of a doctor's suspicions rather than as a tool to reach a specific diagnosis.

POTENCY, see *Impotence*

PPD, see *Skin Reaction*

PRA, see *Renin*

PRECIPITIN, see *Complement Fixation*

PREDICTIVE TESTING, see *Genetic Disorder Screening*

PRE-EJECTION PERIOD, see *Systolic Time Intervals*

PREGNANCY

Although pregnancy is not really a disease, the bodily changes caused by pregnancy are sufficiently complex to be considered a deviation from normal. After fertilization occurs and the fertilized ovum is implanted in the uterus, the newly formed tissue material that attaches the fertilized egg to the uterus produces a hormone substance called human chorionic gonadotropin (HCG). Most pregnancy tests ascertain the presence of HCG in the serum or urine. Formerly, the blood or urine from the patient with suspected pregnancy was injected into a rabbit (A-Z test). If the rabbit's ovaries showed signs of pregnancy, the test was considered positive. The rabbit test is rarely used today; rats, which are easier to obtain than rabbits, have been substituted should this particular version of the test be requested (Friedman).

Most tests for pregnancy depend on **Agglutination.** Either HCG-sensitized red cells or latex particles (which are treated to act like red blood cells) are added to a patient's serum or urine in a test tube. The pregnant patient has antibodies to chorionic gonadotropin that will react (agglutinate) by clumping together and settling at the bottom of the test tube. The same test may be performed on a slide. When a drop of urine is placed on the slide with sensitizing chemicals, agglutinizing can be seen if pregnancy exists. A slide test takes only two to three minutes and is accurate 96 percent of the time. These tests are called DAP, Neocept, Pregnosticon Dri-Dot (or Slide), UCG, and Pregnate, to name a few. Do-it-yourself early pregnancy tests are now as accurate as most tests performed in the doctor's office or laboratory.

The most recent measurements of HCG (now sometimes written hCG) are made by using monoclonal antibodies (see **Agglutination**). This technique allows the detection of pregnancy much earlier than had previously been possible; one can ascertain pregnancy even before the expected (or missed) menstrual period is due. And these more specific, more accurate methods also allow a more precise prediction of the age of the fetus; this can be especially valuable in a woman who cannot remember the onset of the last menstrual period prior to pregnancy. Monoclonal antibodies may be attached to dipsticks, and with the new dipstick-type tests, it is also possible to add a drop of blood serum to the tip of the plastic test strip; it has been reported that this method of testing for pregnancy is almost 100 percent accurate 10 days after conception, or about 2 days prior to the expected menstrual period. And because it is so sensitive, it is considered a good screening test when ectopic pregnancy is suspected. Some trade names of the newer pregnancy tests include: Advance, e.p.t. PLUS, Fact, and Quikstik.

Other ways of determining fetal maturity include the testing of amniotic fluid (see **Amniocentesis**) for the amount of fat in the cells, called the nile blue fat stain test. Testing for fetal lung maturity can reveal the probability of an infant's surviving premature delivery; more than half of all deaths of premature infants come from the respiratory distress syndrome (RDS; or hyaline membrane disease, as it was once known). Some tests for amniotic fetal lung maturity include: amniostat-FLM, which detects the presence of phosphatidyl glycerol; its presence indicates a good possibility of infant survival, and a deficiency is considered a risk factor for RDS. The shake test and the foam stability index (FSI) measure the ability of the amniotic fluid to act as a surfactant to break up fluid surface tension (soap and detergents are surfactants); the more surfactant present, the easier it is for the lungs to breathe. The lecithin/sphingomyelin ratio in amniotic fluid is also a means of assessing the risk of RDS. These tests are usually performed when high-risk pregnancy is under consideration, such as in a mother with diabetes, Rh problems, or one who has had previous difficult pregnancies.

When performed: When there is suspicion, or fear, of pregnancy. Pregnancy tests should be routinely performed on all women of childbearing age (at least from age 12 to age 50) when hospitalized, prior to any X-ray test or treatment, or before embarking on any course of drug therapy.

Normal values: A positive test in the presence of pregnancy is normal.

Abnormal values: False-positive pregnancy tests may occur when certain hormones are temporarily increased (such as after the menopause); when red blood cells or excessive protein are found in the urine; when certain tranquilizing drugs such as barbiturates, Compazine, Phenergan, Stelazine, or Thorazine are present. Even penicillin and methadone can cause false-positive results. In addition to urinary infections, hepatitis and some rare uterine and ovarian tumors can produce false-positive reactions. Menstrual irregularities can also cause abnormal values.

Lower-than-normal HCG levels can indicate an ectopic pregnancy (in which the fetus grows outside the uterus). A sudden drop in HCG levels has been interpreted as signaling the possibility of a spontaneous abortion.

Risk factors: Negligible (see general risk factors for blood testing).

Pain/discomfort: Minimal (see general pain/discomfort factors for blood testing).

Cost: Most do-it-yourself urine test kits average $8 to $12 per test kit. When performed by a laboratory, the charge is usually $5 to $15 in addition to the doctor's fee for an office visit. Blood tests for pregnancy are $10 to $20. A specific measurement of the HCG amount is $20 to $40.

Accuracy and significance: When properly performed, urine and blood tests for pregnancy are considered to be 98 percent accurate. Levels of HCG are detectable within three weeks after one's last menstrual period, or about a week after pregnancy begins. The more sensitive the test, the earlier pregnancy may be detected. When the test is negative, but the possibility of pregnancy is still suspected, the test must be repeated in seven days. When the amount of HCG is measured and followed, the test is considered to be 60 to 80 percent accurate in helping diagnose ectopic pregnancy and predicting spontaneous abortion. Urine pregnancy tests can be inaccurate (give a false-negative result) if the urine's specific gravity is low (see **Urine Examination**); that is why the first morning urine specimen (usually most concentrated) is best. Fetal lung maturity tests are about 75 percent accurate.

PREGNANCY TOXEMIA, see *Rollover*

PREGNANEDIOL, see *Estrogen*

PREGNANETRIOL, see *Cortisol*

PREGNOSTICON DRI-DOT (OR SLIDE), see *Pregnancy*

PREMARIN L-DOPA, see *Growth Hormone*

PREMATURE INFANT HEALTH, see *Electroencephalogram*

PRENATAL DETECTION, see *Amniocentesis; Chorionic Villi Sampling; Chromosome Analysis; Genetic Disorder Screening*

PRESBYOPIA, see *Visual Acuity*

PRISM, see *Strabismus*

PROCTOSIGMOIDOSCOPY, see *Endoscopy*

PROFILE, see *Comprehensive Multiple Test Screening*

PROGESTERONE, see *Estrogen*

PROGESTERONE RECEPTOR (PgR), see *Estrogen Receptor*

PROGESTIN CHALLENGE, see *Estrogen*

PROGRAMMED ELECTRICAL CARDIAC STIMULATION, see *Electrocardiogram*

PROLACTIN (HPRL, hPRL)
Prolactin (sometimes called lactogenic hormone) is a pituitary hormone (see **Pituitary Function**) that causes the breasts to enlarge and secrete milk. It must be present in order for a mother to nurse her child. In addition, prolactin has been reported to act as a **Growth Hormone** under certain conditions. Blood is taken from a vein, and the serum or plasma is tested.

When performed: When a mother who has just given birth is unable to nurse; when certain brain tumors are suspected; when women have menstrual problems; during pregnancy when fetal difficulties are suspected.

Normal values: Prolactin levels range from 5 to 25 ng per ml in both men and women but are normally increased in women during pregnancy and while nursing.

Abnormal values: Increased prolactin is found in both men and women during stressful (anxiety-producing) situations; when brain tumors involve the hypothalamus portion of the brain; in certain pituitary tumors (although if the pituitary is destroyed, prolactin levels may be reduced); and in women taking certain drugs — especially those for high blood pressure and some tranquilizers — that may, in turn, cause the breasts to secrete milk without any relation to pregnancy. Prolactin is usually absent when a mother of a newborn is unable to nurse her child.

Risk factors: Negligible (see general risk factors for blood testing).

Pain/discomfort: Minimal (see general pain/discomfort factors for blood testing).

Cost: From $25 to $50.

Accuracy and significance: Basically, the test's only significance is in helping to determine the reason a mother is unable to nurse her child following pregnancy. However, it is also used to help evaluate a high-risk pregnancy, and it is considered approximately 65 percent accurate in predicting fetal problems. Unfortunately, this predictive value is accompanied by a high false-positive rate. The test helps to diagnose brain tumors in the pituitary-hypothalamic areas of the brain, lung tumors, other hormone disorders, and kidney problems. When evaluating prolactin levels, the doctor must consider the patient's use of tranquilizers, antidepressants, some high blood pressure drugs, and procainamide, all of which tend to lower prolactin values.

Note: Recent observations seem to relate the level of prolactin in men to their sexuality; the greater the amount of blood levels of this hormone, the less the man's sexual desire or libido and the less his sexual activity.

PROSTAGLANDINS

Prostaglandins are probably the newest and most interesting of all tests; some are still in the experimental or research stage. In essence, they are fatty acid products (many are derived from polyunsaturated fats in the diet) that are part of every cell in the body. They act somewhat like hormones, in that they direct countless body organs and functions; however, unlike hormones which originate in one part of the body and usually act in another, prostaglandins act where they originate. They seem to have derived their name from the fact that they were first discovered in seminal fluid (from the prostate gland) but are now known to be produced everywhere in the body. At present, more than a dozen different prostaglandins are known and can be tested for, but this is thought to be but a small portion of all that exist. While some have been given names, they are all labeled with letters, and those letters may well have numerical subscripts; for example, thromboxane is also called prostaglandin A_2. Prostaglandin D_2 causes severe bronchial constriction (it has been linked to asthma), and prostaglandin $F_{2\alpha}$ is also known to cause difficulty in breathing. Prostaglandin A_2 has been used to help confirm the diagnosis of polycythemia vera (see **Red Blood Cell**), a disease characterized by too many red blood cells. They can be found in blood, feces, urine, and other body substances such as peritoneal fluid (see *paracentesis* in

Thoracentesis), heart muscle, and tissue samples from the fetus. Prostaglandin $F_{1\alpha}$, when measured from the blood of infants born of mothers who have diabetes, may help prevent thrombosis (blood clots) in the newborn babies. There are innumerable diseases that may, someday, be detected through testing for the presence of these substances.

PROSTATE ENZYME, see *Acid Phosphatase*

PROTEIN-BOUND IODINE, see *Thyroid Function*

PROTEIN ELECTROPHORESIS, see *Albumin/Globulin*

PROTEIN p30, see *Acid Phosphatase*

PROTEINS, see *Albumin/Globulin*

PROTHROMBIN TIME (Quick Test)

Prothrombin (Factor II) is one of the 12 known factors necessary to stop bleeding (normal body coagulants). Like 4 other clotting factors, it is manufactured in the liver from vitamin K, which is obtained in the diet primarily from green leafy vegetables, fish, and liver. It is important to know a patient's diet when testing for prothrombin time, since an excess of such foods will alter the test. Coumarin anticoagulant drugs such as warfarin (Coumadin) and dicumarol are often prescribed to prevent thrombophlebitis subsequent to surgery or after an injury. Anticoagulants have, on occasion, also been prescribed after heart attacks and to prevent eye problems in diabetes. They interfere with the liver's ability to make clotting factors.

Although the prothrombin time test indicates the level of prothrombin in the blood, it is more a measure of the overall blood coagulation response to the taking of coumarin anticoagulant drugs. When anticoagulants are given, it may take from three to seven days before the prothrombin time test reflects the drug activity. It is important to know what drugs a patient is taking in addition to anticoagulants before evaluating the prothrombin time. Blood is taken from a vein, and the plasma is tested. The test must be performed within an hour after the sample is taken for accurate results, unless the blood sample is immediately frozen.

When performed: Primarily as an indication of the activity of certain anticoagulant drugs (but not heparin); as an indication of how the liver is functioning; as a measure of a patient's dietary intake of vitamin K.

Normal values: Normally, it takes 12 to 14 seconds for a fibrin strand (first sign of clotting) to be seen. The test is always run with control plasma that is known to be normal. The result is sometimes reported as the number of seconds it takes a patient's blood to clot compared with the control; more often, it is reported as a percentage of the control's plasma prothrombin time compared to the patient's prothrombin time, called percentage concentration or percentage of patient's prothrombin activity.

Abnormal values: Any amount of time greater than the control is considered an abnormal value; the longer the patient's prothrombin time in seconds, the lower the percentage of prothrombin activity. When anticoagulants are prescribed, an abnormal value is indicative of the effectiveness of the drug. Ideally, a patient taking a coumarin product should have a prothrombin time 2 to 2½ times longer than the control or show between 12 percent and 20 percent prothrombin activity.

The prothrombin time is affected when anticoagulants are taken with other drugs. Barbiturates, oral contraceptives, mineral oil, and antacids will shorten the prothrombin time, while aspirin, thyroid hormone, insulin, and oral antidiabetic drugs will lengthen it. It is also prolonged with liver disease; when used for this condition, the test is usually repeated after the patient is given a large amount of vitamin K. Eating large quantities of food containing vitamin K (salads, fish) will shorten the prothrombin time and require additional anticoagulant drug for effectiveness. Eating commercial French-fried potatoes made with methylpolysiloxane for crispness (the chemical is listed on the label if bought packaged for home use; it is impossible to know about this when dining out) will cause an abnormally decreased prothrombin time for at least a week afterward and could cause a patient to take a dangerous overdose of an anticoagulant drug.

Risk factors: Negligible (see general risk factors for blood testing).
Pain/discomfort: Minimal (see general pain/discomfort factors for blood testing).
Cost: From $5 to $27.
Accuracy and significance: The test is 80 percent accurate for monitoring the blood level of a patient taking warfarin-type drugs. The more frequently the test is performed, the less the chance of bleeding or clotting problems. Recent research now indicates that the "standard" prothrombin time ratios used to guide therapy have been in error, causing doctors to prescribe excessive amounts of anticoagulants. Revised values are being considered in 1986.

PROTOPORPHYRIN, see *Porphyrins*

PSEUDOCHOLINESTERASE, see *Cholinesterase*

PSEUDOGOUT, see *Synovial Fluid*

PSEUDOPARATHYROIDISM, see *Parathyroid*

PSEUDO-PSEUDOPARATHYROIDISM, see *Parathyroid*

PSITTACOSIS, see *Chlamydia Identification; Complement Fixation*

PSP, see *Phenolsulfonphthalein*

PSYCHOGALVANIC SKIN RESISTANCE AUDIOMETRY, see *Hearing Function*

PSYCHOLOGICAL, see *Cornell Index; Depression; Jenkins Activity Survey; Minnesota Multiphasic Personality Inventory; Rorschach; Thematic Apperception*

PSYCHOLOGICAL HEART DISEASE RISK, see *Jenkins Activity Survey*

PTH, see *Parathyroid*

PTT, see *Partial Thromboplastin Time*

PULMONARY ARTERY PRESSURE, see *Blood Pressure*

PULMONARY FUNCTION

Measurements of how well the lungs take in air, how much they can hold, how well they utilize air, and how well they can expel it are important in diagnosing the many different kinds of breathing problems. (The amount of **Oxygen** and **Carbon Dioxide** in the blood are also important measures of the lungs' effectiveness.) There are two main types of lung disease. The first type can be caused by loss of lung tissue, inability of the lungs to expand properly, or inability to transfer oxygen to the blood. The second type results from obstruction or narrowing of the main passageways of air (the trachea and bronchial tubes) in the lung.

Most lung-function tests are performed by having the patient breathe into a spirometer, an instrument that records the amount of air put through it and the rate of air passage for a specified time, and are called spirometry tests. The various tests for pulmonary function are listed and explained below.

Bronchial inhalation challenge, sometimes called methacholine inhalational challenge because the drug methacholine is commonly used, helps differentiate between asthma and other lung conditions that appear similar. After vital-capacity measurements are established, the patient inhales methacholine, or some histamine preparation, and vital-capacity volumes are again observed. When the patient has asthma rather than a problem of deliberate hyperventilation or a nonallergic disease that affects normal breathing, the drug causes bronchial constriction and a reduction of vital capacity. Patients who wheeze but otherwise have normal pulmonary-function measurements are usually given this test. It also helps to diagnose breathing difficulties that can come from heart failure rather than lung disease, a chronic cough produced by a sinus infection rather than lung irritation, and difficulty in breathing that can come from chest tumors rather than allergies.

Another challenge test is called the cold bronchial provocation test; it is similar to histamine inhalation except that cold air is breathed in to measure the lungs' reaction. Many patients who experience exercise-induced asthma will show severe restriction of air movement in the lungs when exposed to only a little cold air; normal breathers are rarely bothered by a large amount of cold air.

Diffusing capacity shows how well the lungs can transfer oxygen to the blood and eliminate carbon dioxide from the blood at the end points of air passage in the lung (tiny sacs called alveoli). A small amount of carbon monoxide is inhaled, and the amount the blood absorbs is measured; normally it should absorb all of it.

Forced expiratory volume (FEV), sometimes called timed vital capacity, is the same as vital capacity with the addition of a time element: the patient is asked to take as deep a breath as possible and then force out the air as hard and as quickly as possible. The amount of air exhaled during the first second of time (FEV_1) is measured. Sometimes, measurements of exhalation last for two or three seconds (FEV_2, FEV_3). Normally, a person will exhale at least 80 percent of his vital capacity in the first second and 95 percent by the third second.

Maximum expiratory flow rate (the rate during the middle half of forced vital capacity) and *maximum midexpiratory flow* (the average flow during the middle half of the total expired volume) are two additional measurements used to confirm the results obtained by other tests.

Maximal voluntary ventilation (MVV), sometimes called maximum breathing capacity (MBC), measures the greatest amount of air a person can breathe each minute. The patient is asked to breathe as rapidly and deeply as possible for 15 seconds. The total amount of air exhaled is then multiplied by 4, giving the result in liters per minute. The normal amount, like that for the vital capacity, is determined by the individual's body surface area. Someone in good physical condition should have an MVV of almost 20 times the VC.

Pulmonary compliance measures how well the lungs can be stretched or distended and then how well they recoil after a full breath; the normal value is determined by body surface area.

Respiratory rate measurements (how many breaths per minute) can reveal the first sign of a lung infection, especially in the elderly. The respiratory rate can increase even before a temperature rise.

Vital capacity (VC), sometimes called forced vital capacity, is probably the most common test of lung volume. It measures how much air the patient can forcefully exhale after inhaling as much air as possible. Usually, the body's surface area is calculated and the number is multiplied by 2.5 to obtain the number of liters (a liter approximates a quart) of air that a patient should be able to expel at one time. An average-size 150-pound man should be able to take in and breathe out about 5 liters (5,000 ml) with one forced breath; any amount from 4,000 ml to 6,000 ml is considered within normal limits for men of that size. *Flow volume curves or loops,* which relate VC to the lung volume, when plotted on a graph, can help diagnose the degree of obstruction in the bronchi and can often help reveal whether the cause comes from inside or outside the lungs.

Several other measurements may be made of amounts of air the lungs hold. A few of these include the *residual volume* (the air that remains in the lungs after the vital capacity is exhaled), the *tidal volume* (how much air is expired with each normal breath), and the *functional residual capacity* (the sum of the last bit of air that can be exhaled during the vital-capacity test and the residual volume). These tests are performed by having the patient inhale known amounts of certain gases such as nitrogen and helium and noting which of those gases are absorbed and which are exhaled; they can also be performed with the plethysmograph (a special machine that measures changes in the body's overall volume during breathing; the patient sits in an enclosed controlled-air chamber that resembles a diving bell).

One particular pulmonary-function test that is being used quite frequently is the *peak expiratory flow rate* (PEFR), sometimes called peak flow monitoring. It is a measure of the strength of a forcible exhalation—after taking in as much air as possible—using a simple gauge to record the flow, usually as compared to a standard set of values by the doctor. It is most often performed at home as a means of preventing serious asthma attacks and also heart failure (by indicating when the lungs are starting to fill with fluid). The instruments cost from $5 to $60 and can be used repeatedly.

When performed: Whenever there are breathing difficulties such as wheezing, persistent coughing, shortness of breath, repeated episodes of fainting or coma, or difficulties due to exposure to environmental contaminants such as coal dust, asbestos, moldy hay, moldy sugar cane, or compost; when a patient has been working with birds or poultry; following use of certain drugs (especially heroin, methadone, and some antibiotics); with heart failure, chest injuries, and certain nervous system diseases; when there is suspicion of a growth in the lungs; when anxiety causes breathing difficulties; to measure progress in treating lung diseases; to determine when a patient can breathe on his own after being in a mechanical respirator.

Normal values: Most normal values for breathing tests must take into account the age, height and weight (body surface area), and sex of the individual (obviously, the smaller the person, the smaller the lung capacity). After the normal, or expected, values for a person's size are determined, the measurements are obtained and compared against the standard. A deviation of up to 20 percent from expected values is considered within normal limits.

Abnormal values: In almost all the pulmonary-function tests, results showing a person's breathing or lung capacity to be less than 80 percent of the expected value (as determined by the person's body surface area) are considered a sign of disease. In general, the tests, when used together, help diagnose restrictive types of lung disease from obstructive types. If the tests show abnormal results, the usual procedure is to administer a bronchodilator drug such as isoetharine (usually by inhalation) and then repeat the measurements; if the drug produces bronchodilatation and causes marked improvement, the lung disease is usually considered reversible. For example, with asthma, the vital capacity will increase after a bronchodilator drug; with emphysema, there will be no improvement. The vital-capacity measurement is reduced with nerve diseases that affect respiratory muscles (Guillain-Barré disease, myasthenia gravis), edema of the lungs, and conditions that take up space in the lung area such as tumors.

The other lung-function tests will give lower-than-predicted results depending on the specific cause of the disease and the extent of the disease process. In chronic bronchitis (an obstructive type of disease), the vital capacity and the FEV_1 are reduced. In sarcoidosis (where the lung alveoli, which transfer oxygen to the bloodstream, are thickened), the FEV_1 is usually normal because there is no obstruction to the bronchial tubes. The lungs will not recoil normally with emphysema.

Sudden changes in forced expiratory volume measurements may be one of the earliest indications of heart disease.

Risk factors: If an undiagnosed pulmonary disease exists such as weakness in the lungs' air sacs, there is a slight risk of collapsing the lung(s) during the performance of the test.

Pain/discomfort: Wearing a nose-closing piece and having to breathe through a special tight-fitting mouthpiece can be quite uncomfortable, especially for prolonged periods of time. Sitting in the sealed, controlled-air chamber causes anxiety in a number of patients.

Cost: Most doctors measure vital capacity and FEV_1 with a small hand-held instrument and make no charge for the procedure. When more elaborate equipment is employed and three or four pulmonary functions are measured, the fee ranges from $35 to $70. When the complete battery of pulmonary-function tests is performed, and includes functional residual capacity and diffusing capacity, the charge is $100 to $300. It is possible that a health insurance company or government-sponsored medical program will not reimburse the doctor or patient for the cost of a pulmonary-function test used only for screening purposes.

Accuracy and significance: Pulmonary-function studies, when performed in their entirety, are considered 90 percent accurate in helping to diagnose the specific cause of lung disease. The tests are particularly significant in that there are very few false-positive results. When results of a test vary, the patient's best score is the one used.

One way to check the accuracy of these tests is to compare the FEV_1 with the MVV; the MVV should be about 35 times the FEV_1 or something may be wrong with the testing equipment.

PULSE ANALYSIS

The word *pulse* refers to the sudden expansion of the walls of a blood vessel, usually a medium- to large-sized artery, as blood is forced through the artery by each heartbeat. Most people are familiar with "taking the pulse," when the doctor feels for the artery on the inside of the wrist (see **Blood Pressure**). But there are other pulse test measurements that can be made, depending on the blood vessel's location in the body. The pulse of the carotid artery is tested by placing two fingers on either side of the neck, a bit toward the front, and noting the artery's force or pulsations. At times, a stethoscope is used to listen to the sound of the surging blood, and it is not unusual to place a sensitive recording instrument over the carotid area to visualize graphically the carotid pulse—which, in fact, also reflects the action of the heart valves between the heart's left ventricle and the aorta (the body's largest artery). Occasionally, the pulse of the carotid vein, which is adjacent and parallel to the carotid artery, is measured to test the efficacy of the heart's right side (there are no heart valves between the vena cava, the body's largest vein, and the right atrium, the heart's upper right chamber, which first receives venous blood. The right side of the heart directs blood into the lungs.

The brachial pulse is felt for just above or below the collarbone; the femoral pulse is located on either side of the groin; the popliteal pulse is located behind the knees; there are also pulses along the ankle and on the back of the foot that are routinely tested during a physical examination. When pulsations are felt over veins, other than the carotid, they usually signifiy an arteriovenous fistula, a direct opening between an artery and its adjacent vein. Such abnormalities cause the heart to work harder than it should, and the result can be heart failure.

The pulses on both sides of the body are tested, and they should be of equal force; the same pulses are tested while taking deep breaths.

When performed: To help confirm heart and heart valve disease; to detect circulation blockages often caused by another organ compressing the artery (and usually the adjacent nerve, as well); to help diagnose an aneurysm (a ballooning out of a major artery, frequently as a consequence of a weakened arterial wall); to help evaluate decreased circulation to the body, especially to the brain; to help diagnose a coarctation (a constriction or severe narrowing and almost always of the aorta); to help distinguish among a variety of lung conditions such as asthma and emphysema; to help confirm the diagnosis of pericardial disease (the pericardium is the sac around the heart; it can become filled with fluid or tighten from an infection and impair heart function).

Normal values: The pulse should be firm and forceful and equal on both sides of the body; it is normal for the pulse rate to increase slightly when a breath is inhaled and to decrease as air is exhaled.

Abnormal values: The most common abnormality is a diminished pulse beat, usually on one side of the body but at times on both sides. This almost always indicates decreased circulation, which can mean an inadequate supply of oxygen and nutrients is reaching the body tissues. The causes can be atherosclerosis, blood vessel defects, injuries, or congenital malformations. Pulsus paradoxus is an abnormality in which the pulse can disappear when a deep breath is inhaled; it usually signals an obstructive lung problem. Similarly, respiratory sinus arrhythmia—where the pulse decreases, rather than increases, when inhaling—has also been used as a test to indicate heart disease, ostensibly by measuring the "stiffness" of the heart; a "stiff," or unhealthy, heart does not respond to the usual chest pressure of breathing.

Risk factors: None.

Pain/discomfort: None.

Cost: There is usually no fee when the test is part of a physical examination. Should recording instruments be used, the fee is $50 to $70.

Accuracy and significance: In many instances, the measurement of pulsations is subjective and depends primarily on a doctor's training and experience. Graphic records, on the other hand, can document significant characteristic patterns that quite accurately indicate disease. Most often, pulse analysis is a supportive test used in conjunction with more definitive tests for heart and blood vessel pathology; it has no consistent accuracy rating.

Note: Pulse analysis is not the same as the "pulse test," once proposed as a detect-it-yourself allergy test. In the "pulse test," it was purported that the pulse would increase to a specific rate when an offending substance was eaten or inhaled.

PULSE PRESSURE, see *Blood Pressure*

PUNCH BIOPSY, see *Biopsy*

PUPILLARY REFLEX

The pupils of the eye (the openings in the center surrounded by the colored iris) open and close (widen and narrow) when exposed to different amounts of light and when focusing on near or far objects. The smaller the opening, the more clearly objects can be seen at different distances (in photography, this is called "depth of field"). To test pupillary reflexes, first, a strong light is directed into the eye to note the pupil's reaction; second, the patient is asked to look at objects both close up and far away, and the pupil is observed. The consensual reflex test is performed by shining a light in one eye and observing that the pupil of the other eye also contracts; if it does not, this could indicate several eye/brain/**Lead** poisoning problems.

When performed: Whenever brain, nerve, or eye disease is suspected; whenever abuse or overdose of certain drugs is suspected.

Normal values: Normally, when a bright light is directed toward the eye (or when a person is in bright sunlight), the pupils contract and become very small (miosis). As the amount of light diminishes, the pupils widen. When a person looks at an object close up, the pupils usually contract (accommodation). If light is directed to one eye only, normally the pupil of the other eye also becomes smaller, even if it is blocked off from the light source. As people become older, pupil size normally becomes smaller. Both pupils should be round and of the same size.

Abnormal values: In patients with Argyll-Robertson pupil, light will not diminish pupil size, but looking at a close object will. The condition is most often a result of syphilis. In patients who are blind in one eye, the pupil may still respond to light in the other eye, but not to direct light. When the pupil does not react at all, it is usually indicative of nerve-brain disease. Various drugs can cause either sustained dilatation or contraction of the pupil. Narcotic drugs usually cause fixed "pinpoint" pupils.

Risk factors: None.

Pain/discomfort: None.

Cost: There is usually no charge, as the test is part of a routine physical examination.

Accuracy and significance: The test is 95 percent accurate and significant because the measurements are totally objective. Observation of pupil abnormalities, however, cannot necessarily distinguish the particular cause of an abnormal pupillary reflex, nor can it differentiate between the various drugs that cause pupillary changes.

PURE TONE, see *Hearing Function*

PUTATIVE PARENT, see *Parentage*

PYELOGRAM, see *Radiography*

PYRIDOXINE (Vitamin B_6)

Vitamin B_6 (also called pyridoxine) is essential to the metabolism of proteins, carbohydrates, fats, and fatty acids. Brewer's yeast, blackstrap molasses, bran, and organ meats contain large amounts of pyridoxine. Vitamin B_6 deficiency is rare but is seen in pregnancy and with the ingestion of certain drugs (isoniazid, penicillamine). Symptoms of deficiency include dermatitis, conjunctivitis, neuritis, loss of appetite, nausea, vomiting, and lethargy. In addition, B_6 deficiency can cause anemias and oxalate crystals in urine. Recent research seems to show an association between low blood levels of pyridoxal (the active metabolic product of pyridoxine, which is easier to measure) and arteriosclerosis. The urine is usually examined for the amount of pyridoxal. A 24-hour urine specimen is required. Blood from a vein can be tested for pyridoxic acid or pyridoxal.

A more recent, indirect way of detecting pyridoxine deficiency is the tryptophan loading (sometimes called tryptophan tolerance) test. Here, the patient is given large doses of tryptophan in tablet form, and then the patient's urine is collected for the next 24 hours to measure the output of xanthurenic acid (a tryptophan metabolic product that is not usually excreted if an adequate amount of pyridoxine is part of the diet). This method of testing for pyridoxine is particularly valuable when pregnant women show symptoms of a deficiency of this vitamin—symptoms that can be early warning signs of a dangerous pregnancy. When more than 50 mg of xanthurenic acid is found in the urine, it is considered an abnormal result. This version of testing for pyridoxine deficiency is also being applied to patients who use birth control pills regularly, who seem to be alcoholic, who require dialysis; in many instances, replacement of the vitamin also lessens any related dangers. The large amounts of tryptophan needed for this test may cause sleepiness (this protein product has been used as a natural sleep-inducing medicine). (See **Serotonin**.) It may also cause a slowness of movement and reflex actions.

When performed: When symptoms indicate a possible deficiency of vitamin B_6.

Normal values: Excretion of 35 to 55 mcg of pyridoxal per day in the urine is considered normal. Blood levels range from 3 to 20 ng per ml.

Abnormal values: Excretion of less than 35 mcg of pyridoxal per day indicates a deficiency, as do blood levels below 3 ng per ml.

Risk factors: Negligible (see general risk factors for blood testing).

Pain/discomfort: Minimal (see general pain/discomfort factors for blood testing).

Cost: From $40 to $60.

Accuracy and significance: So many symptoms and signs come from a vitamin B_6 deficiency that the test is very nonspecific. Even when no deficiency exists, many drugs and diseases will alter pyridoxine levels. A vitamin B_6 deficiency is usually diagnosed long before a laboratory test confirms it. The test has no accuracy rating.

PYROSIS, see *Gastroesophageal Reflux*

Q

Q-FEVER, see *Agglutination*

QUICK, see *Prothrombin Time*

QUICKSTIK, see *Pregnancy*

QUIZ ELECTROCARDIOGRAM, see *Electrocardiogram*

R

RADARKYMOGRAPHY, see *Radiography*

RADIATION POISONING, see *Nuclear Scanning*

RADIOACTIVE IODINE SCREENING, see *Thyroid Function*

RADIOACTIVE UPTAKE, see *Nuclear Scanning*

RADIOALLERGOSORBENT, see *RAST*

RADIOGRAPHY

Radiography, or the use of X-rays, is an integral part of many different testing procedures. A chest X-ray for a cough, for instance, is no different from a specific screening blood test for anemia or infection; it may not always reveal a specific disease, but it offers clues toward a diagnosis. Much depends on the type of X-ray. There are X-rays of specific parts of the body or specific organs taken from different angles. There are X-rays using a contrast dye (usually, an iodine solution) that cannot be penetrated and that causes great contrast on the X-ray film, silhouetting or imaging whatever tissue the dye fills; the dye reveals organs that normally would not be seen by X-ray alone. The dye may also be used to show concentration in an organ or to follow how efficiently and rapidly an organ eliminates that dye (excretion test).

An X-ray of a bone will show if that bone is broken (or has a slight crack) and thus is essentially a test for fracture. The chest X-ray may show pathology in the lung as well as the size, shape, and position of the heart and, like the standard electrocardiogram, will help diagnose suspected heart problems; in this sense, it is a "test" for coronary disease. A fluoroscopic examination will show heart movement (using X-rays) and, with the use of a contrast dye, will delineate just what happens when a person swallows; the contrast dye outlines the stomach, the intestines, and the large bowel. The gallbladder, joint cavities, spinal canal, uterus and tubes, lungs, and even arteries and veins are also outlined by contrast dye. Dental X-rays are used to check the alignment of teeth, to detect cavities or abscesses, and to help uncover the causes of sinus pain though many doctors consider sinus X-rays useless.

Amniography utilizes X-rays to help outline the fetus within the mother's uterus. A contrast dye is injected into the amniotic sac, which surrounds the developing infant; the resultant shadows can reveal an abnormal physical development such as a tumor or some organ growing outside the infant's body rather than inside. The fetus may swallow the dye and show an abnormality in its digestive tract. (See **Amniocentesis**.)

Angiography is the particular study of the arterial blood vessels by X-rays and contrast media. In cerebral angiography, the dye is injected into the neck arteries, and X-ray pictures are taken of the circulation of the brain. (The dye fills and outlines arteries that normally cannot be visualized by X-ray.) Coronary angiography is similar, except that the dye is injected into the coronary arteries (those that feed heart muscle) via a catheter (thin tube) from the arm or neck through the heart into the aorta; the dye is specifically placed to fill the tiny arteries that supply the heart, the plugging of which seems to cause most heart attacks. Angiography is also performed on the pulmonary arteries leading to the lungs.

Because angiography involves the positioning of cardiac catheters through X-rays, other heart observations can be made without dye, or after the dye is administered. Various pressure measurements are recorded from inside the heart's chambers and in the large arteries leaving the heart (the pulmonary artery, which leads to the lungs, and the aorta, which leads to the rest of the body). The amount of oxygen in the blood can also be recorded. Then, too, intraatrial pacing studies can be done. For these studies, a special sensory electrode placed inside the heart's atrial, or upper, chamber records the origin, direction, and time of the nerve impulse that establishes the pace of the heartbeat. At times, the electrocardiogram is recorded from inside the heart rather than from outside it. Many doctors now feel this test is performed far too often without justification.

Digital subtraction angiography (DSA) is a form of angiography that does not use catheters and, hence, avoids their risks. A computer is employed in this technique to enhance the X-ray images on a TV screen. This test is easily performed and does not require hospitalization. Furthermore, it offers excellent results when surveying the body's major arteries—especially those in the abdomen, extremities, and heart chambers.

Cardiac output (CO) is another angiographic-type test measurement, usually made when the catheters used in angiography or **Nuclear Scanning** are in place. It reveals the amount of blood the left ventricle (heart chamber) pumps into the aorta—either in terms of each heart contraction (pulse beat), and called stroke volume, or when multiplied by the pulse rate (number of beats per minute), as a volume measurement per minute. Normally, the heart's stroke volume is from 4,000 to 6,000 ml (1 to 1½ quarts) per minute; a lower-than-normal CO will fail to supply sufficient oxygen to the body, especially the brain. With activity, depending on how forceful, the CO can normally increase to 15,000 ml. Much also depends on the heart's rhythm (see **Electrocardiogram**). This test is also used to measure the effect certain drugs will have on the heart's activity; it can show whether a drug being considered for treatment will do more harm than good by the way it acts on the heart. Thermodilution cardiac output measurements, where solutions of different temperatures are injected into the heart's chambers, are used as a test to evaluate the treatment of extremely ill patients.

Arthrography refers to X-rays of the joints using a contrast media (dye) or air to outline the joint spaces. Arthrography may be performed on almost any joint. Most frequently the knee is examined, in order to diagnose meniscal injury. (Menisci are the small cartilage cushions in the knee joint that separate the bones of the upper and lower leg.) Fluoroscopy is used after the dye is injected to help locate the area to be studied; then, X-ray films are taken.

Barium enema is described below under "Gastrointestinal (GI) Series."

Bronchography involves dripping contrast media into the lungs through a catheter (tiny tube) inserted into the trachea in order to examine the bronchial tubes—their size (opening), location, and number. The technique, though not in frequent use, is still a fairly definitive test for bronchiectasis (abnormally dilated passages of the bronchial tubes).

Cardiokymography (CKG)—sometimes called displacement cardiography, electrokymography, kymography, or radarkymography—is a means of observing the heart in action. The image of the moving heart is shown on a fluoroscope, permitting observation of the heart's borders, measurement of the size of the heart's contraction (ventricle wall motion), and evaluation of the elasticity of those arteries leading to the lungs and of the aorta, which carries blood to the rest of the body. At times, the beating heart is photographed in motion for a permanent record. This form of radiography is particularly valuable when a heart wall aneurysm (a weakened area of the muscle wall that balloons out) is suspected. Many doctors consider this test experimental.

Cholangiography, sometimes called intravenous cholangiography (IVC), is another test of the functioning of the ducts that carry bile from the liver to the gallbladder and then to the intestine. It is usually employed when two oral cholecystography tests fail to show the gallbladder, or after a patient has had gallbladder surgery and still has symptoms. The dye is injected into an arm vein; X-ray pictures are taken every 15 minutes (usually for an hour) until the bile ducts and the gallbladder can be visualized. It may be valuable when a gallstone is suspected in a bile duct rather than in the gallbladder. Occasionally, this test, too, must be performed a second or third time in order to find the gallstone or to ascertain that the gallbladder is not functioning.

Transhepatic *cholangiography* may be performed when it is impossible to tell whether jaundice is caused by bile stones or by liver damage. A needle is inserted into the liver through the skin, and after a bile duct is located, dye is injected directly into the duct. If the liver is not outlined by the dye, bile stone blockage is indicated, and surgery is usually performed immediately to remove the obstruction.

Oral *cholecystography*, using X-rays and contrast media, will detect gallstones (a plain X-ray of the liver and gallbladder area usually will not). The patient follows his usual diet for several days prior to the test; at dinner the night before and breakfast just prior to the test, no fat is ingested. The patient takes special dye tablets the night before. If the bile ducts and gallbladder are normal, the X-ray (taken the next morning) will show the gallbladder filled with the dye. The patient is then given a fatty meal to eat; X-rays are taken every 15 minutes afterward to determine if emptying of the gallbladder is normal. If stones are present, they usually are seen in contrast to the dye. If the gallbladder does not fill up with the dye the next morning, the test is usually repeated with a double dose of the dye tablets before the results are considered abnormal. An abnormal test can mean gallstones, but it can also mean a sluggish or infected gallbladder or liver disease.

Note: In 1984, it was discovered that the gallbladder reacts no differently to a no-fat or low-fat meal than it does to a high-fat meal; thus, the usual feeding of a high-fat meal as part of this test is outmoded.

Defecography is taking still and motion picture X-rays to evaluate the passage of feces from the colon and rectum through the anal canal (usually part of a barium enema) as a means of diagnosing the cause of fecal incontinence or dyschezia (difficult or painful bowel movements). Anorectal Manometry and Solid-sphere tests are less risky.

Excretory urography is described below under "pyelography."

A *gastrointestinal (GI) series*, or contrast radiography of the gastrointestinal tract, can consist of many different tests. The patient may swallow a mouthful of barium (a compound that resists X-rays and shows up in marked contrast on the X-ray film). As the barium passes down the esophagus into the stomach, the size, shape, and activity of the esophagus can be observed through fluoroscopic examination. When sufficient barium is ingested to fill the stomach, it can be seen both by fluoroscopic examination and by X-ray pictures. Any filling "defect" (a place where the normal outline of barium should be seen but is not) is usually an indication of disease (ulcer, growth, or infection). When barium is in the stomach, it is common to tilt the patient so that his head is lower than his feet; the procedure helps to diagnose a hiatal hernia (a weakness of the lower end of the esophagus and the diaphragm around the esophagus), which can cause consistent heartburn. The barium is then followed into the upper (small) intestines, where the physician searches for other defects. Sufficient barium is usually given to outline the entire small intestine. This is sometimes called an upper GI series.

To test for disease in the large intestine (the colon and rectum), barium is usually instilled by enema until the lower bowel is filled. Again, defects in places where barium should normally be seen can indicate disease. In contrast, visible pouches of barium can indicate polyps or diverticuli. After the barium is expelled, X-rays are again taken to see if any residual barium has been captured by the bowel; this can also indicate a disease process (at times, additional air is introduced to exaggerate the contrast). If a complete gastrointestinal series is to be performed, the barium enema is given first. A barium enema can also help prevent unnecessary surgery for appendicitis by revealing the cause of abdominal pain. This is sometimes called a lower GI series.

Hysterosalpingography is a test to discover whether the fallopian tubes are open to allow passage of the egg, or ovum, from the ovary to the uterus. It is one of many fertility tests conducted when a couple is unable to have children (see **Rubin**). The tubes may be closed as a result of infection (appendicitis, gonorrhea) or other disease or abnormally located uterine tissue.

Lymphangiography is a test to determine the effectiveness of the lymph vessels and lymph glands (lymph is a transparent fatty fluid that goes from body tissues back into the bloodstream). When lymph vessels become obstructed or inoperative, edema (water retention) usually results; cancer tends to be spread via the lymph system. Dye is slowly injected into the lymph vessels to be studied, and the patient is X-rayed at that time and then again in 24 hours.

Mammography is the use of X-rays to visualize breast tissue (mammary glands), primarily to detect a growth and secondarily to distinguish, when possible, a malignant from a benign growth. The test is usually performed prior to any breast surgery and especially on women over the age of 30 who have a family history of breast cancer. Usually, the breast is X-rayed from the top and from the side. Xeromammography is a special X-ray technique that is said to provide greater detail with less X-ray exposure. Many physicians feel the danger of too much X-ray makes this test unsatisfactory. While breast X-rays have some advocates, it is a fact that many "masses" detected through these processes are not always cancerous and that one out of five "lumps" is not detected. Mammography is also used to detect early adult-onset diabetes; should calcification of the breast arteries be observed in the course of the procedure, diabetes diagnostic studies are warranted.

Myelography, sometimes called a myelogram test, involves the injection of contrast dye into the spinal canal (using the **Cerebrospinal Fluid** test technique), in order to study the bones of the spinal column (almost always the lower, or lumbar, spinal column) and especially the spaces, or discs, between the bones. Usually, the patient is placed on a special table so that his position can be changed to distribute the dye better and, of even greater importance, so that as much of the dye as possible can be withdrawn at the end of the test. If it is not possible to withdraw all the dye, the removal technique is repeated the following day.

Pancreatography, a procedure most commonly used to detect stones in the pancreatic ducts, is also combined with **Endoscopy** (sometimes called endoscopic retrograde pancreatography) and allows testing of pancreatic secretions and pancreatic cells directly (see **Pancreas Function**). Usually, it is reserved as a final test when cancer is suspected.

Pneumoencephalography (PEG) is a test to outline the cerebrospinal fluid spaces within the brain. Sterile air or a gas is injected into the spinal column (using the **Cerebrospinal Fluid** test technique) and rises up to the brain area, replacing the fluid normally present and giving a clear outline of the spaces, called ventricles. Should defects be seen (such as a suspected tumor or loss of brain substance), the patient may be moved about to provide better visualization. At times, a cisternal puncture is used instead of the usual cerebrospinal fluid tap in the lower spine, usually when the patient has a vertebral defect. With the cisternal puncture, the needle is inserted at the base of the skull just above the first vertebra. **Computerized Tomography** is being used as a less dangerous substitute for this particular test.

Pyelography may be described by a variety of terms: *intravenous pyelography* (IVP), *excretory urography*, or a *urogram*; it is the study of the kidneys, ureters, and bladder by X-rays and contrast media. When the contrast dye is injected into the bloodstream (usually through an arm vein), it will almost immediately concentrate in the kidneys and then pass down into the bladder. Normally, the dye shows in the kidney within minutes and assumes an expected silhouette. If cysts, tumors, or other diseases are present, the dye will take longer to appear, and abnormal filling defects will be seen. In special circumstances, the dye is injected directly into the kidney arteries (usually by catheters inserted into leg arteries and pushed up to kidney level) to determine if both kidney arteries are of normal size and shape and are not narrowed or blocked. This is called a renal arteriography test and is particularly useful in cases of undiagnosed high blood pressure.

The same test can be performed by inserting a contrast dye through a cystoscope into the urethra and then via tiny tubes into the ureters and watching the dye fill up in the kidneys; it is called retrograde pyelography. This form of the test is usually used when there is some doubt about kidney function and when the cause of the problem is thought to be below the kidneys.

At times, pyelography will not be sufficient to diagnose a blockage in the ureter (the tube that carries urine from the kidney to the bladder). The Whitaker test may then be performed. Here, instruments are used to measure the pressure in the kidney (where urine exits) and the bladder at the same time. This does require insertion of a needle through the back into the kidney as well as a catheter through the urethra (the tube that carries urine from the bladder to the outside) while pyelography is performed. This test can cause bleeding and infection. Many doctors, reluctant to perform the Whitaker test, will instead use the furosemide renogram (furosemide is a diuretic drug) along with a kidney scan (see **Nuclear Scanning**); while not as accurate, it is less dangerous.

Salpingography enables the shape, size, and outline (for irregularities) of the uterine cavity to be visualized after an opaque substance is instilled into the uterus.

X-rays may also be taken of various body cavities such as the sinuses—with or without the use of opaque dyes (contrast media)—the salivary gland ducts (sialoangiography), and the orbits of the eye, as but a few examples.

Venography is similar to angiography except that the dye is injected into a vein instead of an artery. This test is especially valuable for detecting thrombophlebitis (a clot blocking the passage of blood in a vein, usually—but not always—existing along with an infectious process). There are many newer tests to detect thrombosis (using sound waves or air pressure measurements); however, phlebography (X-rays of dye in the vein) is still considered the most accurate for blood clots in veins. Normally, no clot or blockage is seen in veins.

The newest form of radiography is the dynamic spatial reconstructor (DSR), which utilizes a great many X-ray tubes in a half-circle around the patient; each X-ray is detected by a television receiver opposite it. This device allows three-dimensional images of organs in motion, such as the heart beating or the lung breathing. (Also see **Computerized Tomography, Magnetic Resonance Imaging,** and **Ultrasound.**)

When performed: In general, radiography is performed to detect any disease process that cannot be diagnosed by other means. Specific indications are discussed in the descriptions of the procedures above.

Normal values: Each area of the body has a standard photographic pattern. Through training and experience, the physician can determine whether the patterns seen on an X-ray (including minor variations for individual patients) are normal.

Abnormal values: The finding of suggested pathology shadows or the absence of an X-ray shadow that should be visible is considered abnormal, as described in the descriptions of the various procedures.

Risk factors: Even the slightest amount of radiation from X-ray machines can cause some damage to one's body. As more X-ray pictures are taken, or as continuous X-rays are applied (such as with fluoroscopy or other procedures), the risk increases. Radiation damage can also accumulate over the years; small amounts of X-ray exposure will add up, increasing the total amount of body injury. Special attention must be given to pregnant women, young children, and adolescent girls, whose developing breasts are particularly sensitive to radiation's cancer-causing effects; the latter caution is relevant when screening for scoliosis, such as is done in some schools. Routine chest X-rays, such as those taken at schools and colleges, can be equally risky, and there is no justification for such screening in terms of health or economics, according to most medical experts. The consequences of radiation exposure include: cancer, especially leukemia; sterility; premature menopause; destruction of the intestinal lining; anemia; loss of immunity and the inability to fight off infections and other diseases; internal bleeding; ulcers; and inadequate blood supply, especially to the brain.

Radiation sickness—which is not the same as generalized overexposure to radiation and which usually, but not necessarily, manifests itself within a short period of time after a patient receives X-rays—can cause extreme weakness, nausea and vomiting, loss of hair, pigmentation and atrophy of the skin, and dilated blood vessels on the skin surface. The breast and thyroid gland are the organs most sensitive to X-ray damage, but any organ damage may not become evident for several hours to several years following exposure.

Radiation enteritis is a particular form of radiation sickness that can follow X-rays to the abdomen, kidneys, and genitourinary (pelvic) areas. It is often mistaken for forms of colitis or irritable bowel. It can cause bleeding, perforations, and even strictures of and in the bowel—in many instances necessitating surgery. More than half of those with this complication of X-rays die within a few years.

Any radiography test using a contrast dye can cause a reaction in a patient—from minor itching and a rash to a fatality (see general risk factors for contrast substance use). The patient must always be screened for any allergy to the dye to be used; patients with allergic diseases such as hay fever or asthma must be tested with extreme caution for an allergy to the dye. The dye used in intravenous pyelography has been known to lead to kidney failure; the odds of this occurring are highest in patients with diabetes. When contrast medium (the dye injected to enhance the X-ray image) is used, it also appears to cause a 10-fold increase in radiation damage to the body's cells, especially to the cells' chromosomes. Other adverse reactions from the dyes used with radiography include nausea; vomiting; irregular heartbeats; a dangerous lowering of the blood pressure; edema or swelling of the larynx (vocal cord area), which can cut off breathing; inflammation and swelling of the tongue; paralysis; and even death. Manipulative procedures that are part of radiological examinations, such as the use of catheters, greatly increase the risks (see general risk factors for catheter and needle insertion). Whenever catheters are inserted and directed to particularly sensitive parts of the body (heart, brain, and other internal body organs), the risk increases in proportion to the distance the catheter must travel. Catheters in the heart and major arteries, and especially in the lungs, can cause fluctuations in heart rhythm. They have been known to cause cardiac arrest, in which the heart stops beating completely, and to damage the heart valves directly. It has been reported that some of the catheters used in angiography cause hemoptysis (spitting-up of blood). The more complicated the procedure, the longer it takes, and the greater the body area being X-rayed, the greater the risks associated with radiography.

With angiography and its related tests, much depends on the training and experience of the medical team performing the catheterization. Deaths resulting from the test reportedly range from 1 in every 100 tests to 1 in every 1,000 tests. The more times a patient has the test, the greater the risk seems to be. If angiography is performed in an institution doing fewer than 100 of the procedures a year, the risks are some eight times greater than they are when the test is performed in a hospital doing a minimum of 400 of the procedures a year.

As with many medical decisions, the risks in testing must be weighed against the benefits. Too much X-ray exposure, the possibility of sensitivity to dyes, and the use and manipulation of medical instruments such as catheters may well cause problems far worse than the suspected disease for which the patient is being tested. Whether the benefits of the testing outweigh the hazards is something that must be decided solely by the patient and/or his family after a full and frank discussion with the physician.

One indirect risk factor in radiography can come from the technicians who take the X-ray pictures. At the present time, only 11 states require X-ray technicians to be licensed or to demonstrate evidence of their knowledge and ability to operate the radiographic machines properly and safely. In California, even doctors may not take X-ray pictures until they show proof of their skills; only one out of six doctors in California is legally permitted to operate X-ray equipment. Although it is estimated that nearly 200,000 technicians perform X-ray services, fewer than half are known to have had any formal training or to hold proper credentials. The Food and Drug Administration states that "it's reasonable to assume incompetence by some technicians" is partly responsible for the 2,000 to 4,000 annual deaths from cancer attributable to the use of X-ray equipment.

Note: In 1985, newer contrast dyes were introduced; they are said to be less dangerous than the dyes in common use. When employed, however, they can raise the cost of radiography testing by from $50 to $200, depending on the amount used.

Pain/discomfort: When the test involves only a simple X-ray picture, there is no pain or discomfort. When radiography requires multiple pictures over a period of time, the patient can experience some discomfort lying on a hard table. Some patients, too, find unusual positioning uncomfortable (when the search is for a hiatus hernia, the patient must be almost upside down). Many patients find swallowing barium distasteful, and not a few patients are embarrassed by the ordeal of a barium enema. (See general pain and discomfort factors for catheter and needle insertion.) When air is inserted through the uterus to test the patency of the fallopian tubes (that is, whether the tubes are open), a number of women complain of abdominal pain for several hours after the test. The prolonged use of the catheter in angiography can make patients apprehensive and lead them to complain of discomfort, although the catheter itself rarely causes pain. The use of injected contrast material, such as dyes, to outline blood vessels, as in venography, can cause excruciating pain if the injection of the dye misses the vein, and the pain can last for days.

Cost: One or two uncomplicated X-ray views of the chest or an extremity cost from $35 to $80. For areas of the body requiring more detailed X-rays—such as the head, spine, or pelvis—the fees are $50 to $150. In short, the more X-rays taken and the more time required to obtain satisfactory pictures, the higher the cost. When contrast dyes or X-ray-resistant substances such as barium are used, the charge is often from $75 to $500. Arteriography of major blood vessels is $400 to $800. When heart catheterization is part of angiography, the fee runs from $1,000 to $2,500. A few other examples: myelography runs from $200 to $275; a venogram can cost up to $400; mammography ranges from $30 to $165; an upper or lower gastrointestinal (GI) series ranges from $150 to $225. In many instances, especially when tests are performed in a hospital, there can be additional fees for consultants (some hospitals require a cardiologist and/or an anesthesiologist to be present during intricate X-ray examinations). And of course, there are the hospital charges for the length of stay.

In 1984, some doctors began performing angiography on an outpatient basis (the patients walk into the X-ray facility and walk out after about four hours); they resume normal activities after two days. This procedure is reported to be as safe as when the patient is hospitalized, and the cost is greatly reduced.

Some doctors consider pneumoencephalography outmoded, and it is possible that a health insurance company or government-sponsored medical program will not reimburse the doctor or patient for the cost of the test. Cardiomyography is not reimbursable by all health insurance plans.

Accuracy and significance: It should be remembered that the results of almost all radiographic tests are in large measure subjective and depend primarily on a doctor's interpretation of the shadows, or in some instances the absence of shadows, on the X-ray picture, fluoroscopic, or television screen. Despite the impressiveness of all the equipment and procedures used in radiography, it is not as accurate as most people imagine. Unless the pathology is obvious, it is all too easy for the radiologist to miss seeing a fracture, an ulcer, a gallstone, a kidney stone, or a cancerous growth. Many doctors believe **Ultrasound** is far more accurate than intravenous cholangiography in diagnosing gallbladder problems; cholangiography usually reveals specific gallbladder problems in fewer than one out of every five patients. Recent medical journal articles report the accuracy of this test to be from 13 to 30 percent when the contrast dye is taken orally and about 50 percent when the dye is injected, and some articles go so far as to call the test "obsolete." Although pyelography is one of the most frequent of all radiographic tests — almost considered routine whenever a urinary tract problem is being considered — it is relatively valueless when it comes to a urinary tract infection and most other kidney-related conditions. In 1985, a group of radiologists condemned its routine use, reporting that it had virtually no significance in most instances where it is employed and that its dangers far outweighed the few benefits it might conceivably offer. Cardiomyography is considered a qualitative, rather than a quantitative, test; much depends on the radiologist's subjective interpretation.

Mammography has only a fair degree of accuracy. More then 1 out of 10 patients suspected of having cancer who were examined by the best-trained mammographers did not have cancer, while 1 out of 5 known cancers was missed. Only 1 out of 3 existing breast cancers is detected by mammography alone.

Although radiologists specializing in angiology working with heart surgeons might feel cardiac angiography is the best method of diagnosing heart disease, most nonsurgical cardiologists are not too impressed with such diagnostic techniques; they feel there are many noninvasive, far less risky, diagnostic tests that are at least as good as angiography, if not better.

In general, then, radiography — not including **Computerized Tomography, Magnetic Resonance Imaging, Nuclear Scanning,** and other somewhat related tests — is really only about 50 percent accurate; while much of the lack of accuracy comes from poor technique in taking the X-ray pictures, faulty equipment, and relatively untrained interpretation of X-ray shadows, the results of X-ray tests are often more a personal opinion than an objective fact.

One particular study seems to reflect the accuracy of X-ray diagnosis. When highly experienced radiologists were asked to review the chest X-rays of 143 patients known to have lung cancer, 78 of whose X-rays displayed clear-cut evidence of cancer, the doctors missed the obvious diagnosis in 27 cases. The conclusion was reached from this and other published studies that there is an error rate of 20 to 50 percent in the detection of cancers that are visible on X-rays. The chances of accuracy can be increased by having more than one radiologist "read" the X-rays.

Another indication of the lack of accuracy in X-ray testing is the use of radiography allegedly to determine a child's bone age as an indication of whether growth is normal or not. Although such testing is in common use, medical experts for more than 30 years have decried the practice because of its lack of accuracy; medical textbooks have long pointed out that it is virtually impossible to appraise skeletal age by X-rays. As but one example, if both arms and hands are X-rayed, one side can show totally different results from the other, offering no definitive answer. The younger the child, the more inaccurate the test results. And of course, the more X-rays taken, the greater the risk of radiation damage.

RADIOIMMUNOASSAY, see *Nuclear Scanning*

RADIOIMMUNOSORBENT, see *RAST*

RADIOISOTOPE SCANNING, see *Nuclear Scanning*

RADIONUCLIDE, see *Nuclear Scanning*

RADIONUCLIDE TRANSIT, see *Nuclear Scanning*

RAF, see *Rheumatoid Factor*

RAJI-CELL ASSAY, see *Immunology*

RAPE, see *Acid Phosphatase; Semen*

RAPID EYE MOVEMENT (REM), see *Sleep Monitoring*

RAPID PLASMA REAGIN (RPR), see *Syphilis*

RAST

Although skin tests (see **Skin Reaction**) are still the most common way to test for allergy, the newest technique for measuring a potential allergic reaction is called the RAST test (sometimes called radioimmunosorbent assay test or radioallergosorbent test). It begins as a generalized measurement of a patient's serum immunoglobulin E, or IgE (see **Immunoglobulin**), which will react to known allergy-causing substances (the many varieties of grasses, foods, animal danders, molds, house dust and house dust mites, insect stings, trees, weeds, and cosmetics). The test is a form of Coombs' test reaction (see **Agglutination**). If a patient's blood contains antibodies to certain allergy-provoking substances, these antibodies will combine with known nuclear-radiolabeled allergens and can be so detected.

A positive RAST test (one that shows a reaction) is really a qualitative measure of IgE in the body; the test not only detects the allergens but can also show how much of an allergen it takes to cause an allergic manifestation (asthma, hay fever, eczema). The RAST test is much less time-consuming (one day versus several months), less painful (one needleprick versus scores), and less dangerous (no chance of severe allergic reactions) for a patient than skin-scratch tests for allergy.

Blood is taken from a vein, and the serum is examined. Usually, the serum is tested against specific groups of known allergy-causing antigens (such as all the grasses and trees and various weeds, animals, and house dust mites). When a grouping shows a positive reaction, further tests are performed on individual items in the group if known antibodies are available (not all known antibodies have been processed into allergens for testing).

The basophil histamine release test isolates basophils (see **Blood Cell Differential**) and measures the effect of foods on them; if the suspected food causes the cells to release histamine, it is considered a positive test—meaning there is an allergy to the food. Eosinophils (see **Blood Cell Differential**) are usually increased with allergy; they are also measured as a response to an allergy provocation or challenge test (see **Pulmonary Function**), where they almost always increase after a trial exposure and then decrease after a trial treatment.

Another blood test alleged to reveal the specific cause(s) of an allergy is called cytotoxic allergy detection. Here, a patient's **White Blood Cells** are mixed with common food substances to observe whether any reaction (destruction of the white blood cells) occurs; if so, it is reported that the patient is allergic to that substance. The procedure has also been used to test for allergic-type reactions to other substances such as food additives and other chemicals. As of April 1985, the Food and Drug Administration declared cytotoxic allergy testing to be "unreliable" and not recognized by experts as effective.

Two other tests for allergy, at present still considered unproven, are: sublingual provocative testing, where minute amounts of different foods or food extracts are placed under the tongue to see if they provoke an allergic response; and intracutaneous provocative testing, where various food solutions are injected under the skin—also to elicit an allergic reaction as a means of identifying the food at fault. Some doctors will use larger and larger concentrations of foods if weaker dilutions show no reaction; there is no consensus as to what would be a standardized dose.

When performed: To help find the specific cause of an allergy; as a means of measuring progress in the treatment of allergies.

Normal values: A RAST negative reaction indicates that no allergenic antibodies are present.

Abnormal values: A RAST positive reaction, especially in the presence of high serum IgE levels, indicates the presence of allergenic antibodies. Sometimes, a positive test is reported as from class I to class IV, the latter indicating a very large amount of antibodies. Because different laboratories may show different results (some will report a positive reaction where others report negative), it is usual to have RAST tests repeated by more than one laboratory.

Risk Factors: Negligible (see general risk factors for blood testing).

Pain/discomfort: Minimal (see general pain/discomfort factors for blood testing).

Cost: A general RAST survey, which merely identifies the group in which an allergy could exist, is $10 to $15. Once the group is detected, specific tests for different grasses, different molds, different foods, etc., range from $50 to $300 for testing within the entire group and from $15 to $20 for each suspected allergen.

Accuracy and significance: Many doctors consider the RAST test more accurate than traditional skin testing. In patients with true allergic disease, the RAST test is approximately 80 percent accurate in detecting the allergic substance. It reaches its highest level of accuracy when used to uncover food allergies; its level of accuracy decreases when used for pollens and other environmental irritants.

RAT-BITE FEVER, see *Agglutination*

RAYNAUD'S PHENOMENON, see *Cold Pressor*

RBC, see *Red Blood Cell*

RECTILINEAR SCAN, see *Nuclear Scanning*

RED BLOOD CELL

The red blood cells (erythrocytes) contain hemoglobin (about 60 percent of the body's iron), which is the essential carrier of oxygen in the blood. Besides carrying oxygen to all parts of the body, red blood cells pick up certain waste products (such as carbon dioxide) that are given off later by the lungs. In testing, the red blood cells are counted as well as stained to reveal the size, shape, and hemoglobin content. Sickle cells are seen directly this way, as are certain anemias (see **Blood Cell Differential, Red Blood Cell Indices,** and **Hemoglobin**). Blood taken from a vein is most commonly used; a drop of blood, usually from the fingertip or earlobe, can also be collected. The blood is viewed through the microscope and counted manually or by automated machines.

Erythropoietin is a hormone that stimulates the production of red blood cells; its amount can be measured in the blood as a means of confirming polycythemia (in which erythropoietin levels are lower than normal). It is usually increased in anemias that are caused by drugs and other toxic substances and with some brain and kidney tumors.

On occasion, a siderocyte stain will be applied to the slide being examined under the microscope; the presence of siderocytes (abnormal red blood cells whose iron carries no hemoglobin) can help differentiate the cause of an anemia, such as from **Lead** poisoning. It is not, however, considered very accurate.

When performed: When there is suspicion of one of the anemias or polycythemia (a disease where the bone marrow makes too many red blood cells); in certain parasitic diseases; to verify certain poisonings; to help determine blood loss after hemorrhage. Some states require the testing of newborn babies for sickle-cell anemia unless there is parental objection; they are Arizona, Colorado, Georgia, Louisiana, New Mexico, New York, North Carolina, Texas, and Wyoming (see **Hemoglobin**).

Normal values: Normal levels for men range from 4 to 6 million red cells per cubic millimeter (cu mm) of blood. Women may have a slightly lower count, and newborn babies a higher count.

Abnormal values: Higher-than-normal values are usually found with polycythemia, dehydration, certain kidney diseases, and lung conditions where there is difficulty in breathing and the body needs more oxygen. Lower-than-normal values are usually found with anemias, severe infections, certain cancers, **Malaria,** lead poisoning, and after prolonged bleeding.

Risk factors: Negligible (see general risk factors for blood testing).

Pain/discomfort: Minimal (see general pain/discomfort factors for blood testing).

Cost: From $3 to $6. Usually included in **Comprehensive Multiple Test Screening** panels, which range from $7 to $42. Erythropoietin tests average $20.

Accuracy and significance: Although blood cell counting is 90 percent accurate, there is recent evidence that when blood cells are counted by automatic machines, the results can show false lower-than-normal amounts. It is important, therefore, to know whether or not a blood cell count was performed by an automatic machine.

Note: A red blood cell osmotic fragility test is now being used to help detect and differentiate between various anemias. Here, the cells are put in special solutions of various strengths, and the dilution of those solutions at the point at which they cause the cells to be destroyed is noted. The test seems particularly valuable in screening for thalassemia (see **Hemoglobin**) and other inherited red blood cell disorders. The cost varies from $2 to $35, depending on whether it is performed as a screening test or to aid in making a specific diagnosis.

RED BLOOD CELL DISTRIBUTION WIDTH, see Iron

RED BLOOD CELL ENZYME SCREENING, see Glucose 6-Phosphate Dehydrogenase

RED BLOOD CELL HEMOLYSIS, see Haptoglobin; Tocopherols

RED BLOOD CELL INDICES (Red Blood Cell Profile)

New electronic equipment has made determination of the red blood cell (erythrocyte) indices a valuable aid not only in classifying anemia but in determining the basic cause of the anemia and in helping to decide the specific therapy. The three indices are (1) mean corpuscular volume (MCV), a ratio of the hematocrit to the red blood cell count, expressed as the area of cubic microns (cu μ) per cell; (2) mean corpuscular hemoglobin (MCH), a ratio of the hemoglobin to the red blood cell count, expressed as picograms (pg) of hemoglobin per cell; and (3) mean corpuscular hemoglobin concentration (MCHC), a ratio of hemoglobin to hematocrit, expressed as a percentage. (See **Hematocrit, Hemoglobin,** and **Red Blood Cell.**) Blood is taken from a vein (or from a fingertip, earlobe, or heel) and placed in a special indices chamber.

When performed: When the cause or type of anemia cannot be determined; after the cause of an anemia is determined, to follow the progress of therapy; in certain cases of liver disease and suspected vitamin deficiencies.

Normal values: Normal levels for MCV range from 83 to 103 cu μ; for MCH, from 27 to 35 pg; for MCHC, from 32 percent to 36 percent.

Abnormal values: The MCH and MCV are lowered with some genetically caused anemias and with iron deficiency, liver disease, and blood loss. The MCHC is increased with anemias due to inadequate blood formation. The MCV and MCHC are increased with pernicious anemia, tapeworm infestation, and when certain medicines are taken.

Risk factors: Negligible (see general risk factors for blood testing).

Pain/discomfort: Minimal (see general pain/discomfort factors for blood testing).

Cost: The test is commonly part of a complete blood count, which ranges from $4 to $20. Usually included in **Comprehensive Multiple Test Screening** panels, which range from $7 to $42.

Accuracy and significance: The test is of value in helping to differentiate among the various types of anemia and is a significant aid to the doctor in diagnosing hemolytic anemias and anemias from **Folates** deficiency. It is about 80 percent accurate.

RED BLOOD CELL OSMOTIC FRAGILITY, see Red Blood Cell

RED BLOOD CELL PROFILE, see Red Blood Cell Indices

RED BLOOD CELL SURVIVAL, see Nuclear Scanning

RED CELL ADHERENCE, see *Cancer*

REFLEX

A reflex test is a measure of the reaction of the body to stimulation. Most commonly, muscles are measured for their reflex reaction. Testing for the reflex reaction of the eyelid, the cornea (surface of the eye over the iris and lens), the pupils (see **Pupillary Reflex),** and the skin surface can help in the diagnosis of disease. (See **Caloric** test for ear reflex responses.)

In general, a muscle is tested by applying sufficient pressure to cause stretching of its fibers. In the knee-jerk reflex test, for example, the tapping of the patellar tendon just below the kneecap (usually with a rubber hammer) stretches the attached thigh muscle that lifts the lower leg. The muscle reacts by contracting (shortening), and the lower leg lifts suddenly and involuntarily.

Arm and leg muscle reflex tests are called "deep" reflex tests because of the force of the tap necessary to elicit a response. When a reflex is tested by a gentle stroking motion over or near the muscle, it is called a "superficial" reflex test. For example, when the upper abdomen is stroked, the stomach muscles contract and pull the umbilicus (navel) upward. If a gentle stroke is applied just inside the upper thigh, adjacent to the testicle, the scrotum (the sac that holds the testicle) will suddenly rise upward on the same side that is stroked because of contraction of the cremasteric muscle.

Virtually every muscle can be tested this way, but only about a dozen reflex tests are routinely performed. Each muscle reflex represents an area of the spinal cord where the nerves to that muscle arise and, of course, the nerve itself. Thus, testing for a specific muscle reflex can determine the exact area of the nervous system involved. For example, the bicep (the usually large, bulging muscle of the upper arm) is activated by nerves that come from between the fifth and sixth cervical vertebrae (the neck bones of the spine).

Failure to elicit the reflex, or an extremely exaggerated reflex, indicates disease of the nerve from the muscle to the spinal cord, disease of the spinal cord itself, or disease of the nerves from the spinal cord. The knee-jerk reflex is indicative of nerves that come from the lumbar (lower back) portion of the spine. Superficial reflexes also indicate nervous system locations. Pathology in certain nerves that come directly from the brain can be determined by the corneal reflex. When the colored part of the eye is touched with a piece of cotton, both eyes should immediately close as a reflex action. Failure of the eyes to close, or only one eye closing (on either the same side or the opposite), indicates disease inside the brain.

The usual instrument for testing reflexes is the rubber hammer, but the edge of the hand will do as well. When it seems impossible to obtain a positive reflex reaction, the patient may be asked to perform some other muscular act to draw attention away from the area being tested. This will relax the muscle and allow a normal reflex. To obtain a knee-jerk reaction, for example, the physician may ask the patient to interlock his fingers and pull hard with both hands.

The Bender-Purdue reflex test, sometimes called the symmetric tonic neck reflex test, is performed primarily to determine whether an infant will hold his head up high and look forward and up when creeping. The position and use of the arms, hands, knees, and feet are also recorded. The manner of the child's movements is said to be indicative of the child's ability to learn (to be educated).

For pupil reflex test, see **Pupillary Reflex.** The eyelids should close when touched and at the sight of any approaching object; unless the patient is requested to do otherwise, both eyelids should close simultaneously. Blinking should also be simultaneous.

Another specific reflex test is the cold face test (CFT). Some doctors ask patients to hold their breath and then immerse their faces in cold water for 15 seconds. Others cover the patient's face with a large ice bag. The cold face test, while somewhat similar to the **Cold Pressor** test, is a measure of the heart rate's reflex response. Normally, the application of cold slows the heart, but in patients who have had a stroke, or have multiple sclerosis or severe diabetes, the heart rate does not slow as it should. If the heart slows as expected, the possibility of brain disease can usually be eliminated.

When performed: As part of a routine physical examination to ascertain the functioning of nerves, muscles, and spinal cord; whenever nerve, muscle, or brain damage is suspected; after any injury.

Normal values: Pressure or stimulus on any relaxed muscle should cause a contraction of that muscle or at least a reaction indicating that the pressure or stimulus was acknowledged by the body. Experience has taught doctors the expected responses, so that weak or overly strong reactions can be noted. The reflexes on exact opposite sides or parts of the body should be about the same.

Reflex reactions are usually recorded on a "plus" scale from 1 to 4: 4+ means hyperactive; 1+ means weak or inadequate; 2+ and 3+ are average.

Abnormal values: Total absence of a reflex or extreme hyperactivity is considered abnormal. Specific pathological reflexes include the Babinski, in which stroking the sole of the foot causes the toes to point up and separate (normally, the toes turn down as a response). The reaction is indicative of brain disease. The abnormal doll's-eye reflex occurs when the head is rotated from side to side and the eyes follow the movement to each side (normally, they continue to look straight ahead). This is indicative of severe brain disease, but it can also occur with a large overdose of barbiturate drugs.

Risk factors: Negligible, with the exception of the doll's-eye reflex; performing this test on a patient with a neck injury is extremely hazardous.

Pain/discomfort: Minimal, although there are those who find it uncomfortable to immerse their faces in cold water.

Cost: There is usually no charge for reflex testing, as almost all reflex measurements are part of a routine physical examination.

Accuracy and significance: Reflex responses are about 80 percent accurate and assist the doctor in diagnosing nerve, brain, and muscle diseases. They are especially significant in identifying malingerers. The cold face test is valuable because an ice pack can be placed over the face of an unconscious or comatose patient to help determine if brain damage is present.

REFRACTION, see *Visual Acuity*

REM SLEEP, see *Sleep Monitoring*

RENAL ARTERIOGRAPHY, see *Radiography*

RENAL STONE, see *Urinary Tract Calculus*

RENIN

Renin is an enzyme produced by the kidney. (A renin-type substance that acts exactly like renin is also produced by the liver as an adverse reaction when oral contraceptive drugs or other female hormones are taken.) Renin regulates the production of the hormone **Aldosterone,** which, in turn, controls the salt and water balance in the body. It also metabolizes to form other compounds that cause the muscles around arteries to tighten and become smaller in size, thus raising the blood pressure.

The test is really a renin activity measurement, since an angiotensin compound made from renin is actually measured (see **Rollover).** It is important to know how much salt the patient has been eating for at least three days prior to the test (the less salt, the higher the renin values). The patient should be lying down for several hours before the test (standing, and even sitting, increases renin activity). Usually, blood is taken from a vein, and the plasma is tested. It is now becoming common to measure renin activity separately in each of the kidney veins, since the comparative values are important in evaluating the potential success of kidney surgery as a treatment for high blood pressure.

Some doctors will amplify the test for renin activity by having their patients ingest a tablet of furosemide (a diuretic drug) to measure its effect after the patient has been lying quite still for several hours. This helps distinguish whether the aldosterone problem is primary or whether it is secondary to some other condition such as a potassium imbalance.

A more recent test to help diagnose high blood pressure that can come from kidney, or kidney blood vessel, disorders is called the saralasin infusion test. Saralasin is similar to angiotensin II, an enzyme that is part of the renin-angiotensin system. It is given to the patient intravenously, and the blood pressure's response is noted; a drop in blood pressure caused by the saralasin usually indicates that the cause of the patient's hypertension is from within the kidneys.

When performed: To diagnose one cause of high blood pressure and to help ascertain the type of therapy and whether that therapy will be effective; when adrenal disease is suspected.

Normal values: Plasma renin activity (PRA) measures from 0.2 to 4 ng per ml per hour, depending on the amount of salt in the diet and for how long the patient was in an upright position before the test. Normal values are higher in the early morning hours. When renin activity is measured in each of the kidney veins, there should be no significant difference between the left and right vein.

Abnormal values: PRA is increased with high blood pressure caused by kidney disease, sometimes with chronic kidney disease alone, following kidney injury, with certain adrenal tumors, and with chronic liver disease. Increased values can also occur with pregnancy, with certain diuretic drugs, and with a salt-free diet. Values are usually decreased when patients are eating large amounts of salt or foods containing salt, when patients are taking certain steroid hormone drugs, when the adrenal glands secrete excessive aldosterone, and when high blood pressure comes from eating large amounts of licorice.

Risk factors: Negligible (see general risk factors for blood testing).

Pain/discomfort: Minimal (see general pain/discomfort factors for blood testing).

Cost: From $20 to $50. It is customary to test at least three to six blood samples to evaluate the test results properly.

Accuracy and significance: The test is significant for those few patients with high blood pressure resulting from kidney disease, as it helps to pinpoint this particular diagnosis. The test is also useful if there is a suspicion that only one kidney is involved; renin activity can indicate the specific kidney. Because of the many factors that can interfere with renin evaluations, the test is 80 percent accurate only when it is performed with precision.

Note: A somewhat related test is angiotensin converting enzyme activity (ACE, sometimes called SACE—the S stands for serum). This enzyme converts one form of angiotensin to another and the test may help confirm the diagnosis of sarcoidosis (see **Kviem**), excessive blood **Calcium, Thyroid Function** problems and even histoplasmosis (see **Agglutination, Skin Reaction**). In general, it is not considered accurate enough for a specific diagnosis but may be of some value in following the course and treatment of these diseases. It costs from $50 to $100.

RENOGRAM, see *Nuclear Scanning*

REOVIRUS, see *Virus Disease*

REPTILASE TIME, see *Partial Thromboplastin Time*

RESIDUAL LUNG VOLUME, see *Pulmonary Function*

RESPIRATORY DISTRESS SYNDROME, see *Pregnancy*

RESPIRATORY RATE, see *Pulmonary Function*

RESPIRATORY SINUS ARRHYTHMIA, see *Pulse Analysis*

RETICULOCYTE COUNT

Reticulocytes are immature red blood cells. The reticulocyte count is a measurement (though not precise) of the production of erythrocytes (red blood cells). When the production of erythrocytes is increased by a process that stimulates bone marrow, the reticulocyte count also increases. Any bodily process that can limit red blood cell production (infection, renal disease) can limit the number of reticulocytes in the blood. A drop of blood is stained, and the reticulocytes are viewed under the microscope and counted.

When performed: To evaluate the patient's response to therapy for anemia and polycythemia (an excessive amount of red blood cells).

Normal values: The reticulocyte count is reported as a proportion of the red blood cell count. The usual range is 0.5 to 1.5 reticulocytes per 100 red blood cells.

Abnormal values: The reticulocyte count is decreased in severe autoimmune types of hemolytic (blood-cell-destroying) disease. The count is increased when bone marrow cells are made more active (as with recovery from anemia or following hemorrhage).

Risk factors: Negligible (see general risk factors for blood testing).

Pain/discomfort: Minimal (see general pain/discomfort factors for blood testing).

Cost: From $5 to $24.

Accuracy and significance: Although the test is only about 50 percent accurate, it serves as an aid to the doctor in diagnosing anemia and in measuring the progress of anemia therapy. Much depends on the doctor's interpretation of the cells under the microscope and the reticulocytic relationship to the **Hematocrit**.

RETINOL (Vitamin A)

Deficiency of vitamin A (a fat-soluble alcohol) is considered a major problem of nutrition. Usually, vitamin A is supplied in minimal amounts in the average diet. It is found mostly in fish and fish oils, dairy products, eggs, green and yellow vegetables, and polar bear liver. Some health faddists who eat excessive amounts of food high in vitamin A may display symptoms of hair loss, fatigue, irritability, cerebral edema, and yellowish skin color.

Vitamin A deficiency is a major cause of blindness in young children in parts of the world where the diet is inadequate. Night blindness and "dry eye" are early indications of the deficiency. Blood is taken from a vein, and the vitamin A, retinol, or carotene (forms of the vitamin) is measured from the serum. Retinol can also be measured from a liver **Biopsy**.

The vitamin A tolerance test consists of giving a patient a large dose of vitamin A by mouth and measuring serum levels four to five hours later. Normally, vitamin A levels will rise to greater than 150 mcg per 100 ml. Failure to rise indicates improper fat absorption by the intestine.

When performed: With vision problems, especially inability to see at night; when there are teeth and bone growth problems; in certain cases of sterility; with children whose extreme irritability has no obvious cause; as a possible indication of hidden cancer; with patients who have skin rashes and hair loss that has been difficult to diagnose.

Normal values: Serum levels of 30 to 60 mcg per 100 ml or more are indicative of adequate storage and intake of vitamin A.

Abnormal values: Less than 20 mcg per 100 ml indicates decreased absorption of vitamin A, retinol, or carotene and may be found with food absorption problems such as pancreatic and biliary insufficiency, celiac disease (in addition to the associated eye problems), sprue, and excessive use of mineral oil as a laxative. Some patients with vitamin A deficiency have impaired senses of taste and smell. Decreased retinol levels are being found in patients with cancer, especially cancer of the lung and intestines. Increased levels of vitamin A are found in patients with hair loss, unusual skin rashes, and bone pain (children who are given an excess of vitamin A will scream in pain if their crib or bed is shaken). Patients who take oral contraceptives may also have increased blood levels of vitamin A.

Risk factors: Negligible (see general risk factors for blood testing).

Pain/discomfort: Minimal (see general pain/discomfort factors for blood testing).

Cost: From $10 to $20; up to $40 if carotene measurements are included.

Accuracy and significance: The test is 90 percent accurate in detecting hypovitaminosis or hypervitaminosis A and is significant in helping diagnose unusual skin conditions and vision problems. It is particularly significant in helping to detect the excessive consumption of vitamin A, which can produce a host of toxic symptoms.

RETINOSCOPY, see *Visual Acuity*

RETROGRADE PYELOGRAPHY, see *Radiography*

REVERSE T$_3$, see *Thyroid Function*

RF, see *Rheumatoid Factor*

RHEUMATOID FACTOR (RF, RA, RAF, Rheumatoid Arthritis Factor)
The majority of patients suffering from rheumatoid arthritis have an **Immunoglobulin** antibody called rheumatoid factor. The more rheumatoid factor detected in the blood, the greater the possibility that rheumatoid arthritis exists. Unfortunately, a number of other diseases can also elevate RF levels (liver, lung, and heart conditions; syphilis; and some worm infestations). Blood is taken from a vein and tested through various **Agglutination** techniques.

Note: The bentonite flocculation test and the DNA-bentonite flocculation test are similar to **Complement Fixation** tests and are alleged to indicate rheumatoid arthritis. The antibodies (see **Agglutination**) this test is claimed to detect are also found in cases of systemic lupus erythematosus (SLE) (see **Antinuclear Antibodies**). Some questions as to the tests' accuracy have been raised, but they are considered of value in differentiating rheumatoid arthritis from SLE.

When performed: Primarily on patients with arthritic symptoms to help confirm the diagnosis.

Normal values: No rheumatoid factor or very low levels of it (a low titer, or detection of the substance before any substantial dilution of the blood). The older one gets, the greater the possibility the blood will reveal some rheumatoid factor without evidence of arthritis.

Abnormal values: Titers greater than a dilution of 1:160 (RF present in very diluted serum).

Risk factors: Negligible (see general risk factors for blood testing).

Pain/discomfort: Minimal (see general pain/discomfort factors for blood testing).

Cost: From $10 to $30, depending on the particular agglutination test performed.

Accuracy and significance: It is reported that 80 to 90 percent of patients with rheumatoid arthritis have a high titer of RF. However, failure to have any RF in the blood does not indicate the patient is free of rheumatoid arthritis. Thus, elevated levels of RF only help confirm the doctor's diagnosis. There is some disagreement among doctors as to whether the sheep cell or latex agglutination technique is the most accurate; most prefer the sheep cell method.

RH FACTOR, see *Agglutination: Typing and Cross-Matching*

RHINOMANOMETRY, see *Smell Function*

RIA, see *Nuclear Scanning*

RIA-PAP, see *Acid Phosphatase*

RIBOFLAVIN (Vitamin B$_2$)
Deficiency of vitamin B$_2$, or riboflavin, can cause many eye problems (ulceration, cataracts, corneal vascularization, burning and itching) and skin problems (scaling,

inflammation), as well as problems in the blood (leucocytopenia or fewer-than-normal **White Blood Cells**) and the nervous system (neuritis). Riboflavin is found mostly in milk, meat, and nuts. It can be measured in both the urine and the blood.

When performed: With skin, eye, and nervous system problems that cannot be diagnosed.

Normal values: Normal urinary riboflavin excretion is from 30 to 100 mcg in a six-hour sample. In the blood, riboflavin should be greater than 15 mcg per 100 ml of red blood cells.

Abnormal values: Less than 30 mcg in the urine or less than 15 mcg in the blood is indicative of a deficiency significant enough to cause symptoms.

Risk factors: Negligible (see general risk factors for blood testing).

Pain/discomfort: Minimal (see general pain/discomfort factors for blood testing).

Cost: From $35 to $40.

Accuracy and significance: Riboflavin deficiency diseases are on the increase, thanks to many of the fad diets being promoted today. It has been discovered that some disease conditions that are very difficult to diagnose are caused by an inadequate intake of riboflavin—hence, the newfound significance of this test; considered to be 80 percent accurate.

RINGWORM, see *Fungus*

RINNE, see *Tuning Fork*

RISK FACTOR FOR HEART DISEASE, see *Jenkins Activity Survey*

RKG, see *Radiography*

ROBERTSON, see *Cystometry*

ROBINSON-POWER-KEPLER, see *Chloride*

ROCKY MOUNTAIN SPOTTED FEVER, see *Agglutination*

ROLLOVER

Toxemia of pregnancy (more correctly referred to as pregnancy-induced hypertension, since no "toxin" is involved) is probably the most serious side effect of having a baby. It usually develops during the last three months of pregnancy, and unless it is detected at its earliest stage, it can be fatal to both mother and infant. Until the rollover test was devised, there was no easy way to determine which women were more susceptible than others to toxemia. While the test is not considered perfect at this time, it is the best available. The patient lies on her left side, and the blood pressure is tested. Then the patient rolls over on her back and the blood pressure is measured immediately and then again five minutes later. The test seems to be an indication of a pregnant woman's susceptibility to producing angiotensin, an enzyme made in the kidney that can cause high blood pressure (see **Renin** test). The test does not necessarily signify potential eclampsia (the convulsions and coma that rarely accompany pregnancy).

When performed: On all pregnant women, especially those having their first baby; on a regular basis after the third month of pregnancy.

Normal values: The blood pressure readings should not change after the patient rolls over.

Abnormal values: An increase in the diastolic blood pressure, usually by more than 20 mm Hg (see **Blood Pressure),** within five minutes of rolling over is considered a warning sign; the pregnant patient is then watched far more closely for blood pressure changes.

Risk factors: None.

Pain/discomfort: None.

Cost: There is usually no charge for this procedure, as it is part of the routine examination during pregnancy.

Accuracy and significance: Approximately 75 percent of the women with a positive rollover test develop toxemia of pregnancy. Less than 10 percent of those with a negative rollover test develop toxemia of pregnancy.

ROMBERG, see *Caloric*

ROPES, see *Synovial Fluid*

RORSCHACH

The Rorschach test, invented by a Swiss psychiatrist, consists of a series of essentially formless black inkblots (some also containing red spots), which a subject is asked to interpret. Rorschach believed that personality traits could be revealed by the way a person reacted to these abstract shapes. The Rorschach test is scored on the basis of several criteria: whether all or only part of the inkblot is used in description; whether the subject goes into unusual detail (compulsive personalities supposedly respond first to details instead of to the overall blot); whether form or color is more important (people who are upset by color are supposed to be more emotional); and whether motion is read into the blot (human movement is supposed to represent creativeness). Many uncommon responses are assumed to indicate a schizophrenic disturbance.

Rorschach "scores" have demonstrated little validity as indicators of individual behavior and personality. When the test is used by a therapist to help form hypotheses about an individual, there is the danger that the therapist will make highly personalized interpretations that cannot be considered scientifically valid.

The Holtzman inkblot technique is a similar test using different types of blots. The Holtzman allows the subject to give only one response to the inkblot (in the Rorschach, a patient is asked to give as many interpretations of the blot as possible).

When performed: The test is performed ostensibly to aid in the diagnosis of neurotic or mentally disturbed persons. It is usually given as a part of a battery of tests, since recent studies have cast doubt on the value of Rorschach test interpretations for either diagnosis or prognosis.

Normal values: There are certain standard responses to the inkblots that a majority of subjects state.

Abnormal values: In people who are clearly suffering from mental problems, peculiar responses verify the obvious.

Risk factors: None.

Pain/discomfort: None.

Cost: From $25 to $100, depending on whether the test administrator is a psychologist or a psychiatrist.

Accuracy and significance: There is absolutely no way to test the accuracy of such an examination, since all personalized interpretations are kept completely confidential.

ROSE BENGAL, see *Nuclear Scanning*

ROSE GARDENER'S DISEASE, see *Agglutination*

ROSE SHEEP CELL AGGLUTINATION, see *Agglutination*

ROTAVIRUS, see *Virus Disease*

ROUNDWORM, see *Toxocariasis*

ROUTINE URINALYSIS, see *Urine Examination*

RT, see *Nuclear Scanning*

rT$_3$, see *Thyroid Function*

RUBELLA (German Measles)

German measles was once considered a mild childhood disease. It is now known that if a pregnant woman is exposed to this virus infection and contracts the disease, especially during the first three months of pregnancy, she has a 50 percent chance of giving birth to a child with a congenital defect (deafness, cataracts, heart problems, abnormal growth of various organs, blood disorders). The test for rubella, therefore, is primarily one of determining an individual's susceptibility to the disease by measuring the amount of German measle antibodies in the blood. Usually, an attack of rubella causes a lifelong immunity, which can be measured. If no rubella antibodies are detected, however, there is a vaccine that can help bring about immunity and prevent birth defects. Prior to the use of the vaccine, the results of a German measles epidemic could be tragic; in the United States, in 1964 and 1965, in the wake of such an epidemic, more than 20,000 infants were born with congenital malformations; there were in addition 30,000 stillbirths. Blood is taken from a vein for testing.

When performed: Whenever there is some question of whether a woman is immune or susceptible to the disease. Eleven states require women obtaining a marriage license to be so tested: California, Colorado, Connecticut, Georgia, Hawaii, Idaho, Indiana, Montana, Nebraska, Rhode Island, and Vermont. The law does not usually require immunization, however, if susceptibility is found. Some states may require rubella testing as a condition of employment; in New York, for example, a woman employee of the State Health Department may be fired if she is found to lack immunity and refuses rubella immunization. Four states—Maryland, New Jersey, North Carolina, and Rhode Island—require the test for all hospital employees. Every woman should be tested prior to pregnancy so that proper immunization can be obtained where indicated; many doctors suggest routine testing of all young girls at puberty. The test is also administered to help distinguish German measles from other, similar diseases such as regular measles (rubeola), exanthem subitum, or other infections that produce a rash as well as drug eruptions. All 50 states now have laws requiring that children be vaccinated for rubella before attending kindergarten, but this alone will not ensure that all women of childbearing age are protected; thus, the screening tests are of vital importance.

Normal values: In this test, a "normal" value is evidence of immunity to the disease; that is, that the disease once had infected the individual.

Abnormal values: Evidence of susceptibility, or no immunity.

Risk factors: Negligible (see general risk factors for blood testing).

Pain/discomfort: Minimal (see general pain/discomfort factors for blood testing).

Cost: From $8 to $27 for a single test; the price depends on the technique used by the laboratory. From $25 to $50 for a series of tests to follow convalescence.

Accuracy and significance: Although the test is claimed to be 80 percent accurate in detecting immunity in those who had a previous German measles infection, it has also been shown to reveal a false positive result in people known to be susceptible. The test is less accurate in detecting immunity in people who were vaccinated against the disease or who contracted it during pregnancy.

RUBEOLA, see *Virus Disease*

RUBIN

The Rubin test is one of several tests performed in cases of infertility. Specifically, it determines whether the fallopian tubes (which carry the ovum, or egg, from the ovary to the uterus) are open or blocked. Carbon dioxide gas is forced into the uterus under pressure; if the tubes are normal (open), the gas is detected in the abdomen. Occasionally, the test procedure itself acts therapeutically to open blocked tubes.

When performed: When disease of the fallopian tubes is suspected; in cases of sterility.

Normal values: Normally, the carbon dioxide passes easily through the tubes into the abdomen.

Abnormal values: Obstruction of the fallopian tubes may occur in endometriosis and infections (particularly following previous delivery or abortion) or following peritoneal inflammation (appendicitis). Occasionally, the patient may have a spasm of the tubes during the test, giving a false-negative result. Therefore, if the test is negative (tubes blocked), a second test should be performed for verification.

Risk factors: Although it is possible to force an excess of air into the abdominal cavity and cause trauma, this happens very rarely.

Pain/discomfort: After the air is inserted, there is an uncomfortable feeling of fullness in the abdomen and occasionally discomfort around the liver. Once the test is completed, there is almost always an aching sensation in the shoulder resulting from the pressure of gas pushing up against the diaphragm. Actually, this discomfort indicates the fallopian tubes are open.

Cost: From $25 to $50; usually performed in the doctor's office.

Accuracy and significance: The test is quite significant in revealing whether a woman's fallopian tubes are open or blocked. Should air escape from the apparatus during the test, there could be a false-negative result, giving the impression of blockage; thus, about 75 percent accurate.

RUMPEL-LEEDE, see *Capillary Fragility*

S

SAAST, see *Alcoholism*

SABIN-FELDMAN DYE, see *Toxoplasmosis*

SACCADIC VELOCITY, see *Caloric*

SACCHARIN, see *Smell Function*

SALICYLATES

A salicylate is any salt of salicylic acid (prepared synthetically or obtained from wintergreen leaves or the bark of white birch). Aspirin is one of the most common sources of salicylates, as are many other drugs used to minimize pain. Taking an excessive amount causes poisoning. Aspirin is often added to chickenfeed to ease the pain and discomfort of chickens that are bred in crowded conditions. Aspirin also seems to increase the amount of fat in chickens. Eating large quantities of chicken that have been fed aspirin can increase the blood salicylate level. Blood is taken from a vein for testing. Urine may be tested for screening to consider salicylate poisoning.

When performed: When patients are taking large doses of salicylates for arthritis or rheumatic fever; in cases of suspected accidental aspirin poisoning in children; in coma.

Normal values: Normally, there are no salicylates in the blood or urine. Therapeutic levels of salicylates in the blood range from 5 to 12 mg per 100 ml.

Abnormal values: More than 30 mg per 100 ml in the blood is considered toxic. Symptoms of salicylate poisoning include dizziness, nausea, vomiting, tinnitus (ringing in the ears), restlessness, disorientation, rapid breathing, shock, and coma. Salicylate poisoning can also cause abnormally low blood sugar levels.

Risk factors: Negligible (see general risk factors for blood testing).

Pain/discomfort: Minimal (see general pain/discomfort factors for blood testing).

Cost: From $8 to $15 whether tested in blood or urine.

Accuracy and significance: Blood measurements are more specific and are 90 percent accurate; they are better than urine measurements. Although the measurement of salicylate in the blood is quite accurate, there is no significant level that indicates salicylate poisoning. Death has occurred when only very low salicylate levels have been detected in some patients; others with extremely high toxic levels exhibit no symptoms of salicylate poisoning.

SALINE WET MOUNT, see *Wet Mount*

SALIVARY GLAND SCANNING, see *Nuclear Scanning*

SALMONELLOSIS, see *Agglutination*

SALPINGOGRAPHY, see *Radiography*

SALT LOADING, see *Aldosterone*

SARALASIN INFUSION, see *Renin*

SARCOIDOSIS, see *Kveim*

SART, see *Gastroesophageal Reflux*

SAXENA, see *Pregnancy*

SCABIES INFESTATION

Scabies is a dermatological condition caused by a biting, burrowing mite. The incidence of scabies is increasing greatly, even among people who keep themselves fastidiously clean. A skin test in which extracts of the mite are injected is the primary method of differentiating between scabies and other dermatological conditions. Another test is to paint the skin with fluorescein dye and then shine ultraviolet light over the area; the burrowing tunnels then fluoresce. Serum immunoglobulin A is reduced in patients with scabies (see **Immunoglobulin).**

When performed: To differentiate certain rash-causing itching patterns from syphilis or lice infestations; whenever venereal disease is suspected; when a woman has a dermatitis of the nipples or a man has a rash over his scrotum; when a patient has a localized rash over the buttocks.

Normal values: There should be no evidence of the mite on direct examination and no reaction to the skin test.

Abnormal values: A positive skin test reaction (a hard, red nodule forms) confirms the diagnosis of scabies.

Risk factors: Negligible.

Pain/discomfort: Children often find the injection of the solution under the skin uncomfortable.

Cost: The skin test is $20. Customarily, there is no charge for ultraviolet light examination.

Accuracy and significance: The skin test is 80 percent accurate, but direct examination of the skin showing the tunneling is generally sufficient.

SCANNING, see *Nuclear Scanning; Ultrasound*

SCARLET FEVER, see *Skin Reaction*

SCHICK, see *Skin Reaction*

SCHILLER

In gynecological examinations, many doctors "paint" the cervix (entrance to the uterus) with an iodine solution in order to isolate any suspected area of disease. Normal cells contain glycogen (starch), which iodine will stain. Although the Schiller test is not a specific diagnostic tool, it does point out suspicious areas for further study. Before the cervix is stained, the cervical mucus (discharge) is also examined for threadiness (called spinnbarkeit). The time it takes for the thready components of the mucus to be stretched indicates the phase of the menstrual cycle (see **Tackmeter**).

When performed: During a routine gynecological examination; whenever the patient has a persistent vaginal discharge or bleeding or a vaginal infection that is not easily cured.

Normal values: After being painted with iodine, the cervix should show a uniform brown (sometimes slightly bluish brown) color.

Abnormal values: Any area of the cervix that does not take the stain and remains white or pink indicates a lack of normal starch-containing cells (most commonly from infection, cancer, or injury) and a bit of the unstained tissue should then be taken for **Biopsy**. False-positive tests (lack of staining without subsequent disease) occur in one out of three patients, often due to infected or unestrogenated cells.

Risk factors: Negligible, unless the patient is allergic to iodine, in which case there can be irritation.

Pain/discomfort: Usually minimal, if the doctor exercises care. Should the iodine solution touch the vagina's outer edge or other sensitive parts, there can be severe stinging or burning.

Cost: There is usually no charge, as the test is part of a routine gynecological examination.

Accuracy and significance: The Schiller treatment of the cervix is not a specific test, yet it is highly significant, as it directs a doctor's attention to potential disease conditions; it is considered to be about 70 percent accurate.

SCHILLING (Vitamin B_{12})

Vitamin B_{12} (cobalamin) is essential to several bodily functions (tissue growth, nervous system functioning, and red blood cell production). Anemia is sometimes caused by a deficiency of vitamin B_{12} in the diet, but the more common cause is a difficulty in absorbing vitamin B_{12} through the intestine. In pernicious anemia, the "intrinsic factor" (a protein in gastric secretion) does not join with the vitamin B_{12} ingested in the diet; as a result, the vitamin cannot be absorbed through the intestine into the blood.

In the Schilling test, the patient fasts for 8 to 12 hours and is then given radioactive vitamin B_{12} (cyanocobalamin) orally, followed by an intramuscluar injection of nonradioactive vitamin B_{12} in sufficient amount to saturate the body with the vitamin. The amount of radioactive B_{12} that is absorbed and excreted is measured. All the urine over a 24-hour period is collected. Vitamin B_{12}, the "intrinsic factor," and antibodies to the "intrinsic factor" can also be measured directly from blood serum. These tests, although more accurate, are very expensive.

Recent research indicates that pernicious anemia is an autoimmune disease (see **Immunology**), and intrinsic factor–blocking antibodies have been found in the blood of patients with that disease. Testing for these antibodies helps diagnose pernicious anemia where there is some doubt as to the cause of an anemia.

When performed: When the patient has symptoms of weakness and pallor; to aid in the diagnosis of certain anemias; following gastrectomy (surgical removal of the stomach).

Normal values: The total amount of radioactive vitamin B_{12} excreted in the urine is compared with the amount that was given to the patient. It should be from 8 percent to 40 percent, depending on the original amount administered and particular laboratory methods.

Abnormal values: Values between 2 percent and 8 percent are considered borderline. Values of less than 2 percent are seen in malabsorption of vitamin B_{12}, which can cause pernicious anemia and other megaloblastic anemias (characterized by oversized, immature red blood cells). Deficiency of vitamin B_{12} follows gastrectomy. It is also seen with alcoholism and intestinal infections, in people on certain vegetarian diets, in patients taking oral contraceptives or anticonvulsants, and in old age.

Risk factors: Negligible (see general risk factors for blood testing).

Pain/discomfort: Minimal (see general pain/discomfort factors for blood testing).

Cost: Usually $20 to $60; $20 for simple blood vitamin B_{12} measurements. When radioactive B_{12} is used, the fee can be $100 to $200. Generally, **Folates** are tested for at the same time, and there is an additional fee of $20. The intrinsic factor test runs $30 to $40.

Accuracy and significance: While the test is an 80 percent accurate aid in determining the specific cause of an anemia, many patients with pernicious anemia still show normal values. Unless the test is meticulously performed, it is possible to miss a vitamin B_{12} deficiency. The most significant test to help diagnose megaloblastic anemia is a **Bone Marrow** study.

Note: Because this test can show a normal response even in the presence of cobalamine deficiency, a variation of the test reported twenty years ago was finally accepted in 1985. The chemical deoxyuridine acts to block out those factors that can cause a false-negative test result; thus, the deoxyuridine suppression test makes the Schilling test more accurate. An even newer test of vitamin B_{12} deficiency is called the intrinsic factor–blocking antibody assay. If these antibodies are present, it allows a diagnosis of pernicious anemia. No radioactive B_{12}, injections, or urine collections are needed.

SCHIOTZ, see *Tonometry*

SCHIRMER'S

Schirmer's test measures whether the eye produces enough tears to keep it sufficiently moist. Usually, a drop of anesthetic is placed in the eye and then a thin strip of filter paper is placed in the conjunctival sac (just inside the lower lid). The eyes are kept closed for five minutes; the paper is then removed and examined for tears (moisture). Tears normally come from lacrimal glands located in the upper outer corner of the eye and occasionally from the upper inner area. They empty into a tiny duct at the innermost corner of the eye and drain into the nose area. The tears are examined not only for their quantity but also for their **Lysozyme** content. The latter is a particular diagnostic test for Sjögren's syndrome (dry eyes, dry mouth, and rheumatoid arthritis).

Fluorescein Eye Stain is sometimes used to measure tearing; the fluorescein dye should disappear into the nasal duct within two minutes and be seen in the nasal cavity.

When performed: Whenever a patient complains of "dry eye" (most often when wearing contact lenses); whenever the eye waters constantly.

Normal values: The filter paper resting inside the eyelid should show almost half an inch of moisture after five minutes.

Abnormal values: The filter paper fails to show sufficient moisture with certain eye infections (such as conjunctivitis), vitamin A deficiency, and Sjögren's syndrome (now considered an autoimmune disease found primarily in women past the menopause). The failure of tears to leave the eye can come from infection and blockage of the nasolacrimal duct (this condition may also be congenital and is easily treated by dilating the tear duct with a thin metal probe).

Risk factors: Negligible.

Pain/discomfort: Some people find the paper applied to the eye irritating.

Cost: There is usually no charge when performed as part of a routine eye examination. If lysozyme is measured in the tears, there is often an additional charge of $30 to $40.

Accuracy and significance: The test is 80 percent accurate to indicate the amount of tear production. In itself, however, it is only significant in its ability to suggest conditions that cause dry eye.

SCHISTOSOMIASIS, see *Agglutination; Parasite*

SCHIZOPHRENIA, see *Catecholamines*

SCHLICHTER, see *Culture*

SCHWABACH, see *Tuning Fork*

SCINTILLATION, see *Nuclear Scanning*

SCINTOGRAPHY, see *Nuclear Scanning*

SCOTCH TAPE, see *Feces Examination*

SCOTOMA, see *Visual Field*

SCREENING URINE EXAMINATION, see *Urine Examination*

SCROTAL SCAN, see *Nuclear Scanning*

SECRETIN STIMULATION, see *Pancreas Function*

SEDIMENTATION RATE (ESR)

The erythrocyte sedimentation rate, called "sed rate" by most physicians, is a measure in millimeters (mm) of how far the red blood cells (erythroctyes) cling together, fall, and settle toward the bottom of a specially marked test tube in an hour's time. The cells group together and then form a sediment, as mud does in still water. Essentially, it is an indication of any infectious process going on in the body. The various methods of performing the ESR are labeled according to the different sizes and shapes of tubes (Cutler, Westergren, Wintrobe) in which whole blood, usually taken from a vein, is placed.

When performed: With any suspected infection or tissue damage; to detect if an unsuspected disease is present; to follow the progress of disease (an increased ESR that begins to return to normal is considered to be a good prognostic sign).

Normal values: Normal values differ slightly depending on the tubes used: Cutler, 2 to 10 mm fall in one hour; Wintrobe, 0 to 20 mm fall in one hour; Westergren, 1 to 12 mm fall in one hour. In general, a fall of up to 10 mm in one hour in men is considered normal; in women and elderly people, rates of up to 20 mm in one hour are still within normal range.

Abnormal values: The ESR is increased (falls faster) with certain infections (not with typhoid fever or with most virus diseases); tissue damage, as with a heart attack (not with angina); rheumatic fever; rheumatoid arthritis (not degenerative arthritis); kidney disease; thyroid disease; and some other hormone disorders, some cancers, and many connective tissue diseases or autoimmune conditions. It is also increased after poisoning, during menstruation, and in pregnancy.

Risk factors: Negligible (see general risk factors for blood testing).

Pain/discomfort: Minimal (see general pain/discomfort factors for blood testing).

Cost: From $3 to $24.

Accuracy and significance: Because the test shows abnormal values in such a wide range of conditions, it is basically a screening device that has no intrinsic accuracy rate; it suggests the possibility of an illness when it is elevated. Although the test is still performed in doctors' offices, it has been replaced in most laboratories by various enzyme measurements (ALT, AST, CPK, LDH) as part of **Comprehensive Multiple Test Screening** panels. (Also see **C-Reactive protein.**)

Note: If the sedimentation rate results do not seem to agree with the doctor's clinical impression (tentative diagnosis), the zeta sedimentation ratio may be employed. Here, the **Red Blood Cells** are centrifuged (as opposed to letting them fall by gravity) to measure their rate of descent. This version of the test is supposed to correct the sedimentation rate for the effect of any anemia that might be present. It is reported as a percentage figure and, in general, should be less than 60 percent to be normal.

SEIDEL, see *Tonometry*

SELENIUM

Selenium is a trace mineral (required by the body in very minute amounts) and is essential for heart and other muscle function; it acts as a coenzyme (necessary for certain enzyme activity). It also seems to act on, and with, vitamin E as a protective antioxidant (prevents cell destruction) in the body. Selenium is found particularly in onions, garlic, meats, eggs, seafood (especially shellfish), leafy green vegetables, and most grains; the amount varies with the amount of selenium in the soil. No more than 150 mcg of selenium is needed in the daily diet, and if 1,500 mcg or more are eaten on a regular basis, toxic symptoms may develop. Whole blood taken from a vein may be tested, but more often, selenium is measured in the urine. Recently, selenium measurements have been made in hair (see **Hair Analysis**) and toenail clippings; the results are reported to be as reliable as blood studies for epidemiological (survey) purposes. If selenium-containing shampoos are used, hair samples are useless.

When performed: With hair loss or brittle fingernails; when there is unusual irritability that cannot be explained; with certain liver diseases; when amyotrophic lateral sclerosis (degeneration of part of the spinal cord, causing paralysis) is suspected; in people whose occupation requires contact with certain electronic equipment containing selenium.

Normal values: Selenium levels of up to 0.2 mg per 100 ml of blood and 0.1 mg per liter of urine are considered normal.

Abnormal values: Decreased values are found in people with heart disease, in early aging, and in some cases of muscular dystrophy. Increased values are found in patients with liver disease, fatigue, irritability, and excessive, early hair loss. Markedly increased amounts have been found in patients with amyotrophic lateral sclerosis.

Risk factors: Negligible (see general risk factors for blood testing).

Pain/discomfort: Minimal (see general pain/discomfort factors for blood testing).

Cost: From $60 to 75 whether tested in blood or urine.

Accuracy and significance: A 70 percent accurate test, the significance of which is not completely understood at this time. It can be valuable in testing people whose occupations expose them to the possibility of selenium accumulation in the body.

SELF-ADMINISTERED ALCOHOLISM SCREENING, see *Alcoholism*

SEMEN

The semen, seminal fluid, or ejaculate is the single most important test of testicle function and fertility. (Fertility has nothing to do with potency.) In barren marriages, 30 percent of the husbands are infertile; more than half of these men can be helped to become fertile. Besides sperm (spermatozoa), normal semen contains spermatocytes, Sertoli cells, sperm nutrients, red and white blood cells, macrophages, lecithin crystals, and secretions from the prostate as well as other glands (fructose, citric acid, proteins, prostaglandins, and hormones).

Semen is usually examined for volume, viscosity (thickness), **pH** (acidity), motility (movement: whether sluggish or quick), morphology (form and structure of sperm), amount of sperm (sperm count), and fructose level (deficient fructose levels in semen seem to parallel testicular hormone, or androgen, deficiency).

It takes approximately 10 weeks for sperm to form, so that the sperm sample analyzed is actually indicative of bodily functioning over the preceding 10 weeks. Thus, a single examination that indicates irregularities cannot be considered valid. If any abnormality is noted, at least three more specimens should be examined for verification.

After sexual abstinence for four to six days, the patient collects a specimen either by masturbation or by coitus interruptus. Masturbation is preferable so that none of the sample is lost. Semen should be examined immediately, but no later than two hours after collection. The one exception is the postcoital (after-intercourse) test, where, because of religious convictions or extreme embarrassment, the woman reports to her doctor as soon as possible after normal intercourse and the specimen is removed from the vagina.

The Huhner test is an examination of the sperm in the semen, which is taken from the vagina after intercourse to determine if the sperm can penetrate the cervical mucus to fertilize the egg.

The most recent test to evaluate male fertility is called the sperm penetration assay (SPA). It is based on the ability of human sperm to penetrate the ova (egg) of a hamster; the test can be performed in the laboratory. Because hamster eggs are used, and because the egg first has its enveloping layer (called the zona pellucida) removed, the test is also referred to as the hamster zona-free ovum test (HZFO). In essence, the test shows the ability of a man's sperm to survive all the many factors required to cause pregnancy. The sperm of infertile men usually cannot penetrate the hamster's egg, and where less than 20 percent of the sperm penetrate, it is considered a sign of subfertility. Many doctors now consider this test far more accurate than semen fluid analysis.

Yet another way of testing the degree of sperm penetration is to note how far the man's sperm can travel through bovine cervical mucus (as a substitute for the man's partner's cervical mucus); failure to migrate to a specified distance within 90 minutes is considered to be diagnostic of sterility.

A different cause of infertility is the presence of sperm antibodies in the semen, which can be found by testing the blood of men (antibodies to sperm have also been found in the blood of women). Some consider these to be autoantibodies (see **Immunology**) made by the body as a yet unexplained defense reaction to sperm, but they are also found in association with testicle disease as well as with unexplained infertility. Several newer tests allow for the direct examination of sperm for antibodies (as opposed to blood serum) and can be performed on cervical and vaginal fluids, as well; the tests take only 30 minutes. They are thought to be more accurate than blood testing, which must be repeated several times.

Note: It is now possible to test for semen in or on clothing and bedding related to rape, and new tests allow authorities to determine the blood group and type of a man's semen (saliva and bloodstains can also be tested for genetic marker typing, as this form of identification is called). Semen contains three different genetic markers; in addition to blood groupings, there are two enzyme markers that can help identify an accused assailant (see **Acid Phosphatase**).

When performed: As a test of gonadal function; in suspected infertility; after vasectomy to measure success of the surgery; when rape is suspected.

Normal values:

Volume: The normal ejaculation is 2.5 to 5 ml of seminal fluid (about one teaspoon). A low-volume ejaculation (1 ml) may still be normal and may contain a high sperm count.

Viscosity: Semen seems to gel just after ejection but normally liquefies in 15 to 30 minutes. It should not be examined until it has liquefied.

pH: Normally, the pH level ranges between 7.2 and 8.0 (slightly alkaline).

Motility: At least 70 percent to 90 percent of normal sperm are motile (active) in the first hour after ejection, and 50 percent should still be motile up to 10 hours after ejection.

Morphology: In a sample, 80 percent to 90 percent of sperm should appear to have a normal form. The normal sperm has head, neck, and tail. Slight variations in the size and shape of the head (tiny, large, round, elongated, and double heads) may be normal.

Sperm count: The normal semen sample contains 60 to 120 million sperm per ml. Patients who have more are not considered more fertile than others.

Fructose level: Normal fructose is 315 mg per 100 ml.

Abnormal values:

Volume: A low volume of semen (less than 2.5 ml) may be, but is not always, associated with fertility problems unless accompanied by a low sperm count. An exceptionally high volume (more than 5 ml) can also be an indication of infertility.

Viscosity: Failure of the semen to liquefy from its gel form after 15 to 30 minutes may be associated with infertility.

Motility: Immobile or sluggish sperm are abnormal and usually indicate infertility.

Morphology: Variation from the normal size and shape in more than 20 percent of sperm is indicative of infertility problems. The different ways the sperm takes up stain are significant. Frequency of senile or juvenile forms, diffuse staining, or lack of staining are abnormal variations. Usually, the fewer the sperm, the more abnormal forms that are seen.

Sperm count: A sperm count below 60 million per ml is considered abnormal. Organic disease of the genitals (mumps, prostatitis, occlusion of ducts), endocrine or other systemic disease, spinal cord injury, hypopituitarism, and even a form of anxiety (anorexia nervosa) can cause low or no sperm count.

Rape test: When there is a question of sexual intercourse, an examination for semen (especially sperm) may be performed. The presence and activity of sperm taken from the vagina may indicate the approximate time intercourse took place. If no sperm are found, suspected semen and/or vaginal fluid are sometimes examined for prostatic **Acid Phosphatase,** the presence of which usually indicates intercourse. Sperm can live for up to six days after intercourse within the cervix portion of the uterus, but evidence of sperm has been found as long as four months after a rape-murder.

Abnormal sperm have been found in men who are heavy cigarette smokers with no evidence of other testicle dysfunction.

Risk factors: None.

Pain/discomfort: The collection of sperm can embarrass some patients.

Cost: The most common test is for sperm motility; when performed alone, the cost is $8 to $12. A complete semen analysis is $20 to $35. Fructose testing runs from $70 to $90.

Accuracy and significance: Most semen testing is totally objective and hence 85 to 95 percent accurate. However, men with completely normal values can still be infertile, and men with some abnormal values can still father a child. The significance of the test, after several examinations at different times, is that when a cause for infertility is found, it can be corrected in at least half the men with testicle dysfunction.

Note: A new, computer-assisted analysis system called CellSoft-CASA now allows much more accurate measurements of the motility, velocity, and linearity of forward motion of the sperm cell that can be of great value in diagnosing male infertility. Using multiple-exposure photography through the microscope, it is also less expensive than extensive professional direct observations.

SEMEN GLYCOPROTEIN p30, see *Acid Phosphatase*

SEMINAL FLUID, see *Semen*

SENILITY, see *Cognitive Capacity Screening*

SENSITIVITY, see *Culture*

SENSORY

Many different tests measure a patient's ability to perceive various sensations (pain, a light touch, temperature differences, vibrations, etc.). Discovering the exact locations where sensations are decreased (or at times increased) can help indicate the area in the nerves or spinal cord where disease originates. In addition, when patients complain of unusual sensations (burning, tingling, pins and needles), tests must be performed to isolate the area involved.

In most sensory tests, the patient is asked to keep his eyes closed so that the sensitivity of the skin area being tested can be measured directly. Various objects (cotton, pins, tubes) are touched to or pressed on the skin to elicit a response. Sensory ability is affected by a great many conditions (injuries, tumors, drugs, poor nutrition, infection, and inherited diseases).

When performed: Whenever nerve, muscle, spinal cord, or brain disease is suspected; when patients complain of an inability to feel normal sensations or experience unusual sensations.

Normal values: A patient should be able to locate and discriminate between a pinprick on the skin, a touch with a piece of cotton, pressure from the doctor's hand, tubes containing warm and cold water applied to the skin, and a vibrating **Tuning Fork** touched to any bone area. The patient should be able to tell if a toe is being pushed up or bent down as well as which fingers and toes are being touched. These feelings should be equal on both sides of the body.

More discriminating types of sensory tests measure the ability of the brain to interpret sensation. For example, the skin may be touched at two points at the same time; normally, a patient can describe the touching and how far apart the points are. Normal patients can also distinguish different materials that touch them (cotton versus silk), specific shapes, and letters or numbers that the doctor outlines with a finger on the palm of their hand or other skin area.

Abnormal values: Although any absence or diminution of sensory ability usually indicates disease, the area affected must always correspond to a specific nerve distribution, called a dermatome. For example, if the patient complains of loss of feeling in the knee area, a definite area above, below, and alongside the knee should also be affected. If the loss of feeling does not correspond to the anatomical distribution of the nerve, other causes for the complaint (hysteria, attempting to mislead the physician, etc.) must be considered.

Risk factors: None.

Pain/discomfort: None.

Cost: There is usually no charge for the sensory tests, which are part of a routine physical examination.

Accuracy and significance: The tests are of value in diagnosing the existence of nerve and spinal cord disease, but they are not sufficiently precise to distinguish between the possible causes of an illness. They are particularly significant in detecting malingerers.

SEQUENTIAL MULTIPLE ANALYZER, see *Comprehensive Multiple Test Screening*

SEQUENTIAL TESTS OF EDUCATIONAL PROCESS, see *Learning Disability*

SEROLOGICAL, see *Agglutination; Complement Fixation*

SEROTONIN (5-HIAA, HIAA)

Serotonin (hydroxytryptamine) is manufactured in the blood from tryptophan (one of the amino acids in the protein we eat) and is then metabolized into 5-hydroxyindolacetic acid (HIAA), a compound that can be tested for in the urine. Serotonin acts to transmit nerve impulses and also constricts blood vessels. An excess of serotonin seems to be implicated in both flushing and blueness of the skin, rapid heartbeat, diarrhea, precipitation of asthma attacks, and increased blood clotting (it is also found in the platelets). Exposure to the sun seems to increase serotonin production. Blood from a vein may be tested for serotonin, but it is more common to test a 24-hour urine sample for HIAA. Recently, the test has been performed on mentally retarded patients (usually, those whose retardation resulted from inherited developmental disabilities) and on patients with **Depression.**

In 1985, it was reported that serotonin antibodies (see **Agglutination**) were found in more than half of a group of children with autism; none were found in normal children. It has been postulated that higher-than-normal levels of serotonin can be a diagnostic lead to that abnormal behavioral condition and that the test finding could also be evidence that autism is either an autoimmune disease (see **Immunology**) or a marker for a genetic-type problem (see **Genetic Disorder Screening).**

When performed: Primarily when a carcinoid tumor (usually in the intestinal tract) is suspected; when there is unexplained cyanosis (bluish color to the skin) and an enlarged liver; on patients with inherited metabolic deficiencies; on mentally ill patients; and as a means of detecting the possibility of suicide.

Normal values: Serotonin in whole blood ranges from 0.05 to 0.20 mcg per ml. HIAA in urine ranges from 2 to 8 mg per 24-hour sample.

Abnormal values: With a carcinoid tumor (called an argentaffinoma), values of HIAA may go up to 1,000 mg per 24-hour urine specimen. Certain tranquilizers, antidepressant drugs, and foods that contain serotonin (such as avocados, bananas, pineapples, and eggplants) may cause elevated levels. Decreased serotonin levels are found in patients with Down's syndrome and in those with depression who are not being treated with lithium.

Risk factors: Negligible (see general risk factors for blood testing).

Pain/discomfort: Minimal (see general pain/discomfort factors for blood testing).

Cost: Measurements of blood serotonin range from $60 to $90. Urine testing is $20 to $40.

Accuracy and significance: The test is 90 percent accurate and is particularly significant in helping to diagnose a carcinoid tumor; it is equally important in helping to eliminate this tumor from diagnostic considerations. The accuracy of the test in mental retardation and mental illness is still under study.

SEROTONIN ANTIBODIES, see *Serotonin*

SERUM ANGIOTENSIN-CONVERTING ENZYME, see *Kveim*

SERUM BACTERICIDAL ACTIVITY, see *Culture*

SERUM COMPLEMENT, see *Complement*

SERUM ELECTROPHORESIS, see *Albumin/Globulin*

SERUM GLUTAMIC OXALACETIC TRANSAMINASE, see *Aspartate Aminotransferase*

SERUM HEPATITIS, see *Hepatitis*

SERUM PROTEINS, see *Albumin/Globulin*

SERUM TRYPSINLIKE IMMUNOREACTIVITY, see *Pancreas Function*

SET, see *Cognitive Capacity Screening*

SEVENTEEN KETOSTEROIDS (17-KS), see *Cortisol*

SEX CHROMATIN, see *Chromosome Analysis*

SEX DETERMINATION, see *Amniocentesis; Testis Function*

SEXUAL IDENTITY, see *Chromosome Analysis*

SEXUALLY TRANSMITTED DISEASES, see *Acquired Immunodeficiency Syndrome; Agglutination; Chlamydia Identification; Complement Fixation; Cytomegalovirus; Frei; Gonorrhea; Hepatitis; Herpes; Parasite; Scabies; Syphilis; TORCH*

SEXUAL POTENCY, see *Impotence*

SGOT, see *Aspartate Aminotransferase*

SGPT, see *Aspartate Aminotransferase*

SH, see *Hepatitis*

SHAKE, see *Pregnancy*

SHINGLES, see *Herpes*

SHK-STI SYSTEM, see *Electrocardiogram*

SIA, see *Macroglobulin*

SIADH, see *Vasopressin*

SIALOANGIOGRAPHY, see *Radiography*

SICKLE CELL, see *Red Blood Cell*

SICKLE-CELL HEMOGLOBIN (HEMOGLOBIN S), see *Hemoglobin*

SICKLEDEX, see *Hemoglobin*

SICKLE-I.D. SYSTEM, see *Hemoglobin*

SICKLEQUICK, see *Hemoglobin*

SIDEROCYTE STAIN, see *Red Blood Cell*

SIGMOIDOSCOPY, see *Endoscopy*

SINGLE-BEAM PHOTON ABSORPTIOMETRY, see *Bone Mineral Density Analysis*

SINGLE-PHOTON EMISSION COMPUTED TOMOGRAPHY, see *Computerized Tomography*

SINUS CULTURE, see *Culture*

SINUS X-RAYS, see *Radiography*

SJÖGREN'S SYNDROME, see *Schirmer's*

SKINFOLD THICKNESS, see *Anthropometric Measurements*

SKIN GRAFT, see *HLA*

SKIN REACTION

Many diagnostic tests measure the allergic sensitivity of the skin as an indication of either susceptibility to or previous contact with disease-producing substances. Common skin reaction tests (also called intracutaneous, intradermal, or subcutaneous tests) include the tuberculin or Mantoux test, the Tine test (application of tuberculin-sensitive substance to the surface of the skin), the Pirquet test, and the purified protein derivative (PPD), which is similar to the tuberculin test. A new modification of the tuberculin test uses the Tine surface application with PPD rather than the traditional tuberculin substance. There is the Schick test for susceptibility to diphtheria; the Dick test for sensitivity to the Streptococcus toxin (scarlet fever); specific tests for tularemia, mumps, aspergillus, candida, tricophyton, coccidioidomycosis, histoplasmosis, and trichinosis; and the various tests that measure allergic sensitivity to foods and pollens.

About 0.1 ml (much less than a drop) of the testing material, usually a treated antigen, is injected just under the top layer of the skin, producing a small, whitish bump. (If no bump is raised, the material has been injected too deeply.) The usual sites are the inner hairless portion of the lower arm and the back, but the injection can be made anywhere on the body. If the testing substance is mixed in a solution that in itself could cause an allergy, the mixing solution alone—without the testing element—is injected in the opposite arm as a control measure. Sometimes, a tiny bandage soaked in the testing solution is placed on the arm and covered with adhesive tape; this is called a patch test. The newest test for allergies is called the radioimmunosorbent assay test (see **RAST**).

It should be noted that the Food and Drug Administration considers a number of commonly performed skin tests to be ineffective—specifically, those to test for trichinosis, histoplasmosis, lymphogranuloma, diphtheria, and the "old tuberculin" test for tuberculosis (the PPD is accepted by the FDA). The federal government is trying to remove the substances used in these tests from the market.

Skin reaction testing is also used to assess the state of a patient's immunity (how well an individual can ward off an infection or possible cancer; see **Acquired Immunodeficiency Syndrome, Agglutination, Immunoglobulin,** and **Immunology**). When antigens of several diseases are injected under the skin, more than 95 percent of all people will show at least one positive skin reaction (see "Abnormal Values," below) within 48 hours. The reaction is a reflection of antibodies from a previous exposure to the bacteria, fungus, etc., as expressed by the presence of T-cells (see **Lymphocyte Typing**) attracted to the antigen injection as an immunological response. Failure of the skin to show a reaction, or a less-than-usual reaction that does not appear for 72 hours or more, is considered an indication of immune deficiency and is called anergy or cutaneous anergy. This form of delayed or absent hypersensitivity also occurs in **Malnutrition,** and skin reaction testing is frequently used on patients after surgery as a means of monitoring nutritional needs.

When it comes to skin testing for tuberculosis, many doctors now perform the two-step tuberculin technique. If the first skin test, with regular-strength reagent, is negative or only shows a very weak reaction, a second test with a stronger dose of the reagent is administered. Such testing is more commonly performed in the southeastern part of the United States, where certain bacteria, different from those that cause tuberculosis, can provoke false-positive reactions. It is also used with elderly patients, who sometimes need a stronger solution to induce a positive reaction, and on medical personnel, who are more apt to be, or have been, exposed to patients with the disease.

Note: Many health organizations that test for tuberculosis—because of the increased opportunity for exposure—will only accept the Mantoux test (where the test substance is actually injected under the skin) and not one of the multiple-pressure tests such as the Tine because of the inability to standardize the application and amount of the test substance.

When performed: When allergy is suspected; to diagnose certain specific infections; in dermatological conditions that are difficult to diagnose; to measure immunological sensitivity. In 1985, the County of Los Angeles, California, required that all kindergarten pupils, as well as students in all other grades entering a California school for the first time, have a tuberculin skin test or be excluded from attending classes (certain personal beliefs and medical contraindications would be excepted).

Normal values: There are really no normal values for skin tests, since positive responses do not always indicate the presence of disease. For example, a person who was once exposed to tuberculosis but who has no infectious activity whatsoever may still have a positive skin reaction. A person who has had diphtheria may have lost his immunity and thus have a positive reaction. With allergy tests, it is not unusual for the skin to react positively to certain substances that have no direct effect on the nose or lungs and that therefore may not be causing allergic disease in other parts of the body.

Abnormal values: Since a positive test may not necessarily be abnormal, any positive reaction must be interpreted in light of a patient's medical history and physical findings. A reaction is positive when the site of the injected material turns red and/or a raised bump (wheal) at least ¼ inch in diameter can be felt. The reaction generally appears 24 to 72 hours after the injection but may last for several days.

Risk factors: Although mostly negligible (see general risk factors for catheter and needle insertion), the risk of an infection (e.g., AIDS, hepatitis) must be reiterated. Doctors who reuse the same syringes (and sometimes needles) for different patients — even with sterilization — can transmit disease this way. An indirect risk is a false-positive reaction. A few years ago, more than 41,000 people were unnecessarily treated for tuberculosis because of a faulty test solution. Any positive skin reaction should be confirmed by a second test using a different test solution.

Pain/discomfort: Minimal (see general pain/discomfort factors for catheter and needle insertion).

Cost: The tests are generally performed in a doctor's office and range from $5 to $10 per test. Allergy testing may require scores of skin tests and can range from $100 to $200. Skin tests for unusual infectious diseases are more often performed in a public health laboratory, where the testing may be free, or there may be a charge of $5 to $20. Hospitals average $27 for a single skin test.

Some doctors feel that skin reaction tests for brucellosis, cat-scratch disease, certain fungus infections, lymphogranuloma venereum, mumps, psittacosis, and trichinosis are so ineffective that many health insurance plans and government-sponsored medical care programs will not reimburse the doctor or patient for the test.

Accuracy and significance: Although the efficacy of many skin tests is questionable, they can help to eliminate certain disease possibilities. The Tine test is probably the most commonly used screening test for tuberculosis, but it gives false-negative as well as false-positive results. The PPD test, given by injection just under the skin, is the most accurate, although it is reported that up to 30 percent of patients with known tuberculosis will have a negative tuberculin skin test. Once a patient has been adequately treated for tuberculosis, a positive tuberculin skin test may become negative. However, it should be emphasized that a positive tuberculin skin test does not necessarily mean the existence of active tuberculosis. Recent studies in Sweden and other countries have shown the Schick test as a poor predictor of diphtheria immunity; it is believed that previous tetanus vaccinations and other factors can cause false Schick results.

Many doctors do not consider the skin reaction tests for food allergies of value; too often, the tests cannot be judged significant, as there are many false-positive reactions to food testing. Allergy specialists acknowledge that there are many variables that can affect the accuracy of skin testing for hay fever, asthma, and other sensitivity illnesses. For instance, the particular area of the body on which the test is performed can affect the results; different parts of the arm react to the testing material in different degrees, and the skin on certain parts of the back can prove twice as reactive as the skin on the arms. Then, too, the time of day can alter a skin test result; for some people tests performed in the morning are three times as reactive as those performed in the afternoon; others have a totally opposite reaction response. If skin reaction tests are placed too near one another on the body, a positive reaction in one site may trigger a false-positive reaction in the adjacent site. False-positive reactions also occur when the same needle is used to inject different test materials without being adequately cleaned between tests. A false-negative result, or lack of reaction, may occur if a patient has been taking an antihistamine drug for up to three days prior to testing (antihistamine drugs do not seem to interfere with RAST testing), and there are many false-negative results when the testing material is more than one month old. Thus, it is difficult to give skin reaction tests any accuracy rating.

SKIN-SURFACE TOUCH PRINT, see *Fungus*

SLEEP MONITORING

Insomnia or hypersomnia (too much sleeping, as opposed to not enough) are well-known symptoms of many different illnesses, but it is only recently that sleep laboratories have been established to observe patients during their usual sleeping hours. Direct observation of the individual, along with mechanical measurements including the **Electrocardiogram, Electroencephalogram,** electronystagmography (see **Caloric), Electromyography, Pulmonary Function** along with various **Plethysomography** studies of breathing, esophageal pressure studies (see **Gastroesophageal Reflux),** blood gas studies (see **Oxygen, Carbon Dioxide, pH)** to mention only a few; when several or all of these tests are performed at the same time during sleep, they are referred to as polysomnography and may help in uncovering the cause of many sleep disorders, such as nighttime breathing difficulties. An annoying problem such as loud snoring can be the key to an underlying severe heart or lung disease that was previously undetected. Measurements of various hormone levels—especially those related to blood pressure, kidney function, and the **Catecholamines**—may also be performed while the patient is sleeping.

Severe breathing difficulties during sleep are called sleep apnea syndromes. Some doctors feel that they are the cause of, or at least reflect, a great variety of illnesses. Anatomical deformations, such as a deviated septum in the nose, abnormally large tonsils, tongue malformations, and tumors in the upper respiratory tract have been found to cause sleep apnea. Brain and nerve disease may also be responsible for the temporary cessation of breathing during sleep. Sudden death as a consequence of sleep apnea is being reported in medical journals with increasing frequency.

Apnea monitoring—measuring heart and lung activity during sleep—while usually performed in a hospital setting, can now be performed in the home. In particular, it is applied to infants within the first six months of life as a means of preventing sudden infant death syndrome (SIDS), believed by some to be caused by sleep apnea and said to occur in from 1 to 2 out of every 1,000 babies (also see **Botulism).** When an infant has a momentary cessation of his heartbeat and/or breathing, the monitor sets off an alarm so that the parent or person in attendance can restore the vital functions. Apnea monitoring is also available for adults; the most common warning sign of sleep apnea is the sudden onset of loud snoring. Some monitors record the sounds of the snoring; at times, they alone can help make the diagnosis. Common causes of adult apnea include: a respiratory tract obstruction (the tongue folding back on itself), respiratory infections, irregular heart rhythms, brain disorders, hypoglycemia, allergic reactions, and endocrine gland (hormone) disease. Smoking on the mother's part during pregnancy is suspected as a cause of infant apnea. Most often, the devices for apnea monitoring are rented for from $100 to $200 per month (they can be purchased) and used under the strict guidance of a physician specializing in these disorders.

Specialists in sleep disorders describe several stages of sleep. First, there is REM sleep (*REM* stands for "rapid eye movements," where, under closed lids, the eyes shift to and fro sideways quite involuntarily). This is the deepest stage of sleep. Lifting the eyelids will reveal this movement, but it is usually detected by applying electronic sensing devices over the eyes. NREM, or nonrapid eye movements sleep, is how sleep starts; it ranges from very light (easily awakened) to deep in four stages; the eyes do not move during these stages. Measuring the time it takes after falling asleep to the onset of REM sleep can help indicate whether a state of **Depression** is biological (physical, such as from a nervous system chemical imbalance or from drugs) or psychological.

Some other applications of sleep monitoring are helping to distinguish Alzheimer's disease (see **Cognitive Capacity Screening**) from depression; excessive daytime sleeping—as distinguished from narcolepsy, which is an uncontrollable desire to sleep at any time; biological clock problems, where regular day and night activities are difficult to perform; and even **Gastroesophageal Reflux** problems that are limited to nighttime attacks. In some instances, sleep monitoring has helped cure enuresis, or bed-wetting.

Most sleep monitoring takes place at sleep disorder centers. As of April 1985, there were 41 accredited and 56 provisional centers throughout the United States; the locations of these and newly accredited centers can be obtained from the Association of Sleep Disorder Centers, P.O. Box 2604, Del Mar, California 92014. Some of these centers will only test patients referred by a physician, but others do accept self-referral. In addition to attempting to uncover the cause of sleeping difficulties, testing is also performed for problems of staying awake and even for troublesome behavior during sleep.

When performed: When insomnia becomes a disability—with or without the use of sleep-inducing medications, especially if those medications have been used for several months; when obstructive sleep apnea occurs (even when nothing more than snoring becomes an annoyance); when unexplained chest pains occur during the night; when the cause of high blood pressure cannot be determined; when there are breathing difficulties during sleep; when patients sleep too much during the day or cannot keep themselves from dropping off to sleep at inappropriate times.

Normal values: Each of the various monitoring devices that can be utilized at a sleep center shows normal or usual patterns during sleep (the heart rate decreases, blood pressure falls, some hormone activity increases while other hormones decrease in amount, brain waves change their pattern, etc.); specialists in sleep disorders know what to expect and can distinguish normal from abnormal findings.

Abnormal values: Deviations from normal or expected body activities and responses.

Risk factors: While, in general, the risks are negligible (see general risk factors for blood testing and electrical instrument use), there have been reports of deaths and electrical burns involving some home apnea monitors. One cause was a parent erroneously plugging electrode leads into the wrong places (electrical outlets); the monitors themselves were not to blame. Such a risk emphasizes the need to have expert supervision with such devices.

Pain/discomfort: Minimal (see general pain/discomfort factors for blood testing).

Cost: Much depends on where the testing is performed. Some hospitals add an extra fee for the room; others limit the cost to the testing laboratory only. In general, the costs range from $300 to $2,000 a night, depending on how many measurements are made, and sometimes the testing must be repeated for two or three days. Some health insurance plans will pay for sleep monitoring; some allow reimbursement only if the testing is performed at an accredited center.

Accuracy and significance: Sleep monitoring, or polysomnography, while still considered a relatively new field of medical testing (it came of age in 1974), is now accepted as a 70 to 80 percent accurate means of diagnosing, and preventing, several possibly fatal conditions. It is also being applied to help uncover the cause of other conditions such as **Impotence**, enuresis, and hormone disorders in addition to the usual sleep-related problems. In a recent survey of medical experts, about half felt that apnea monitoring was an established procedure, while half felt such testing to be still in the investigational stage or still indeterminate. And so far, no sleep studies have been able to evaluate the relationship between sleep and a patient's well-being.

SLIT LAMP, see *Fluorescein Eye Stain*

SMA, see *Comprehensive Multiple Test Screening*

SMELL FUNCTION

Smell function, or olfactory perception, refers to the ability to distinguish different odors. Before smell function can be determined, nasal airway resistance must be measured—usually with a pneumotachometer, an instrument that electronically indicates how much forced pressure is required to allow air to pass through the nasal cavity as well as the volume of air passed per second. At first, both sides of the nose are measured together; then, each side is measured separately. If resistance is found, a decongestant drug is instilled to shrink the nasal membranes, and the test is repeated.

Once nasal resistance is eliminated, specific, familiar odors are introduced directly into one side of the nose and then the other. The Elsberg apparatus is used to ensure strict control of odor administration time. Tobacco, cloves, coffee, vanilla, and lemon are some characteristic odors used. (Other odors such as ammonia and menthol, while characteristic, should not be used because of their irritability; they will cause a "reaction" in the nose that the patient wrongly interprets as smell.) Smell function is usually tested along with **Taste Function**.

It is believed that most people normally begin to lose their ability to smell after the age of 60; the loss seems to become more severe with increased aging. Men lose the ability to distinguish odors and aromas much more than women. The importance of smell function cannot be overestimated when considering elderly people living alone or with others of the same age; the capacity to notice escaping gas or to identify bad food may be gone to the point of danger.

Another means of seeing how well the mucociliary clearance system functions is called the saccharin test. *Mucociliary* refers to the effectiveness of the tiny hairs (cilia) lining the nose and lungs that help push mucus (phlegm) out of the bronchial and nasal passages (mucus usually increases with infection and other respiratory tract irritations such as asthma, bronchitis, or even smog). With this test, after clearing the nose as well as possible, a tiny amount of saccharin is placed inside each side of the nasal opening (one side at a time). The time it takes for a patient to notice the sweet taste of the saccharin (it should happen within one hour) indicates how well the mucociliary clearance system functions. The test is used to help decide the best treatment for patients with respiratory diseases that do not respond to the usual therapies. Since this test is commonly performed in the doctor's office, as part of the standard nose examination, there usually is no charge.

Although rhinomanometry testing is more than 100 years old, it is only recently that doctors have been routinely performing this test in their offices; in the past, it was usually limited to research studies in medical colleges. By using devices similar to the pneumotachometer, such as a peak nasal inspiratory flow meter, the doctor can confirm the patient's complaint that "my nose is all stuffed up" and can then go on to try and differentiate between an allergy, an infection, or a psychological basis for the nasal obstruction. Rhinomanometry may also aid in locating the exact area of obstruction (front or back part of the nose), and it has also been used to measure the reaction of the nose to irritants (dust, smoke, pollens) as well as the therapeutic effect a particular medicine will have on the affliction.

Rhinomanometry is also used to test for an allergic reaction to fungi that may exist in automobile air conditioners. An increase in nasal airway resistance within 30 minutes after turning on the car's air conditioner could mean one's allergy is exacerbated by that device. At least one out of every five people with known allergies reacts to one of the many molds that can grow in car air-cooling systems.

When performed: Whenever a patient complains of the loss of aroma perception, especially the aroma of foods; whenever brain disease is suspected; following brain injury; in sinus infections; prior to rhinoplasty (plastic surgery on the nose); and to record the degree of deviation of the nasal septum in interfering with smell function.

Normal values: Most patients can perceive the smallest trace of a familiar odor when it is mixed with air and forced directly into the nose.

Abnormal values: Anosomia, or the total absence of smell, most commonly comes from brain tumors or injury to the nerve from the brain to the upper, inner portion of the nose. A loss of smell on only one side of the nose is even more suggestive of brain disease. People who have a disease of one particular area of the brain hallucinate smells but do not actually lose the sense of smell. Naturally, any condition (such as infection) that prevents odors from reaching the area of the nose that detects smell will also cause a false-negative reaction (once the condition is cleared, normal smell returns). A false-abnormal value may result if rhinomanometry is performed at the same time a patient is taking, or has recently used, aspirin; this drug is known to cause nasal congestion in some people.

Risk factors: None.

Pain/discomfort: None.

Cost: There is usually no charge for this test when it is performed in the doctor's office as part of a neurological examination. Some doctors now use a scratch-off set of various odors that costs them $20 and add that charge to the patient's bill.

Accuracy and significance: The test is one of many used to help diagnose brain disease. It is significant as a confirmation of the patient's complaint of loss of the sense of smell, and it helps to identify which side of the brain might be affected. When properly performed, the tests are considered to be 90 percent accurate.

SMOKING, see *Hemoglobin*

SNELLEN, see *Visual Acuity*

SOBRIETY, see *Alcohol*

SODIUM

Sodium is one of the blood electrolytes. (Atoms or ions of **Bicarbonate, Chloride,** and **Potassium** are the other major electrolytes.) It is essential to maintaining the body's normal water metabolism and acid-base balance and to keeping the proper amount of fluids in the bloodstream and in the tissues *around* the cells (potassium holds the water *in* each cell). On a typical diet, the average adult takes in about 6 g (about 0.2 ounce) of sodium a day. The ingestion of excess sodium from salt (sodium chloride), monosodium glutamate (MSG), and the many heavily sodium-based flavor enhancers (such as disodium inosinate and disodium guanylate) found in processed foods can cause water retention (edema), headache, and several other symptoms. A loss of body sodium (from excessive sweating, vomiting, or fever) produces dehydration. Blood is taken from a vein, and the serum is tested. Sodium is also measured in the urine, in **Sweat,** occasionally in the spinal fluid, and in saliva.

When performed: When there is persistent water retention; to help diagnose various hormone disorders; to determine the cause of coma; to confirm suspected cystic fibrosis of the pancreas (it has been suggested that all patients with chronic lung disease be sodium-tested for cystic fibrosis).

Normal values: Normal sodium levels range from 135 to 150 mEq per liter in serum and 40 to 200 mEq per liter in a 24-hour urine sample.

Abnormal values: Increased sodium levels (hypernatremia) are found in some endocrine disorders, especially those of the adrenal glands (Addison's disease); in dehydration; and in patients taking certain hormones and drugs such as steroids, contraceptive pills, and sodium-formulated medicines. Kidney disease, heart disease, and high blood pressure can also cause increased amounts of sodium in the blood. Decreased serum sodium (hyponatremia) can accompany out-of-control diabetes, the use of diuretic drugs, adrenal gland disease (see **Cortisol**), excessive alcohol use, impaired **Pancreas Function,** and kidney diseases and can follow vomiting or diarrhea. It can be a common finding accompanying a great many illnesses but rarely requires any specific treatment.

Urine sodium usually parallels serum sodium, except with dehydration or with certain hormones or drugs that cause the kidney to excrete excessive amounts in the urine.

Sodium is greatly increased in sweat and in saliva (as are chlorides) with cystic fibrosis of the pancreas (mucoviscidosis), a congenital condition that usually expresses itself through repeated lung infections.

Risk factors: Negligible (see general risk factors for blood testing).

Pain/discomfort: Minimal (see general pain/discomfort factors for blood testing).

Cost: From $4 to $25 for blood measurements. The test is generally included in **Comprehensive Multiple Test Screening** panels, which range from $7 to $42. Measurement of sodium in the urine is $6 to $25; and in other body fluids, $6 to $50.

Accuracy and significance: While sodium measurements are 90 percent accurate, a deviation from normal occurs in such a variety of conditions that, basically, the test serves only to confirm a doctor's suspicions.

SOMATOMEDIN, see *Growth Hormone*

SOMATOTROPIN, see *Growth Hormone*

SONOGRAPHY, see *Ultrasound*

SOUND, see *Hearing Function*

SOUND CARDIOGRAM, see *Phonocardiogram*

SOUND SCANNING, see *Ultrasound*

SOUTHERN BLOT, see *Chromosome Analysis*

SPA, see *Bone Mineral Density Analysis*

SPATIAL ELECTROCARDIOGRAPHY, see *Vectorcardiogram*

SPECIFIC GRAVITY (URINE), see *Mosenthal; Urine Examination*

SPECT, see *Computerized Tomography*

SPECTRAL BRUITS ANALYSIS, see *Ultrasound*

SPEECH, see *Language Function*

SPERM, see *Semen*

SPERM ANTIBODIES, see *Semen*

SPERM PENETRATION ASSAY, see *Semen*

SPINAL FLUID, see *Cerebrospinal Fluid*

SPINAL FLUID CULTURE, see *Culture*

SPINAL FLUID SCAN, see *Nuclear Scanning*

SPINAL TAP, see *Cerebrospinal Fluid*

SPINAL THERMOGRAPHY, see *Thermography*

SPINNBARKEIT, see *Schiller*

SPIROCHETE, see *Syphilis*

SPIROMETRY, see *Pulmonary Function*

SPLEEN SCAN, see *Nuclear Scanning*

SPODICK-HAFFTY-KOTILAINEN: SYSTOLIC TIME INTERVALS, see *Electrocardiogram; Systolic Time Intervals*

SPOROTRICHOSIS, see *Agglutination*

SPOT, see *Mononucleosis*

SPUTUM

Sputum is the mucous secretion (phlegm) from the lower respiratory system (the lungs, the bronchi, the trachea, and the larynx). The sputum examination usually does not include the nose or sinus secretions, which are part of the upper respiratory tract. In infections and other inflammatory conditions, sputum volume and viscosity (thickness) increase.

Sputum is collected for microbiologic **Culture** or **Cytology** examination. Some is placed on culture plates to check for bacterial growth, some is placed on slides for microscopic study, and some is examined by the Papanicolaou stain for tumor study. Most clinicians request a specimen of all the sputum a patient produces in a 24-hour period; a few find a single specimen sufficient for diagnostic study. Usually, sputum is obtained by coughing. It can also be aspirated (suctioned) through a bronchoscope (see **Endoscopy**).

When performed: With suspected respiratory tract disease, when there is a persistent cough that cannot be explained, or with an undiagnosed general infection.

Normal values: Unless there is a disease process (infection, irritation, allergy, or cancer), very little sputum is produced. Any minute amounts of sputum produced should be clear, colorless, and odorless and should reveal no bacteria and very few cells or crystals under the microscope.

Abnormal values: An increased amount of yellow to greenish sputum indicates a lung infection. Reddish or brown sputum accompanies lung congestion with or without infection (pinkish, watery, foamy sputum is considered diagnostic of pulmonary edema).

In lung infections, there is a great increase in the white blood cells and fat crystals. With coliform bacteria and anaerobic infections, the sputum has an unpleasant odor. With allergy such as asthma, there is an increase in one particular white blood cell, the eosinophil, along with Curschmann's spirals and Charcot-Leyden crystals, which are quite different from the crystals seen in infection. With irritation of the lung (from dust, smog, etc.), an increase in the cells that line the bronchial passageways is seen. Elastic fibers found in the sputum on microscopic examination suggest a destructive process such as pneumonia, tuberculosis, cancer, or lung abscess.

Risk factors: None when obtained while a patient has a productive cough. If a bronchoscope is used to obtain the specimen, see **Endoscopy**.

Pain/discomfort: None, unless the specimen is obtained by bronchoscopy.

Cost: Much depends on which tests are performed on the sputum. When a **Culture** test is performed for microorganisms, the fee is $10 to $30; a **Cytology** is $5 to $50; a **Gram Stain** or an allergy examination is $5 to $15.

Accuracy and significance: Sputum examinations are 90 percent accurate and can be extremely valuable in the diagnosis of lung disease, particularly in identifying the cause of infection. If cancer cells are detected, the test can be very significant when it leads to early treatment.

SPUTUM CULTURE, see *Culture*

SQUINT, see *Strabismus*

STABILE FACTOR, see *Fibrinogen*

STAMP, see *Impotence*

STANDARD BICARBONATE, see *Bicarbonate*

STANFORD ACHIEVEMENT, see *Learning Disability*

STEATORRHEA, see *Pancreas Function*

STENGER, see *Hearing Function; Tuning Fork*

STEP, see *Learning Disability*

STEREOPSIS, see *Visual Acuity*

STEREOTACTIC BIOPSY, see *Biopsy*

STERILITY, see *Body Temperature; Semen*

STI, see *Systolic Time Intervals*

STOMACH CONTENTS, see *Gastric Analysis*

STOMACH HORMONE, see *Gastrin*

STOOL CULTURE, see *Culture*

STOOL EXAMINATION, see *Feces Examination*

STRABISMUS

Strabismus is a condition in which the two eyes do not see the identical image simultaneously; usually, one eye is pointed in a slightly different direction from the other. Most often, this condition is the result of an eye muscle weakness (eye movement is controlled by six different muscles); it can also come from brain and nerve involvement. By having the patient look at fixed points in certain directions, the physician can determine the specific external ocular muscle at fault. Forms of strabismus include heterotropia (squinting); esotropia (cross-eyes), where one or both eyes look inward; exotropia (walleyes), where one eye always looks outward; and diplopia (double vision).

Diplopia is detected when a red glass is placed over one eye and the patient, looking at a light with both eyes, sees both a red and a white dot. In the Worth four-dot test, a red glass is placed over one eye and a green glass over the other; the patient looks at a special light that shows one red, one white, and two green dots. Depending on what the patient sees, the doctor can determine which eye is affected and whether the two eyes can work together.

In the Wirt stereopsis test, polarized-lens glasses are used to ascertain the degree and possibility of fusion (the ability to use both eyes together for three-dimensional viewing). In the cover-uncover test, a patient looks at an object 20 feet away, first with one eye covered and then with the cover removed. The Hirschberg test, similar in technique, is used on young children who do not easily cooperate; movement of corneal light reflex is noted. The Maddox rod test uses cylinders to measure eye deviations. All the tests help confirm the specific cause of strabismus and help determine prognosis. About 1 in 20 children has a form of strabismus.

When performed: Whenever patients have cross-eyes, walleyes, squinting, or double vision; following head or eye injury; with all cranial nerve diseases; in patients with diabetes or vascular diseases.

Normal values: When both eyes look at the identical spot or object, they should see it is one rather than two distinct spots or objects, without blurring (in this instance, blurring would be due to double vision rather than loss of **Visual Acuity).** The patient should be able to control each of the six muscles of the eye so that they move in perfect harmony.

Abnormal values: Deviations are measured in units of prisms. With strabismus, a prism lens must be placed in front of the eye to correct muscular weakness or nerve defect. One prism diopter (diopter is a unit of measurement in ophthalmology) means that at a distance of one meter (a bit more than three feet), the eye sees an image one centimeter away from its true location. In the Worth four-dot test, a patient with double vision will see five dots instead of four; whether the extra dot is red or green determines which eye is affected. In the cover-uncover test, when the cover is removed, the weak eye will suddenly move instead of focusing in the direction in which the uncovered eye is looking.

Risk factors: None.

Pain/discomfort: None.

Cost: Generally, there is no charge, as these tests are part of a routine eye examination.

Accuracy and significance: The tests are 95 percent accurate as an aid to determining the cause of strabismus; if the cause is muscle imbalance, the tests help to identify the specific muscle. The significance of the tests lies in their ability to indicate which strabismus conditions can be corrected and to what degree.

STREPTOCOCCAL INFECTION, see *Antistreptolysin O Titer*

STREPTOCOCCUS, see *Skin Reaction*

STREPTOCOCCUS LATEX AGGLUTINATION, see *Antistreptolysin O Titer*

STRESS (NERVOUS), see *Electromyography*

STRESS CARDIOGRAM, see *Electrocardiogram*

STRESS-INDUCING CIRCUMSTANCE, see *Jenkins Activity Survey*

STRING

At times, a patient may present vague symptoms of bleeding from the esophagus, stomach, or first part of the small intestine, usually indicative of an irritation, an ulcer, or a parasitic infestation. A simple test to detect such bleeding, and to help justify subsequent expensive and complicated examinations, is the string test. It is so named because all the patient must do is swallow a string (usually of the same material as that used to tie the umbilical cord at birth). At times, the string is weighted at the end with a small capsule that may or may not dissolve. The distance the string travels is noted; it is then pulled back up, and the stains from blood, bile, or mucus are observed. In addition, material adhering to the string can be examined microscopically to observe the types of cells that make up the linings of various organs (see **Cytology**). The presence of crystals of cholesterol, bilirubin from bile, or segments of parasites or their eggs can also be noted (parasitic infestation can exist so high up in the intestinal tract that it is difficult to diagnose through a feces examination). Finally, certain fungus overgrowths that can interfere with the effectiveness of antibiotics can be detected by the string test. Today, there are commercial products that are much-improved versions of the traditional string; some use nylon and have fast-dissolving capsules and color markers in the string to make diagnosis easier and quicker.

When performed: As a screening test when there is a suspicion of bleeding or other pathology in the upper digestive tract; when a patient's **Feces Examination** is normal, but there is a suspicion of worms or other parasites; in cases of anemia when the source of bleeding has not been isolated; in malabsorption syndrome (food is not properly digested); when particular medications are not properly absorbed; when pernicious anemia is suspected; to note the presence or absence of bile.

Normal values: No evidence of blood, parasites, fungi, abnormal cells, or bile crystals. Normal acid in the stomach.

Abnormal values: Evidence of bleeding, irritation, parasites, abnormal bacteria (such as those that cause typhoid), abnormal pH (acid) values in inappropriate locations (see **Gastroesophageal Reflux**), and any abnormal (cancerous) cells. Lack of stomach acid.

Risk factors: Virtually none; swallowing the string will cause no real complications.

Pain/discomfort: Some patients find it difficult to swallow the string, while others tend to vomit when swallowing the string or when it is retrieved.

Cost: The fee ranges from $10 to $50, depending on how many different tests are performed on the string and the material that adheres to it.

Accuracy and significance: The test is considered 90 percent accurate in detecting bleeding in the esophagus, stomach, or first portion of the small intestine; approximately 85 percent accurate in detecting parasites in the upper intestine; approximately 50 percent accurate in noting malabsorption problems; quite accurate in measuring the presence or absence of stomach acid and its pH. Although this test is simple and relatively painless, the use of a gastroscope (see **Endoscopy**) is far more accurate (endoscopy can necessitate hospitalization).

STROKE VOLUME, see "Angiography," in *Radiography*

STUART FACTOR, see *Fibrinogen*

SUBCUTANEOUS, see *Skin Reaction*

SUBLINGUAL PROVOCATIVE, see *RAST*

SUCCINYLCHOLINE REACTION, see *Cholinesterase*

SUCROSE HEMOLYSIS, see *HAM*

SUDDEN INFANT DEATH SYNDROME, see *Botulism; Sleep Monitoring*

SUGAR, see *Glucose*

SUGAR WATER, see *HAM*

SULFHEMOGLOBIN, see *Hemoglobin*

SULFITES, see *Allergy*

SULFOBROMOPHTHALEIN, see *Bromsulphalein*

SULKOWITCH, see *Bone Mineral Density Analysis; Calcium*

SUPERFICIAL REFLEX, see *Reflex*

SUPERFICIAL TACTILE SENSATION, see *Sensory*

SURFACE BIOPSY, see *Biopsy*

SUSCEPTIBILITY, see *Culture*

SWAN-GANZ CATHETER, see *Blood Pressure*

SWEAT

Testing for the chemicals in sweat (see **Sodium**) helps to detect many different diseases. Measuring the ability to sweat is a particular test for physical as well as mental disease. A very weak iodine solution (in alcohol) is painted on the skin area under study and allowed to dry; the area is dusted with starch powder. The patient is then made to sweat (by administration of direct heat, hot liquids, or certain drugs). If the sweat glands are functioning properly, the white starch powder will turn dark blue. Vapor pressure osmometry is a new sweat collection procedure that uses a heated cup to help eliminate false results. One simple sweat test is to kiss a baby to find out if the skin seems particularly salty. Many pediatricians urge parents to use this test to detect early signs of cystic fibrosis in their infants.

There is also a sweat patch test for **Alcoholism.** The patient wears a sweat patch from two to eight days; the concentration of alcohol in the sweat collected by the patch determines alcohol consumption.

Recently, sweat testing, after stimulation with pilocarpine (a drug also used to dilate the eyes for a better eye examination), has been used to help evaluate the autonomic nervous system (see **Finger Wrinkle** and **Cold Pressor** tests). Assuming the sweat glands are present (this is a test to determine their presence), a normal sweat reaction is a reflection of a working autonomic nervous system. At times, quinizarin green (a dye used in cosmetics) is applied to the skin instead of iodine; it turns from blue-green to purple in the presence of sweat.

The newest test to detect cystic fibrosis during pregnancy consists of measuring three isoenzymes of **Alkaline Phosphatase** through **Amniocentesis.** The test is indicated for women who are considered to be undergoing high-risk pregnancies (see **Nonstress Fetal Assessment).**

Another new test for detecting cystic fibrosis is called the immunoreactive trypsin assay. Trypsin is a digestive enzyme produced by the pancreas (see **Pancreas Function);** with cystic fibrosis, the same mucus that blocks the lungs' air passages also blocks the pancreatic ducts. When this happens, trypsin backs up into the blood and can be detected there. An advantage of this test is that it can be performed on infants only a few weeks of age. The test costs just $10 to $20, as compared to the newer sweat collection tests, which now cost around $50.

When performed: Most often, the test is performed to ascertain excessive sweating, such as with "night sweats" (which occur only during sleep and suggest chronic infections); to differentiate malnutrition from certain specific diseases such as lupus erythematosus; to measure a spontaneous sweating reaction to anxiety; to collect sweat for cystic fibrosis screening; to distinguish alcohol drinkers from nondrinkers.

Normal values: It is normal for sweat glands to function when exposed to direct heat, exercise, or excessive alcohol or when the body is excessively warmed by clothes or blankets. Sweat may have a color if the body is exposed to certain chemicals (as in some occupations) or if the sweat is accompanied by color-producing bacteria. Excessive bacteria can normally cause bromidrosis, or unpleasantly scented sweat, but this is usually limited to areas with skin folds. Sweat normally contains chloride, from 0 to 40 mEq per L, but up to 65 mEq per L still may not be indicative of cystic fibrosis; sodium values are similar.

Abnormal values: Hyperhidrosis, or excessive sweating under inappropriate conditions (as in a cool room), may be caused by vitamin deficiencies, hyperthyroidism, brain and spinal cord disease, blood vessel disease, and following surgery where certain nerves have been severed. Psychological problems usually cause excessive sweating on the palms of the hands and the soles of the feet. The inability to sweat is usually an inherited condition. Patients with cystic fibrosis have increased sodium and chloride concentrations in their sweat. Patients who drink alcohol but deny it can be identified with this test.

More than 50 to 60 mEq per L on two separate days is considered to be an abnormal amount of sodium and chloride in sweat.

Risk factors: None.

Pain/discomfort: None.

Cost: The charge for alcohol evaluation is $20 to $30; the charge for sodium and chloride evaluations, $5 to $25 each.

Accuracy and significance: Sweat measurements are not considered precise tests (about 70 percent accurate). They are reasonably significant as a confirmation of cystic fibrosis; however, false-positive results occur with enough frequency to warrant blood **Sodium** testing. The inaccuracies found in sweat tests are, in large measure, due to carelessness in performing them.

Note: Many doctors believe the sweat test is of no real value until an infant is at least 6 weeks of age. A new test, called immunological reactive trypsinogen (IRT), based on pancreatic secretions (see **Pancreas Function),** may help detect cystic fibrosis within the first week of life (at the same time tests for **Phenylketonuria** and **Thyroid Function** should be made on all newborns).

SWINGING VOICE, see *Hearing Function*

SYMMETRIC TONIC NECK REFLEX, see *Reflex*

SYMONDS PICTURE STORY, see *Thematic Apperception*

SYNCOPE (FAINTING) TESTING, see *Carotid Sinus Massage*

SYNCYTIAL, see *Virus Disease*

SYNDROME OF INAPPROPRIATE ANTIDIURETIC HORMONE SECRETION, see *Vasopressin*

SYNOVIAL FLUID

All body joints contain a small amount of straw-colored syrupy liquid called synovial fluid that helps lubricate the bone or cartilage surfaces. Three dozen different tests can be performed on joint fluid. The usual examination consists of measuring sugar levels and white blood cells, as well as searching for crystals, immunoglobulins, anti-gamma globulins, various forms of complement, and lupus erythematosus cells (see **Antinuclear Antibodies**). In the ropes test, the fluid is mixed with a mild acid to see if it forms a good mucin clot (a small, ropy-looking mass that stays together even with shaking).

In most instances, the patient is asked to fast the night before and the morning of the test so as not to abnormally alter the sugar level. The synovial fluid is obtained by inserting a small needle into the joint cavity (a process called arthrocentesis). Absolute sterility precautions must be observed to make sure that infection is not introduced into the cavity when the fluid is withdrawn. A joint cavity can contain up to half an ounce of fluid, but only one drop is needed to arrive at certain diagnoses.

Another test, the limulus assay (limulus is a unique chemical substance derived from the horseshoe crab), is now being performed whenever synovial fluid is suspected of being infected with Gram-negative bacteria (see **Gram Stain**); it can give a fairly reliable indication of infection within an hour, as opposed to the several days needed to culture bacteria. The limulus test can also be used on blood to indicate the presence of small amounts of endotoxin (poisons from certain bacteria that can cause blood poisoning, sometimes called toxemia or sepsis). The limulus amebocyte lysate test is a rapid procedure that has been used to diagnose **Gonorrhea** in the male and has also been of value in detecting an intestinal perforation when used on peritoneal fluid.

When performed: Primarily, when there is a swollen joint, whether hot and inflamed or not; to differentiate the different types of arthritis (from infectious to traumatic); to aid in the diagnosis of systemic lupus erythematosus; to follow the progress of any joint disease; when certain bleeding disorders are suspected.

Normal values: Normal synovial fluid is slightly yellow and clear with very few white blood cells (less than 200 per ml), no crystals, and a good mucin clot. Sugar levels and other chemical test values should approximate those found in normal plasma.

Abnormal values: With arthritis, synovial fluid tends to become more yellow or yellowish green and turns somewhat cloudy. The white blood cells increase markedly (over 10,000 per ml), and with certain diseases, various types of crystals appear: uric acid crystals with gout, calcium crystals with pseudogout. With arthritis, the mucin clot is "poor"—that is, fragile and easily breakable on shaking; with gout, it is even more fragile. With infectious arthritis, synovial fluid sugar levels are reduced, and the fluid is given a **culture** test.

Risk factors: An ever-present risk in extracting joint fluid is the subsequent possibility of osteomyelitis or prolonged bone infection. When sterile conditions are meticulously observed, this risk is reduced. When the test itself is correctly performed, the remaining risks are negligible (see general risk factors for catheter and needle insertion).

Pain/discomfort: Minimal (see general pain/discomfort factors for catheter and needle insertion).

Cost: The most common tests performed on synovial fluid are the **Red Blood Cell** count, **White Blood Cell** count, and **Blood Cell Differential,** at a charge of $5 to $20; crystal examination is $10 to $25; the chemical tests are $5 to $20; **Complement** testing is $30 to $45; and **Culture,** $10 to $30. If the battery of tests is done concurrently, the fee ranges from $30 to $50.

Accuracy and significance: Synovial fluid tests are from 20 to 65 percent accurate depending on the condition being looked for, but are significant in their ability to differentiate between joint infection and other noninfectious conditions (arthritis, gout, pathology secondary to an injury). Synovial fluid examinations are done routinely in conjunction with **Radiography.** It is these two tests, supporting the doctor's physical findings, that can help make a diagnosis of joint disease.

SYPHILIS

Many tests help to determine if syphilis is present in the body. These tests may be of the treponemal variety (looking for Treponema pallidum, the corkscrew-shaped organisms that cause the disease, commonly referred to as spirochetes because of their shape) or the nontreponemal variety of serological (blood) tests (see **Agglutination; Complement Fixation),** which give passive evidence of the disease if antibodies are present. The nontreponemal antigen tests include the Hinton, Kolner, Kahn, Kline, Mazzini, Wassermann, rapid plasma reagin (RPR), automated reagin (ART), and Venereal Disease Research Laboratory (VDRL). The VDRL is the most common test, but it is not completely accurate: one patient out of four with early syphilis will have a false-negative reaction. These tests are not as expensive and are more easily performed than the treponemal tests, but they all may give false-positive results in conditions other than syphilis (lupus erythematosus, malaria, leprosy, acute infections, and after smallpox vaccination).

The treponemal organisms are so narrow that they cannot be seen by ordinary microscopic light and need a "darkfield"; that is, they must be illuminated by reflected light in order to be observed. The darkfield examination is performed during the primary stage of syphilis; fluid from the lesion is placed on a glass slide and examined under the microscope for direct, living evidence of Treponema pallidum.

The Treponema pallidum immobilization test (TPI) takes serum from a suspected syphilis patient and adds it to complement (special serum antibodies); when both are then added to a virulent strain of live Treponema pallidum, the organisms become immobilized.

The Fluorescent Treponemal Antibody Absorption (FTA-ABS) test has been found to be more sensitive for syphilis than the TPI. It is easier to perform and therefore used more often, but 1 patient out of 10 with very early syphilis will still be missed (have a false-negative reaction). False-positive reactions may occur when the patient's serum contains antinuclear factors (see **Antinuclear Antibodies**), **Rheumatoid Factor,** or increased globulins (see **Albumin/Globulin** and **Immunoglobulins**). Blood from a vein is tested. Spinal fluid is also tested to detect latent syphilis and to follow the progress of treatment.

When performed: Whenever there is a mystifying infection (syphilis is known as the great masquerader, since it imitates many illnesses); when a skin disease does not heal; with other symptoms that cause suspicion of syphilis; when certain tropical diseases are suspected; when pregnancy is diagnosed.

In most states, a syphilis test is required by law before a marriage license can be issued. (The exceptions are Idaho, Maine, Maryland, Minnesota, Nevada, South Carolina, and Washington; in Colorado, men are exempt.) In Alabama, Alaska, Colorado, Kansas, Louisiana, New Mexico, North Carolina, North Dakota, Oklahoma, Utah, Wisconsin, and the territory of Puerto Rico, applicants for a marriage license must also present a certificate certifying they are free of *all* known sexually transmitted diseases.

In all states other than Alabama, Minnesota, Mississippi, Tennessee, Wisconsin, and the territory of Puerto Rico, the law requires a pregnant woman to be tested for syphilis on her first visit to a doctor or clinic; in California, a woman can be excused from the test if she objects for any reason.

Normal values: Normally, there is no evidence (reaction) of syphilis in the body.

Abnormal values: The test is positive when there is active or even inactive (old) syphilis. Other conditions that can cause a positive reaction include malaria, Hansen's disease, rat-bite fever, pellagra, infectious mononucleosis, pneumonia, tuberculosis, and lupus erythematosus. Following treatment for syphilis, tests such as the VDRL may show a lessened titer (an indication of the degree and duration of the disease) as compared to those who receive no therapy; the test rarely returns to normal, however.

Risk factors: Negligible (see general risk factors for blood testing). Also see **Biopsy**.

Pain/discomfort: Minimal (see general pain/discomfort factors for blood testing). Also see **Biopsy**.

Cost: The simple nontreponemal screening tests such as the RPR, VDRL, Hinton, and Wassermann range from $3 to $50. The more specific treponemal FTA-ABS test is $15 to $100. Direct microscopic observation of material from a sore is $20 to $100. Some, but not all, states requiring syphilis tests provide them at no charge.

Accuracy and significance: Nontreponemal tests are used primarily for premarital and prenatal screening; while they serve this purpose adequately, they are not of sufficient accuracy to confirm a diagnosis. Such a variety of conditions other than syphilis produce a positive nontreponemal test that the finding of an abnormal value requires extensive follow-up. Positive treponemal and microscopic tests are necessary before a specific diagnosis can be made; they are from 80 to 95 percent accurate. All positive test results, regardless of the technique, must be reported to local public health authorities.

Note: Although the FTA-ABS test is in itself quite accurate, there are reports in the medical literature citing an increasing number of false-positive results due to laboratory carelessness (as opposed to those false results that can come from biological factors such as antinuclear antibodies). Therefore, even a positive treponemal test must be repeated—preferably by a different laboratory—before it is accepted as a sign of syphilis.

SYSTEMIC HYPERTENSION, see *Blood Pressure*

SYSTEMIC LUPUS ERYTHEMATOSUS, see *Antinuclear Antibodies*

SYSTOLIC PRESSURE, see *Blood Pressure*

SYSTOLIC TIME INTERVALS (STI)

The word *systole* refers to the time during which the heart contracts and pumps blood into the aorta and the rest of the vascular system (*diastole* is the time the heart relaxes between contractions). An electronic instrument is placed on the side of the neck so that the carotid artery pulse can be felt. The device records the pulse waves (pressure from the heart's contraction and forcible outflow of blood) in the form of specific waves that can be measured and timed.

Many cardiologists consider the STI to be the most accurate of all tests of heart muscle and vascular system functioning. It is usually performed along with a standard **Electrocardiogram (ECG)** and a **Phonocardiogram** (PCG). The first part of the STI measures the left ventricular ejection time, or how long it takes the left side of the heart to empty itself. The second part of the test measures the pre-ejection period (PEP), or the exact time the heart muscle is activated to the time the blood begins to leave the heart. The two parts of the STI can reveal heart disease that is not detected by other tests.

The most recent innovation for measuring systolic time intervals is the Spodick-Haffty-Kotilainen ear pulse wave recording (performed as a part of the 24-hour Holter-type **Electrocardiogram).**

When performed: When suspected heart disease patients have a normal stress electrocardiogram; to check the effectiveness of certain drugs on the heart as well as to uncover toxic effects of other drugs; to follow the progress of patients who have heart attacks.

Normal values: The left side of the heart should empty completely in less than 0.35 second; the pre-ejection period is even less.

Abnormal values: Prolonged systolic time intervals are seen with heart valve disease, with damaged heart muscle (usually after a heart attack), and with heart damage caused by certain cancer-treating drugs.

Risk factors: None.

Pain/discomfort: None.

Cost: From $20 to $50, depending on the method employed. When used with the Holter-type electrocardiogram, the fee is $100 to $200.

Accuracy and significance: There is no unanimity of opinion about the most effective technique for measuring the heart's performance through systolic time intervals. Most radiologists prefer a form of **Nuclear Scanning,** while some cardiologists think the **Echocardiogram** is best. All agree, however, that systolic time intervals are a significant measurement of the heart's function, especially when the standard electrocardiogram is unrevealing and inconsistent with the doctor's suspicions. About 80 percent accurate.

T

TACKMETER

The tackmeter (tackiness viscometer) measures the cohesiveness or stickiness of the mucous secretion of the cervix by noting how much strength it takes to pull it apart. It is a particular test for ovulation time—that is, the exact moment when the ovary releases an egg ready for pregnancy. (Ovulation time is also measured by the **Body Temperature** test.) A version of this test can be performed by women at home. The latest means of determining ovulation time is a dipstick urine test that can be performed at home; several brand name products are available.

When performed: To determine if a woman is fertile and does in fact ovulate, or produce fertilizable eggs; after a woman stops taking birth control pills (to learn when she can become pregnant); as a means of birth control (to inform a woman of her "safe" days).

Normal values: Cervical mucus becomes thinner (less viscous) at the time of ovulation and thickens both before and afterward. Patients using the mucus examination as a means of birth control need to know only the difference between thick and thin; an expert in the field can evaluate the degree of viscosity accurately enough to predict ovulation time within a few hours.

Abnormal values: Failure of the cervical mucus to thin out during the menstrual cycle usually indicates failure to ovulate.

Risk factors: None.

Pain/discomfort: None.

Cost: There is usually no charge for this test when it is part of a routine gynecological examination. When a tackmeter is leased for home use, the charge ranges from $10 to $20. If the tackmeter is purchased, it can cost $50 to $100. The dipstick test costs about $10.

Accuracy and significance: The test is considered a reasonable (70 percent accurate) but not precise measure of ovulation time. Hence, it is not considered a perfect method of birth control. The dipstick test is said to be 90 percent accurate.

T AND B CELLS, see *Lymphocyte Typing*

TANGENT SCREEN, see *Visual Field*

TARTRAZINE SENSITIVITY

Urticaria (hives), sinus problems, and asthma can be caused by reactions to different foods, drugs, and plants. A common cause of these symptoms is sensitivity to tartrazine, a substance that is often added to foods as a coloring (Yellow Dye No. 5). Tartrazine is commonly used as a coloring in ice cream, candy, desserts, commercial pastries, certain vegetable oils, and butter. For many of these foods, federal law does not require that the coloring be listed among the ingredients; state laws require only an indication that the coloring has been added (the specific name of the color need not be mentioned).

Most people who are sensitive to tartrazine are also allergic to aspirin and show this allergy by the same symptoms. Since it can be dangerous to test for aspirin allergy directly, the tartrazine test is used. The patient eats a tartrazine-free diet and takes no pills coated with the coloring for 7 to 10 days. If the usual allergic symptoms go away, the patient is given dose of tartrazine; if sensitivity exists, the allergy will return within three hours. Also see **Allergy**.

When performed: Whenever a patient has repeated episodes of urticaria, asthma, or sinus allergies.

Normal values: There should be no skin or respiratory passage reaction to a large dose of tartrazine.

Abnormal values: A positive skin or respiratory reaction to a dose of tartrazine usually means the patient is also allergic to aspirin and products that contain or act like aspirin (certain drugs for arthritis and sodium benzoate, a food preservative).

Risk factors: The test should always be performed in the presence of a physician with the equipment to treat a severe allergic reaction.

Pain/discomfort: An allergic reaction such as itching skin and/or wheezing can be uncomfortable.

Cost: There is usually no charge for this test when it is part of a routine office visit.

Accuracy and significance: A positive test is definitive evidence (95 percent) of sensitivity to tartrazine and related products. In large part, the significance of the test is measured by the patient's willingness to eliminate all foods and drugs containing tartrazine.

TASTE FUNCTION

The ability to taste four distinctive flavors on both sides of the tongue equally is important to the diagnosis of certain brain lesions. Nerves of taste located on the front of the tongue connect to a different part the brain than nerves of taste located on the back of the tongue. Standardized solutions of 5 percent glucose (sweet), 5 percent salt, 1 percent quinine (bitter), and 1 percent vinegar (sour) are placed directly on both sides of the tongue from the front to the back with a dropper. Usually, **Smell Function** tests are performed at the same time. In the Franklinic test, a small electric current is applied to the tongue and should cause a sour taste. The **Circulation Time** test makes use of the ability to taste a bitter substance.

The loss of taste, or changes in the sense of taste, can be early signs of cancer. It is now thought that a change in the sense of taste reduces the desire to eat and this, rather than the cancer, may lead to the weight loss associated with cancer.

When performed: When brain disease is suspected; following brain or neck injury; with severe tooth problems; with liver, lung, heart, and stomach disease; when cancer is suspected.

Normal values: All four standard flavors should easily be detected. The sweet taste is predominant at the tip of the tongue; the bitter taste, on the back surface. Sour tastes are detected along the sides, and salty flavors are picked up all over the front half of the tongue as well as along the sides.

Abnormal values: The most common cause of taste loss is Bell's palsy (paralysis of one of the main nerves to the face). Total loss of taste (ageusia) can also be the result of a brain or nerve tumor. It may occur, temporarily, with migraine attacks and in lung and liver disease. Hallucinations of taste, but not loss, can come from brain lesions and tongue infections, and during pregnancy.

Risk factors: None.

Pain/discomfort: None.

Cost: There is usually no charge when the test is performed as a part of a regular office physical examination.

Accuracy and significance: The test is valuable in detecting facial nerve disease (Bell's palsy); in confirming the suspicion of brain disease; in helping distinguish among hallucinatory illnesses. If patients who have lost their sense of taste become aware of this loss, they can be more cautious about eating strange foods—especially foods that may have become spoiled. Taste tests are considered to be 80 to 90 percent accurate.

TAT, see *Thematic Apperception*

TAY-SACHS DISEASE (Gangliosidosis)

Tay-Sachs disease is an inherited disorder that seems to occur primarily in Jewish people from Eastern Europe. (Its occurrence in those of non-Jewish origin is rare.) Children born with the disease have little or no active hexosaminidase enzyme, the lack of which causes fat to accumulate in the brain's ganglions (bundles of nerves). The consequences are mental retardation, paralysis, blindness, and cherry-red spots on the retina of the eye; the disorder is usually fatal before the child reaches the age of 4. There are two tests for the disease. The first is a blood test, performed prior to pregnancy (on both parents), that helps detect carriers of the disease. The second, performed during pregnancy, is **Amniocentesis,** which can identify a fetus with the disease.

When performed: As a screening test for parents-to-be, especially among Central and Eastern European Jewish people (also known as Ashkenazi), who have a 1-out-of-30 chance of carrying the disease genes. Before or during pregnancy when there is even the remotest possibility that some distant forebear might have come from Eastern Europe or when a family member, no matter how remote the relationship, once had a child with a genetic defect.

Normal values: Evidence of the presence and activity of the enzyme hexosaminidase.

Abnormal values: Lack of any hexosaminidase enzyme or decreased activity of the enzyme in a carrier.

Risk factors: Negligible for blood testing (see general risk factors for blood testing). See **Amniocentesis** if applicable.

Pain/discomfort: Minimal (see general pain/discomfort factors for blood testing). See **Amniocentesis** if applicable.

Cost: Some community and volunteer health organizations provide the screening test without charge or for a token fee; if performed in a commercial laboratory, the fee is $15 to $25.

Accuracy and significance: The test is considered 95 percent accurate in detecting carriers of the disease. A patient must inform the doctor or laboratory of the presence of diabetes and diseases of the liver or pancreas, as these conditions, along with pregnancy and the use of birth control pills, require a modification of the test procedure for accuracy. The obvious significance is to identify those couples who run the risk of bearing a child with the disease.

TBG, see *Thyroid Function*

TEA, see *Caffeine*

TEAL, see *Tuning Fork*

TEAR, see *Schirmer's*

TEAR DUCT PATENTCY, see *Fluorescein Eye Stain*

TEMPERATURE, see *Body Temperature*

TENSILON, see *Edrophonium*

TERMAN, see *Intelligence Quotient*

TESTICULAR SCAN, see *Nuclear Scanning*

TESTIS FUNCTION

There are several different tests to determine if the testicles (male gonads) are functioning normally (also see **Semen).** Two tests in particular indicate whether the testes are performing their two basic functions: producing the male hormone testosterone and producing sperm. One is the direct measurement of testosterone in blood plasma or in the urine; the other is measurement of gonadotropin (chorionic gonadotropin) in both the blood and the urine.

Testosterone is also manufactured in small amounts in the liver and by the adrenal glands (women normally produce a very small amount of testosterone in their ovaries and adrenals). Thus, testosterone testing is not an absolute measurement of testicle function; however, it is a reasonable approximation. Testosterone is the hormone responsible for secondary sex characteristics such as hair distribution, voice pitch, hip configuration, and muscle development (primary sex characteristics are the sex organs themselves).

Another test of testicle function (and at times, a test for ovary function in women) is measuring luteinizing hormone. While related to follicle-stimulating hormone (see **Estrogen),** for both come from the pituitary, the two hormones can be confused with each other by the testing laboratory. The tests can also be used as an indication of failure of the gonads (testicle and ovary) to perform properly.

In the past, the 17-ketosteroid (17-KS) test was used to evaluate testis function. It has since been learned that almost all 17 ketosteroids come from the adrenal glands and not the testicles, as was once believed; thus, the test is no longer considered to be a measure of male organ activity.

Human chorionic gonadotropin (HCG) measurements in the urine seem to be the most significant indicator of testicular activity. Gonadotropin measured in blood taken from a vein is a confirmatory test. The measurement of human chorionic gonadotropin is also used to determine if a woman is pregnant (see **Pregnancy**).

When performed: Whenever a tumor of the reproductive glands (testis or ovaries), adrenal glands, pituitary gland, or hypothalamus is suspected; whenever congenital (inherited) sex defects are being considered; with hypogonadism (testicles that do not function adequately or failure of the testicles to descend), a condition that is usually not detectable until after puberty and at times not until 21 years of age; with suspected prostate trouble; with **Impotence;** as a possible indication of heart disease. Increased testosterone levels in women may explain hirsutism (excessive body hair) from ovarian tumors.

Normal values: Serum or plasma testosterone averages from 500 to 1,200 ng per 100 ml in men and from 25 to 50 ng per 100 ml in women. Men usually excrete up to 200 mcg in the urine every 24 hours; women and children excrete no more than 10 mcg per 24 hours. There should be no measureable gonadotropins in the blood or urine of men or women (except during pregnancy). At times, a 24-hour specimen of urine may contain from 5 to 50 mouse-uterine units of pituitary gonadotropins. (The test is measured by an increase in the weight of a mouse's uterus after the mouse has been injected with the human specimen; pituitary gonadotropins are slightly different from chorionic gonadotropins.)

Abnormal values: Testosterone levels are decreased in hypogonadism and indicate inadequate or absent testis function, such as can be caused by stress (crowding, military training, threats, etc.) and by alcohol and many other drugs. Urine and blood pituitary gonadotropin levels are increased when hypogonadism originates in the testicle rather than the pituitary gland or hypothalamus. They are usually decreased when hypogonadism is caused by pituitary problems. Chorionic gonadotropins are increased with testicular tumors. Low testosterone levels, only in conjunction with elevated estradiol (female hormone) levels, have been implicated in susceptibility to heart disease (see **Estrogen).** Severe dieting can elevate testosterone levels.

Risk factors: Negligible (see general risk factors for blood testing).

Pain/discomfort: Minimal (see general pain/discomfort factors for blood testing).

Cost: From $33 to $66 whether blood or urine testosterone is tested. Screening for HCG is $10 to $20. When precise amounts of HCG are measured, the fee is $20 to $40; luteinizing hormone testing averages $15 to $30.

Accuracy and significance: Although measurements of testosterone and HCG are 90 percent accurate and are fairly precise, abnormal values are not significant for specific diseases. However, they help to narrow the diagnostic possibilities to abnormal endocrine gland dysfunction.

Note: It is now possible to test for free testosterone as opposed to total testosterone, which is the usual assay for this hormone. Although still not very precise, this test is considered three times more accurate a measure of the hormone's activity; it costs twice as much as total testosterone testing ($50 to $100).

TESTOSTERONE, see *Testis Function*

TESTS OF ACADEMIC PROGRESS, see *Learning Disability*

THALASSEMIA, see *Hemoglobin*

THALLIUM SCAN, see *Nuclear Scanning*

THEMATIC APPERCEPTION (TAT)

The thematic apperception test is a projective (information-provoking) technique in which the subject projects or reads into a series of pictures his own feelings and interpretations. The test was developed by the psychologist H. A. Murray in 1938. It is based on the hypothesis that an individual will view each of the pictures in the light of his own experience and that the themes of the stories the individual tells about each picture will reveal much about his social and emotional adjustment as well as his attitudes toward sex, authority, and aggression.

The examiner shows the subject one picture at a time and asks him to tell a complete story about the picture, the characters in the picture, how they feel, and what the outcome will be. The examiner records the stories and then discusses them with the subject. Later, he makes interpretations from the material developed.

Scoring techniques are based on a number of criteria: whether the subject uses the whole picture or only part of it to develop his story; the characters and emotional tone of the story; and the type of ending. Interpretation of the data is usually based less on the formal scoring than on the interpreter's previous experience with personality patterns that have been suggested by the themes of the stories. As with other projective tests, there is always the danger of the examiner's making arbitrary judgments that conform to his personal experience and beliefs. The examiner, therefore, will often tend to validate preconceived notions through such tests.

A number of variations on the TAT have been developed for specific purposes, such an evaluating handicapped children or ethnic groups and for vocational counseling. The children's apperception test (CAT) uses pictures of animals in social situations in the belief that young children will respond more readily to animals. The CAT-H, a version for older children, uses human figures in the same social situations as the animals in the CAT. The Bellak TAT uses the CAT pictures with a different concept of interpretation.

The Symonds Picture Story uses pictures especially oriented to adolescents.

The Blacky Pictures have a psychoanalytic or Freudian orientation. The child is shown pictures of a dog named Blacky and his family and is encouraged to tell the therapist about his own family and relate the pictures to them. Proponents of this test believe that it demonstrates the validity of psychoanalytic concepts. The Make-a-Picture Story (MAPS) uses a miniature empty stage (with various settings to choose from, such as bedrooms and bathrooms). The subject is offered mounted, cutout figures (young, old, nude, animals, etc.) to place on the stage and explain why the particular figures were chosen and who and what they represent.

When performed: The TAT is used with normal subjects to study thinking processes, family relationships, attitudes toward sex and authority, cultural differences in minority and ethnic groups, and general levels of intelligence. It is also performed when there is suspicion of neurosis or other mental problems, as a measure of the emotional component of some physical illnesses (asthma, ulcers, headache), and as an indicator of progress during psychotherapy.

Normal values: Normal responses are generally those given most commonly by subjects. The test may furnish leads about the individual that the individual would find difficult to express in other ways.

Abnormal values: There is an assumption that evidence of emotional conflict, depression, aggression, phobias, fears, suicidal tendencies, or homosexuality will be revealed by the subject's interpretations of the pictures.

Risk factors: None.

Pain/discomfort: None.

Cost: From $25 to $100, depending on the particular test used and the time required.

Accuracy and significance: As with many psychological tests requiring subjective evaluations, there is no way to measure their accuracy or scientific significance.

THERMODILUTION CARDIAC OUTPUT, see "Angiography," in *Radiography*

THERMOGRAPHY

Thermography measures the slightest variations in temperature of soft tissue in the body using infrared heat sensors. The technique is often used in mammography (breast examination) to detect any growth in the breast (the mass will have a different temperature from other breast tissue). Today, there is a specially constructed bra connected to a measuring device that, when it is worn for 10 to 15 minutes, can reveal differences in temperature on a graph. Thermography may also be used on an extremity, particularly the leg, to help diagnose a thrombus (clot) in a vein. The inflammation usually associated with the thrombus raises the temperature in the area of the clot. Measuring temperature changes of the penis, especially after showing a patient sexually stimulating illustrations, can help differentiate physical from psychological **Impotence**. The area of the body to be tested is usually placed on a heat-detection device that reacts to specific temperatures, either by color changes or by a direct display of temperatures.

Liquid crystal thermography is a different form of testing veins for thrombosis; it seems to be almost as accurate as **Radiography** (albeit the X-ray test is considered the more dangerous). Here, sheets of latex embedded with crystals that change color depending on the temperature they contact are placed over the calf or thigh. There is no pain, discomfort, or risk, and the test usually takes about 15 minutes; it may take longer if readings are obtained from all four sides of the leg being tested.

A somewhat related test for breast cancer screening is called diaphanography (transmission spectroscopy). Here, in a dark room, the breast is transilluminated with a special light, and the shadows are photographed on infrared film or displayed on a video screen. While many doctors say it is as accurate as mammography, others feel the two tests should be used together, since one can detect tumors the other does not. This test, too, does not use ionizing radiation, eliminating that risk factor. At the present time, many health insurance plans will not reimburse a patient for this test.

Recently, thermography has been applied to the evaluation of spinal cord, muscle, and nerve damage. It has been used in legal disputes to offer "objective" evidence of a claimed injury—especially one involving soft tissue (muscles, ligaments, etc.) and "whiplash." The heat patterns are also claimed to help diagnose hidden infections, arthritis, and spinal slipped disks. Thermography has also been used to graphically demonstrate areas that a patient perceives as painful or irritated, based on blood flow patterns. And it is used in allergy testing of black patients in whom **Skin Reactions** are sometimes difficult to identify.

When performed: To aid in diagnosing breast masses; when thrombus is suspected; when other vascular conditions exist such as arterial circulation deficiencies, either from a nerve problem or as a direct defect (blood clot); to ascertain skin and adjacent tissue status (as in instances of possible gangrene).

Normal values: There are no strictly normal values except in relation to other tissue; temperature response should reflect the type of tissue and the blood supply of the tissue being tested.

Abnormal values: Any unexpected change in tissue temperature in relation to surrounding tissue is considered abnormal.

Risk factors: None.

Pain/discomfort: None.

Cost: The fee is $25 to $100, depending on the part of the body tested and the time required for temperature evaluation.

Accuracy and significance: Although many doctors believe breast thermography is more accurate than mammography (see **Radiography**), the general conclusion, at this time, is that thermography alone is not a substitute for other, more suitable tests. It only measures the temperature of the breasts, and almost 90 percent of women with normal breasts will show a change, or increase, in temperature in one breast. It is, however, considered a significant screening device for breast disease. When used to test other parts of the body, its chief value is as a confirmation of other, related test results. Another significant fact is that thermography has been used by judges and juries as a basis for awarding money to individuals claiming pain from injuries. In general, thermography is considered to be about 75 percent accurate.

THIAMIN (Vitamin B_1)

Vitamin B_1 (thiamin or thiamine) deficiency occurs most commonly in people with alcoholism and whose diet consists mainly of polished rice. High-carbohydrate diets may also cause vitamin B_1 deficiency. Thiamin is found in large amounts in yeast, meats, eggs, whole grains, and beans. Because this vitamin is not stored in the body, it must be replenished daily.

Beriberi is a specific disease caused by vitamin B_1 deficiency. Symptoms include cardiovascular irregularities (palpitation with gallop rhythm, abnormal electrocardiogram, venous pressure elevation, shortness of breath, edema), emotional irritability, loss of memory, anxiety, sluggish gastrointestinal activity, weakness, loss of ankle-jerk and knee-jerk reflexes, and inflammation of peripheral nerves. Both urine and blood can be analyzed for thiamin levels. Red blood cell enzymes can also indicate thiamin levels.

When performed: Whenever there is nervous system disease—loss of sensations (touch) or muscle problems; with undiagnosed heart disease or unexplained edema (water retention).

Normal values: The normal range of thiamin in whole blood is 1.5 to 4 mcg per 100 ml. Normal urine levels range from 25 to 75 mcg per 100 ml.

Abnormal values: Lower-than-normal values in either blood or urine indicate vitamin B_1 deficiency. Vomiting and diarrhea can also cause temporary B_1 deficiency.

Risk factors: Negligible (see general risk factors for blood testing).

Pain/discomfort: Minimal (see general pain/discomfort factors for blood testing).

Cost: From $30 to $50.

Accuracy and significance: Although the test can show abnormal values in a variety of conditions, its particular significance lies in helping a doctor diagnose the cause of neuritis, irritability, and hallucinations by linking them with poor dietary habits and/or alcoholism. It is about 80 percent accurate.

Note: Until recently, biotin, one of the B-complex vitamins, was rarely tested for; it is abundant in food, and should it be lacking, the normal bacteria in the intestine could manufacture it. But a lack of this vitamin has lately been noticed in people taking large doses of antibiotics (which kill the intestinal bacteria) and in those eating a large amount of egg whites (a substance in egg whites prevents biotin from being utilized). Its presence is now tested for in infants with convulsions, in alcoholics, and where metabolic imbalance cannot be explained by routine testing.

THORACENTESIS

Thoracentesis is the removal of fluid from the space around the lungs. Normally, no fluid is present. When evidence of fluid is found, usually after **Radiography** (X-ray) or **Ultrasound** testing of the chest, a small needle is inserted between the ribs (the X-ray shows exactly where), and the liquid is removed for further study to isolate bacteria, to look for blood cells, to perform a **Cytology** test, and to perform various chemical tests for enzymes, glucose, and proteins. Because coughing can cause difficulty, a cough-suppressant medicine is usually given to the patient just prior to the test. At times, thoracentesis is also performed to remove large amounts of fluid and thus make breathing easier. Afterward, another chest X-ray is taken to make sure the lung did not collapse as a result of the test.

Pericardiocentesis is the removal of an abnormal amount of fluid from the sac around the heart as a means of uncovering the causes of this condition (e.g., cancer); it has a 75 percent accuracy rate and is considered more risky than thoracentesis.

Arthrocentesis is the removal of fluid from a joint space (see **Synovial Fluid**).

Paracentesis is the removal of fluid from the peritoneal cavity (the sac in the abdomen that holds the intestines). Normally, an accumulation of fluid does not exist in the peritoneal cavity, but when it does (called ascites), it indicates disease. A needle is inserted through the abdominal wall and the fluid withdrawn. Studies similar to thoracentesis are performed; ascites usually results from cancer, liver disease, and infections.

When performed: Whenever a patient has breathing difficulties; when a chest X-ray shows fluid around the lungs; when chest infection, fungus, or cancer is suspected; with heart or kidney failure causing edema; in certain forms of arthritis and rheumatoid disease; in certain bleeding-tendency diseases.

Normal values: There should be no measurable amount of fluid in the lung area.

Abnormal values: Any amount of fluid, called an effusion, is abnormal. Very low glucose levels in pleural (lung) fluid indicate rheumatoid diseases. Increased white blood cells in the fluid are found with cancer and infections. Increased **Lactic Dehydrogenase (LDH)** is almost always found with lung cancer. Increased **Amylase** suggests disease of the pancreas. Increased protein usually signifies an infectious or hemorrhagic process. Decreased protein usually indicates heart, kidney, or liver failure.

Risk factors: See general risk factors for catheter and needle insertion. When performing thoracentesis, especially when testing for fluid around the heart, the needle must be connected to an electrocardiograph in order to observe that the needle does not touch the heart.

Pain/discomfort: See general pain/discomfort factors for catheter and needle insertion.

Cost: A simple thoracentesis for removal of fluid is from $35 to $100. When chemical studies are performed on the fluid, the cost depends on the particular tests.

Accuracy and significance: The test is 80 percent accurate, the presence of any fluid is a positive indication of disease. It is not always significant enough, however, to diagnose a specific disease condition.

THORN, see *Cortisol*

THROAT CULTURE, see *Culture*

THROMBIN TIME, see *Partial Thromboplastin Time*

THROMBOCYTE, see *Platelet Count*

THROMBOPLASTIN, see *Partial Thromboplastin Time*

THROMBOSIS, see *Plethysmography; Radiography*

THRUSH, see *Agglutination*

THYMOL TURBIDITY (Thymol Flocculation)

Thymol turbidity is a test of liver function. The patient should avoid fatty foods and fatty liquids (milk, ice cream sodas) for at least 12 hours before the test. Blood is collected from a vein, and the serum is added to thymol, a phenol chemical from the oil of thyme; the degree of turbidity (cloudiness) is then measured. The **Cephalin Flocculation** test is usually performed along with thymol turbidity to discriminate between various liver diseases.

When performed: When there is suspicion of liver disease; to distinguish between the various causes of jaundice; to follow the progress of treatment for liver disease.

Normal values: Normally, the serum exhibits less than 5 measurable units of turbidity.

Abnormal values: Thymol turbidity is increased in certain liver diseases such as hepatitis (it may be normal in cirrhosis).
Risk factors: Negligible (see general risk factors for blood testing).
Pain/discomfort: Minimal (see general pain/discomfort factors for blood testing).
Cost: From $5 to $8.

Some doctors consider this test outmoded, and it is possible that a health insurance company or government-sponsored medical program will not reimburse the doctor or patient for the cost of the test.

Accuracy and significance: While a positive test may indicate liver disease, the test is only about 50 percent accurate and not sufficiently significant to diagnose a specific form of liver dysfunction. There are more effective and specific tests to detect and identify liver conditions.

THYMOSIN, see *Acquired Immunodeficiency Syndrome*

THYROCALCITONIN, see *Calcitonin*

THYROID FUNCTION

There are a great many ways to assess how the thyroid gland is functioning. The primary tests consist of measuring the amounts of triiodothyronine (T_3) and thyroxine (T_4), both of which comprise the thyroid hormone. The hormone is made by the thyroid gland from tyrosine (an amino acid from protein) and iodine (which can enter the body through the skin and lungs as well as by diet). T_3 is four times as powerful as T_4, and only about half as much T_3 as T_4 is made each day. It is believed that T_3 is the "true" thyroid hormone, while T_4 may be a precursor of it.

Thyroid hormone is essential for normal growth and development, control of oxygen metabolism (energy), and production of other hormones such as the sex hormones and insulin. Thyroid hormone components are usually bound to serum proteins, but unbound, or free, T_4 is sometimes measured; free T_4 parallels T_4 except when certain drugs (oral contraceptives) are taken. T_3 and T_4 concentrations are measured directly in the serum. T_3 is also measured by its "uptake" (T_3U), which also shows how much thyroxine is already bound to serum proteins. A reverse T_3 test (rT_3) to detect a third thyroid hormone can be performed to determine if an abnormal thyroid-function finding might come from drugs or a serious illness unrelated to thyroid function. Another commonly performed test of thyroid function is thyroxine-binding globulin (TBG), a measure of the major serum proteins to which T_3 and T_4 attach themselves. At least two different tests must be performed to understand the specific cause of thyroid disease so that appropriate treatment may be prescribed.

Other thyroid-function tests that may be performed, usually when the tests described above are not conclusive, include the long-acting thyroid stimulator test (LATS), now also known as the thyrotropin-binding inhibitory immunoglobulin test, which is performed on babies whose mothers have thyroid disease, and various tests to detect thyroid autoantibodies (antithyroglobulin antibody, or ATA, and thyroid microsomal antibody, or TMA), which are produced when the thyroid gland acts as if it were infected and the body's immune protection system turns against itself in response.

When cancer or nodules are suspected, a radioactive iodine screening test is performed (see **Nuclear Scanning**).

In the thyroid stimulation test (TSH), the patient is given pituitary gland thyroid-stimulating hormone; by observing its effect on the thyroid, the physician can determine if thyroid problems are coming from the pituitary gland rather than the thyroid itself. An older test, rarely used today, is the protein-bound iodine (PBI), which essentially measures thyroxine (T_4) amounts (but not as accurately as the newer direct T_4 measurements). The simplest routine chemical confirmation test of thyroid function is **Cholesterol**.

The **Basal Metabolic Rate** (BMR), one of the first tests devised for thyroid function, is based on a different measurement principle from the usual thyroid-function tests (oxygen consumption rather than measurement of chemicals in the blood). The BMR is used when the more sophisticated thyroid-function tests cannot be performed (for example, when laboratory facilities are not available or when the patient has taken, or been in contact with, too much iodine to allow proper chemical measurement).

In the Achilles reflex (ankle-jerk) test, or photomotography, the heel tendon that moves the foot downward is struck with a rubber hammer. The force of the reflex activity of the foot and the time it takes the tendon to react are considered measures of thyroid gland activity.

The neonatal hypothyroidism test measures the amount of thyroid hormone in the newborn infant. Diagnosis of cretinism at birth allows treatment to prevent one form of mental retardation.

Blood is taken from a vein for the chemical tests, and the serum is tested. Certain tests may be performed by using a drop of blood from the fingertip or earlobe. The tests can give false values if the patient has had any sort of iodine test in the six previous months (gallbladder X-rays, kidney X-rays; bronchograms, etc., using contrast dye) or has had excessive iodine in the diet for the previous month. Previous radioactive tracer tests can also cause erroneous results. Some thyroid-function tests (PBI, radioactive iodine) may be performed on urine, saliva, and feces.

When performed: Whenever there is suspicion of a thyroid disorder; when other hormone disease is suspected; in all cases of depression; to follow the progress of treatment of thyroid disease; to screen newborn children for cretinism, or congenital hypothyroidism, which can cause mental retardation, nerve problems, and growth inhibition. All states now require thyroid testing at birth, but some states do not enforce the law when parents object.

Normal values:
Free T_3: 100 to 250 ng per 100 ml.
rT_3: 30 to 60 ng per 100 ml.
T_3U: 25 percent to 35 percent.
T_4: 2.8 to 6.4 mcg per 100 ml.
Free T_4: 3 to 5 ng per 100 ml.
TBG: 10 to 26 mcg of T_4 per 100 ml.
PBI: 3.5 to 8.5 mcg per 100 ml.
LATS and thyroid antibodies are not normally present in the serum. Radioactive

iodine uptake should range from 10 percent to 20 percent in the first hour and no more than 50 percent in 24 hours.

Abnormal values: Hyperthyroidism (Graves' disease, thyrotoxicosis, toxic goiter) usually shows increased T_3, T_4, radioactive iodine, and PBI; low cholesterol values; a normal amount of TBG; and low TSH (see **Exophthalmometer**). Hypothyroidism (goiter, cretinism, pituitary disorder) usually shows decreased T_3, T_4, radioactive iodine, and PBI; high cholesterol values; an increased amount of TBG; and an elevated TSH. Thyroiditis (inflammation of the gland) may exist with hyperthyroidism or hypothyroidism, and the tests reflect the way the thyroid is (or is not) functioning. Tumors of the thyroid (cancers, cysts) may also alter the tests, depending on how the growth affects function. Certain drugs such as estrogens and contraceptive pills will increase T_4, TBG, and PBI. Male hormones and other steroid drugs, as well as Dilantin, will cause low T_4, TBG, and PBI. While T_4 changes with some drug use, free T_4 stays normal. Pregnancy can cause false-abnormal values such as elevated T_3, T_4, and TBG. Chronic kidney disease causes low T_3, T_4, and TBG along with an elevated T_3U. Excessive exposure to iodine increases PBI and decreases the radioactive iodine uptake. The taking of thyroid preparations usually increases all values. Large doses of aspirin, antiarthritic drugs, and anticoagulant drugs can alter thyroid function tests, as can many other pharmaceuticals such as oral contraceptives.

Risk factors: Negligible (see general risk factors for blood testing).

Pain/discomfort: Minimal (see general pain/discomfort factors for blood testing).

Cost: T_4 and T_3 uptake tests are $5 to $50 per test. One, and sometimes both, are occasionally included in **Comprehensive Multiple Test Screening** panels, which range from $7 to $42. Tests for free T_3 and free T_4 are $20 to $40 each. The TBG test is $22 to $50. A thyroid stimulation hormone test is $25 to $61; the PBI, from $10 to $27. Other specialized thyroid tests range from $20 to $100, with the LATS test averaging $150. Antithyroid antibodies testing averages $150; reverse T_3 averages $30.

Some doctors consider the protein-bound iodine test outmoded, and it is possible that a health insurance company or government-sponsored medical program will not reimburse the doctor or patient for the cost of the test.

Accuracy and significance: Most doctors believe that more than one abnormal thyroid function test result must be obtained to help diagnose thyroid dysfunction. They also find that the most accurate single screening test for overall thyroid function is the serum free thyroxin (T_4); the most sensitive test for hyperthyroidism (overactive thyroid gland) is the triiodothyronine (T_3); and the most sensitive test for hypothyroidism (underactive thyroid gland) is the thyroid-stimulating hormone test (TSH). Furthermore, the majority of doctors believe that thyroid function tests have no real significance in patients without two or more clinical signs of thyroid disease (heat intolerance, tremor, dry skin, hair loss, changes in heart rhythm). Thyroid-function tests are positive in less than half of one per cent of those patients without signs and symptoms. The remaining thyroid-function tests are merely more sophisticated measurements to confirm or support a diagnosis. In general, thyroid tests are 85 percent accurate.

THYROID SCAN, see *Nuclear Scanning*

THYROTROPIN-BINDING INHIBITORY IMMUNOGLOBULIN, see *Thyroid Function*

THYROXINE (T$_4$), see *Thyroid Function*

THYROXINE-BINDING GLOBULIN (TBG), see *Thyroid Function*

TICK FEVER, see *Complement Fixation*

TICKING WATCH, see *Hearing Function*

TIDAL VOLUME, see *Pulmonary Function*

TIMED VITAL CAPACITY, see *Pulmonary Function*

TINE, see *Skin Reaction*

TOCOPHEROLS (Vitamin E)

Deficiency of vitamin E (really a group of related tocopherol oil compounds, with the alpha form the most active) is rare in the healthy adult who eats a normal diet. However, people who have increased their consumption of polyunsaturated oils (corn, safflower, cottonseed, or soybean) often are found to have vitamin E deficiency, which can cause the destruction of red blood cells. Vitamin E deficiency is known to cause anemia in infants and can cause infertility problems (inability to become pregnant). The vitamin does not have anything to do with sexual performance or potency, as has been erroneously reported. Vitamin E seems to help prevent tissue damage from smog. Blood is taken from a vein, and the plasma is examined.

The erythrocyte (red blood cell) hemolysis test is an indirect, but easier-to-perform measure of vitamin E in the body. Red blood cells are destroyed in proportion to the lack of vitamin E. When newborn infants show anemia, especially if it is associated with jaundice, a peroxide hemolysis test (using hydrogen peroxide to measure the amount of **Red Blood Cells** that are destroyed by the peroxide) may be performed to see whether a vitamin E deficiency is the underlying cause.

When performed: When anemia is present; when smog is a severe lung irritant; when unexplained infertility exists; in malnutrition; when patients are on diets containing excessive polyunsaturated fatty acids.

Normal values: The tocopherol level is normally 0.5 mg per 100 ml of plasma.

Abnormal values: Less than 0.5 mg per 100 ml of plasma causes red blood cell destruction. Higher-than-normal values may also produce symptoms. People who take excessive amounts of vitamin E supplements have been reported to have swelling, particularly of the face and the breasts. Many plastic surgeons prohibit the taking of vitamin E supplements for a month prior to cosmetic surgery.

Risk factors: Negligible (see general risk factors for blood testing).

Pain/discomfort: Minimal (see general pain/discomfort factors for blood testing).

Cost: From $25 to $30.

Accuracy and significance: Although the test is about 85 percent accurate for the body's vitamin E content, the chance of there being a disease causing a deficiency of vitamin E is extremely rare, other than in premature infants or full-term babies who are markedly underweight. The test is a significant aid in diagnosing a cause of anemia in infants.

TOMOGRAPHY, see *Computerized Tomography; Radiography*

TONE DECAY, see *Hearing Function*

TONOMETRY

Tonometry is the specific measurement of the intraocular pressure (pressure of the fluid within the eyeball). It is used primarily to test for glaucoma, although there are rare instances of intraocular hypertension without glaucoma. Most glaucoma is of the chronic open-angle type, which does not occur until late in life and can generally be treated medically. The typical symptoms of glaucoma are poor vision (blurring), usually in only one eye at first, followed by gradual restriction of the **Visual Field.**

A Schiotz tonometer is placed on the pupil after a drop of anesthetic has been applied to the eye, and a gauge records the resistance of the eye to the slight pressure applied. The tonometer translates the resistance into millimeters (mm) of mercury (Hg). The procedure is similar to applying a contact lens to the eye. In another technique, called applanation, a drop of dye is placed on the eye, and the slight pressure is applied and measured while the eye is observed through a special microscope. Tonometry should always be performed in a cool, dark room or false-negative values will be recorded, missing the patient with glaucoma.

When the routine test result is equivocal, procedures to increase eye pressure are performed. In the water provocative test, the patient drinks a full quart of water at one time; the intraocular pressure is measured 30, 45, and 60 minutes later. If the pressure rises more than 8 mm Hg during that time, glaucoma is a reasonable diagnosis. In tonography, constant, gentle pressure is applied to the eye (using a special tonometer) for four minutes; the pressure should cause a decrease in the measured tension in normal individuals. If it does not decrease, glaucoma is considered to be the most likely diagnosis.

Proper technique also calls for measuring ocular pressure in response to posture; there may be a change in pressure values when going from a sitting to a lying-down position and vice versa. Pressure is usually greater when reclining, and variations can help confirm or refute a diagnosis of glaucoma.

The Seidel test places the patient in a dark room for one hour. An increase in eye pressure during that time means that the ocular fluid does not escape when the pupils are dilated, as it normally should. A somewhat similar test is performed by dropping the drug homatropine into the eye. Homatropine causes the pupil to dilate. After an hour, the eye is checked for any increase in pressure; an increase indicates glaucoma.

The latest method of tonometry uses the projection of an inert gas on the pupil; this device not only records the pressure within the eyeball but also records, on a graph, the pulsations within the eye. The graphic changes are also recorded with the patient in different positions. This technique is painless and seems to cause the least amount of apprehension in patients. Each reading takes only five seconds. Differences in pressure between each eye are more readily apparent.

Another measure of pressure within the eye is called ophthalmodynamometry; in this test, the blood pressure of the ophthalmic artery (which supplies the retina of the eye) is measured with an instrument that applies pressure to the eyeball—similar to tonometry. While pressure is being applied (an anesthetic is used so there is no pain or discomfort), the arteries inside the eye are observed, first for pulsations and then for cessation of those pulsations (similar to measuring **Blood Pressure**). The test is used to help diagnose stroke (decreased circulation to the brain) as well as vision problems limited to one eye.

When performed: Tonometry is routinely performed on individuals over 40 years of age and on younger people whenever there is any vision difficulty (especially blurring) or any history of glaucoma in the family. It is also performed after any eye infection, after eye injury, with diabetes, and when there are thyroid problems.

Normal values: Normally, the intraocular pressure measures between 10 and 20 mm Hg. Many physicians, through experience, can place fingers over the closed eye and the bony ridge above the eye and accurately detect normal intraocular pressure (less than 20 mm Hg).

Abnormal values: Lower-than-normal intraocular pressure (less than 10 mm Hg) is rare and is usually due to an infection or sometimes follows surgery. A false lower value may occur in patients taking diuretics. Repeated pressure readings between 20 and 30 mm Hg (these readings must be taken several times; one or two tests are insufficient for diagnosis) indicate ocular hypertension and a presumption of glaucoma. Readings greater than 30 mm Hg are almost always diagnostic of glaucoma, especially when accompanied by certain changes in visual field. Many drugs can cause increased intraocular pressure, which can then lead to glaucoma. Drugs that dilate the pupils, steroids, anticholinergics (such as used for bowel and bladder relaxation), antidepressants, antihistamines, muscle relaxants, and oral contraceptives are particularly dangerous, especially with patients who have a family history of glaucoma.

Risk factors: There is the possibility of scratching the surface of the eye should the test be performed carelessly, but this happens very rarely. There is also the remote possibility of an eye infection should the instrument not be absolutely sterile.

Pain/discomfort: Although the eye is usually anesthetized prior to testing, many patients find the touching of the eyeball quite uncomfortable.

Cost: Generally, there is no charge for the test when it is part of a routine physical examination.

Accuracy and significance: Although tonometry testing is 90 percent accurate in determining the pressure inside the eyeball, research has shown that, as with **Blood Pressure**, any apprehension caused by being in the doctor's office or any nervousness elicited by the test procedure itself can raise eye pressure to the point of causing a false-positive result. Thus, this test must be performed several times and after the patient has become at ease while the measurements are being taken before a positive diagnosis of glaucoma can be made. Other studies have revealed that close to 90 percent of people who do show higher-than-normal intraocular pressure do not have glaucoma; and one-third of all patients with a proven diagnosis of glaucoma do not have persistent abnormal eye pressure. The tests can be significant when, properly performed, they do detect glaucoma in its early stage, allowing treatment to prevent vision impairment.

TORCH

TORCH is not a specific test but an acronym for a group of blood tests performed on a pregnant woman and/or a newborn child to ascertain the presence of antibodies to five conditions: **Toxoplasmosis, Rubella** (German measles), **Cytomegalovirus,** and **Herpes** simplex virus **I** and **II.** These infections are known to cause a variety of physical and mental impairments in babies—blindness, blood abnormalities, deafness, enlargement of the spleen, hepatitis, mental retardation, and other birth defects. The principle of the tests is related to **Agglutination, Complement Fixation,** and fluorescent antibody studies. Many physicians feel that all the tests comprising TORCH are unnecessary and that many laboratories performing the tests have produced unreliable results. With most women, the rubella test is sufficient. Should TORCH tests be advised, the doctor should be assured that the kits used to perform the tests have been tested and approved by the Centers for Disease Control (CDC) of the Public Health Service. All the tests together can cost from $50 to $150.

TOTAL BILIRUBIN, see *Bilirubin*

TOTAL CHOLESTEROL, see *Cholesterol*

TOTAL LIPIDS, see *Lipids*

TOTAL PROTEINS, see *Albumin/Globulin*

TOURNIQUET, see *Capillary Fragility*

TOURNIQUET TEST FOR VARICOSE VEINS

The varicose vein incompetency tests are performed to determine if leg varicosities are caused by diseases of the deep veins as opposed to problems of the superficial veins (which can be seen on the surface). The patient's leg is elevated to empty the veins, and a tourniquet is applied in various areas (above and below the knee, thigh, and calf). The patient stands (Trendelenberg test) and/or walks (Perthes test), and the leg is observed to ascertain how long it takes for the superficial veins to fill.

When performed: When varicose veins cause fatigue and discomfort; when there is lower-leg dermatitis or ulcer; to discover whether the varicosities are from some condition other than vein disease (such as pregnancy or abdominal tumor); when surgery is anticipated on the surface veins (to ascertain that after surgery the deep veins will be competent, or able to carry blood).

Normal values: When the deep veins are normal, the superficial veins fill 30 seconds after the leg is lowered (with the tourniquet still in place).

Abnormal values: If, when the leg is lowered and the veins fill immediately, the connecting veins between the deep and superficial systems are not adequate, surgery will be deemed to be of no help. If, while the tourniquet is on, there is cramping or immediate filling while walking, there will probably be no benefit from surgery.

Risk factors: None.

Pain/discomfort: None.

Cost: There is usually no charge for this test when it is part of an office examination.

Accuracy and significance: The tests are 90 percent accurate in helping a doctor diagnose the cause of varicose veins; they are particularly significant in predicting the success of surgery.

Note: Although it has the same name, this test is not the same as the tourniquet test for **Capillary Fragility**.

TOXEMIA OF PREGNANCY, see *Rollover*

TOXIC CHEMICAL EXPOSURE

Exposure to industrial chemicals (such as paints, polishes, disinfectants, cleaning fluids, deodorants, glues, and inks), pesticides (such as DDT, chlordane, and dieldrin), herbicides, and chlorinated phenols (such as PCB and one of its related compounds, dioxin) is increasingly causing disease, disability, and even death. Until recently, it was very difficult to diagnose the specific cause of bizarre symptoms that—while seemingly related to diseases of the liver, kidneys, heart, and bone marrow—did not conform to the usual pathology of those organs. It is now known that exposure to toxic chemicals—at times, after brief contact, but more likely after prolonged proximity, albeit involving minute quantities—can be the cause of many different illnesses; some are new diseases, unrecognized in the past, and some, such as cancer, are old diseases that are initiated by the chemicals.

PCBs stands for polychlorinated biphenyls, the chemicals used in the manufacture of electrical transformers, hydraulic fluids, plastics, paints, inks, and adhesives, to name but a very few. Two mass PCB poisonings from food have already occurred in two cities. New York City has warned against the eating of striped bass from adjacent waters and, in 1985, banned striped bass commercial fishing in the area because of the large amounts of PCB found in the fish. A particular danger from this chemical is the possibility of stillbirths, abnormal fetal skin pigmentation, and other fetal problems when pregnant women are exposed to it. Signs and symptoms that have been observed in people after eating food contaminated with PCB include headache, weakness, numbness, joint pains, eyelid edema and vision problems, jaundice, menstrual changes, anemia, and acnelike skin rashes. Some insecticides can cause a decreased immunity (similar to **Acquired Immunodeficiency Syndrome**) that allows infections and even cancers to take hold much more easily than usual. Almost all cause some form of skin disease.

It has only been in the recent past that doctors have begun looking to cigarette smoke, motor vehicle exhaust fumes, see **Carbon monoxide,** and the various chemicals that are part of food processing and the manufacture of other consumer products as a common cause of sickness. Few people can avoid some detrimental environmental contact—whether in air, water, food, as part of housing construction, or related to waste disposal—and the dangers associated with toxic chemicals are even greater to those who are employed in or have direct contact with industries that manufacture, transport, or apply those chemicals. Now, when a doctor does think about a toxic chemical as the cause of an illness—and this is still altogether too rarely, unfortunately—it is possible to test a patient's blood to detect if trace amounts of a chemical are present. This information, coupled with the patient's signs and symptoms,, may be the revealing factor to explain a previously unexplainable disease. Some of these chemicals can cause ill health when they are present in the body in only one part per trillion (equivalent to one tiny grain of salt being dissolved in all the water contained in an olympic-size swimming pool).

The first testing facility to develop the means of uncovering toxic chemical exposure illness, Enviro-Health System, now offers the medical profession four different test batteries: the general volatile screening test, which can reveal the presence of 12 different organic chemicals in the body; the chlorinated pesticide screening test, which detects 19 pesticides; the chlorinated phenols screening test for PCP and some other fungicides and defoliants; and the phenoxy acid screening test for herbicides (there now are other toxic analysis laboratories). Testing for malathion (an organic phosphate insecticide) can be performed by measuring **Cholinesterase;** some doctors also use this test to see if carbamates (a herbicide that can cause skin and kidney disease) are the reason for a mysterious illness. In many states, a pesticide-related illness must be reported to the health authorities. This is because the recognition of one individual with such a condition could be the clue to uncovering the cause of illness in others who may have been exposed to the same toxic chemicals. (Also see **Mercury**.)

When performed: Primarily when there is evidence of exposure—employment within an exposed environment; improperly performed insecticide spraying in home or commercial settings; proximity to chemical-manufacturing, mining, or construction sites. Patients who are worried about possible chemical exposure should know that the law in many states requires that the chemical names of all potentially toxic substances used in any locality be made public. When a patient has signs and symptoms that cannot be explained by the most common causes, the physician must consider toxic exposure as a possibility.

Normal values: It is not normal for any amount of a toxic chemical to be found in the blood. The problem is that so many people have been exposed to so many of these chemicals that it is now usual, if not normal, for traces to be detected. Therefore, when testing, the testing facility must take into account the effect of prevailing expected exposure in reporting its "normal value."

Abnormal values: As explained above, while any evidence of a toxic chemical is not normal, the reporting facility attempts to evaluate the amount found in light of the habitual prevalent exposure, when known. The goal is to rule in, or rule out, toxic exposure as the sole cause of the illness; only the doctor can come to that conclusion—using toxic chemical screening tests as a guide.

Risk factors: Negligible (see general risk factors for blood testing).

Pain/discomfort: Minimal (see general pain/discomfort factors for blood testing).

Cost: At the present time, the doctor is billed from $80 to $132 for one screening test group, depending on which of the four screening batteries he orders; he may add on an additional charge for drawing the blood and sending it to the test facility.

Accuracy and significance: The quantity of toxic chemicals reported to be found in the blood is considered 90 percent accurate despite the miniscule amounts of such chemicals. Usually, the doctor is also told the levels of the chemical found in most people the laboratory has previously tested and, if possible, the same figures for individuals in the patient's area. In addition, the laboratory reports the levels considered to be dangerous—both in the environment and in the individual. Blood must be submitted in special collection kits, and the results are usually available within 48 hours. The significance of the test result depends solely on the doctor's interpretation when applied to the patient's problem.

TOXICOLOGY, see *Drug Abuse; Drug Monitoring*

TOXIC SHOCK SYNDROME—ASSOCIATED STAPHYLOCCUS, see *Agglutination*

TOXOCARIASIS

The larvae of the common roundworm of the dog, whose scientific name is Toxocara canis, produce the disease called toxocariasis, also called visceral larva migrans (VLM) because the worm larvae migrate throughout the body (to the brain, eyes, heart, kidneys, liver, lungs, intestines). Generally, the infestation is found in young children who play on the ground, in grass, or in dirt where dogs, especially puppies, defecate. The animal's feces can contain the eggs of the worms, which contaminate the ground. When the child plays in the area and puts his fingers in his mouth, the eggs enter the digestive system, become larvae, and subsequently infect the child's organs. The most common symptoms are a pneumonialike illness, sometimes imitating asthma, an enlarged liver, and an extremely elevated number of white blood cells called eosinophiles (see **Blood Cell Differential**). The symptoms can last for years before being diagnosed; the disease can cause nerve damage, blindness, and even death. Until recently, it was extremely difficult to diagnose toxocariasis; at the very least, it required a liver **Biopsy.** Now there is an **ELISA,** a test similar to **Agglutination,** which can prove the diagnosis when the untoward symptoms appear. Blood from a vein is tested.

When performed: Whenever a patient, particularly a very young child has a chronic cough, recurrent fever, and the neurological signs associated with an enlarged liver; in patients with an extremely high eosinophile-type white blood cell count that cannot be explained; in children whose symptoms imitate asthma but who do not respond to asthma treatment.

Normal values: No antigen-antibody reaction to the worm eggs should be noted.

Abnormal values: Evidence of antibody reaction with a titer greater than 1,000 (a positive reaction in a very weak, dilute solution).

Risk factors: Negligible (see general risk factors for blood testing).

Pain/discomfort: Minimal (see general pain/discomfort factors for blood testing).

Cost: From $15 to $20.

Accuracy and significance: The test has been shown to be at least 90 percent accurate when performed on those suspected of having the disease. It is particularly significant now that the infestation is known to be more prevalent than once believed. It is also valuable as an aid in identifying other eye problems that imitate toxocariasis. Furthermore, it can help to differentiate among other worm infestations, such as those from dog hookworms, which enter the body through the feet and migrate to the lungs and intestines.

TOXOPLASMOSIS

Toxoplasmosis is an infection caused by a parasite. A number of doctors consider it the most common infectious disease, although another parasitic infestation, *giardiosis*, is at least as common. For unexplained reasons, the domestic cat is the primary source of the microorganism, and infected cats, while showing no symptoms of the condition, will still excrete the parasite in their feces. Should people or animals have contact with contaminated ground, they, too, can become infected. Raw or partially cooked meat from infected animals—steak tartare, for example—can also transmit the disease. (Sufficient cooking kills the parasite.) Symptoms and signs include nerve and muscle damage, lymph gland swelling, eye problems, and heart muscle damage. The most serious complication comes when a pregnant woman contracts the disease, shows no symptoms, and passes it on to her fetus. The consequences include spontaneous abortion, stillbirth, or a child born with the disease and all its complications, including encephalitis or physical birth defects. Tests to detect the disease include **Complement Fixation,** fluorescent antibody (see **Agglutination**), and the Sabin-Feldman dye test performed on blood taken from a vein.

When performed: As part of the TORCH screening panel for pregnant women and newborn infants; when the disease is suspected because of specific unexplained symptoms (especially those pertaining to the eye, brain, or heart); when a condition resembling infectious mononucleosis (persistent lymph gland swelling) remains undiagnosed.

Normal values: Ideally, no antibodies should be detected; however, because hundreds of millions of people have had some contact with the parasite, small amounts of antibodies can be considered "normal." Therefore, a low antibody titer can be considered within normal limits. It is also considered normal when the measurable antibodies do not increase over a period of time.

Abnormal values: Usually, a titer of 1:256 or more (the higher the titer value, the more antibodies present); titers greater than 1:1,000 are believed to signify active disease. A rise in antibody titers over a period of months, especially in the newborn, is also considered abnormal.

Risk factors: Negligible (see general risk factors for blood testing).

Pain/discomfort: Minimal (see general pain/discomfort factors for blood testing).

Cost: From $25 to $50 for one test. Generally, the test is repeated in two to three weeks; the fee then ranges from $40 to $50 for the pair.

Accuracy and significance: Considered 90 percent accurate in the detection of antibodies. The significance of the test is not quite as high because of the variation in titers found in numbers of people and because different manifestations of the disease produce a broad range of titer levels. The most significant observation is of a child or pregnant woman whose negative titer is suddenly positive; a negative test (a failure to detect any antibodies) usually indicate a lack of the toxoplasma parasite. The Sabin-Feldman test, considered 95 percent accurate, is rarely performed today except in special laboratories because of the dangers to laboratory personnel of working with a live antigen—which is what makes that test so precise.

TPI, see *Syphilis*

TRACER, see *Nuclear Scanning*

TRACHOMA, see *Chlamydia Identification; Complement Fixation*

TRANQUILIZER, see *Barbiturates; Drug Abuse*

TRANSAMINASE, see *Aspartate Aminotransferase*

TRANSAXIAL TOMOGRAPHY, see *Computerized Tomography*

TRANSFERRIN (IRON-BINDING CAPACITY), see *Iron*

TRANSFUSION, see *Typing and Cross-Matching*

TRANSHEPATIC CHOLANGIOGRAPHY, see *Radiography*

TRANSMISSION SPECTROSCOPY, see *Thermography*

TREADMILL, see *Electrocardiogram*

TRENDELENBERG, see *Tourniquet Test for Varicose Veins*

TREPONEMAL PALLIDUM IMMOBILIZATION, see *Syphilis*

TRICHINOSIS, see *Agglutination; Parasite; Skin Reaction*

TRICHOMONAS, see *Parasite; Wet Mount*

TRICOPHYTON, see *Skin Reaction*

TRIGLYCERIDE, see *Lipids*

TRIIODOTHYRONINE (T_3), see *Thyroid Function*

TRIOLEIN, see *Nuclear Scanning*

TRIOLEIN BREATH TEST, see *Lactose Tolerance*

TRUE CHOLINESTERASE, see *Cholinesterase*

TRYPSIN, see *Pancreas Function; Sweat*

TRYPSINOGEN, see *Pancreas Function*

TRYPTOPHAN LOADING, see *Pyridoxine*

TSH, see *Thyroid Function*

T_3/T_4, see *Thyroid Function*

TUBAL PATENCY, see *Rubin*

TUBE DILUTION SUSCEPTIBILITY, see *Culture*

TUBELESS GASTRIC ANALYSIS, see *Gastric Analysis*

TUBERCULIN, see *Skin Reaction*

TULAREMIA, see *Agglutination*

TUMOR MARKERS, see *Cancer*

TUNING FORK

Tuning forks are metal instruments that vibrate when struck, giving off a pure tone of a predetermined number of cycles per second (cps). They are commonly used to tune pianos or other musical instruments. In medicine, tuning forks are used primarily to measure the ability to hear sounds by both air and bone conduction (see **Hearing Function**); they are also used to measure bone conduction sensitivity in other parts of the body as part of a neurological examination. The base of the vibrating tuning fork is placed against a bone area (elbows, knees, ankles), and the sensation is noted by the patient as well as the equalness of the sensation on opposite sides of the body. There are five basic tuning-fork tests for hearing.

Weber: The base of the vibrating tuning fork is placed in the center of the forehead at the hairline, and the patient is asked if he hears the tone better in one ear than the other. Normally, the tone is heard equally in both ears.

Rinné: The tuning fork is vibrated and placed next to each ear opening (for air conduction) and then against the mastoid bone behind the ear (for bone conduction) to see which tone is heard longer. Normally, the tone will be heard much longer via air conduction (through the ear canal).

Schwabach: The physician vibrates the tuning fork and compares his perception of the tone with that of the patient. Assuming the doctor has normal hearing, the perceptions should be about the same.

Stenger: With the patient blindfolded, two tuning forks of the same tone are vibrated about an inch from each ear at the same time. The forks are then moved away from the ears. Normally, the tone is heard in each ear from similar distances. If one ear is bad, the tuning fork will not be heard when it is placed close to that ear.

Teal: When a patient says he cannot hear the tuning fork via air conduction, the Weber test is again performed with the patient blindfolded. On the second trial, a nonvibrating fork is placed against the bone behind the ear and a second, vibrating fork is held a short distance away from that ear. If the patient is really deaf, he will not hear the tone; if he is simulating deafness, he will claim to hear the tone, although he is really hearing the second tuning fork.

Two additional tuning-fork tests that are occasionally performed are, first, the Bing, in which, after the tuning-fork base is applied to the center of the forehead and the patient says it sounds louder in one ear, the outer ear canal of that ear is covered to see if the sound becomes louder or softer. Normally, it becomes louder. The second is the Gelle, in which, after the tuning fork is placed against the mastoid bone, pressure is applied to the eardrum to note if there are any sound changes. Normally, the sound lessens with increased pressure.

When performed: To test hearing function, nerve function, bone conduction; to detect malingering.

Normal values: Each tuning-fork test should be felt or heard equally on both sides of the body. Normal, or expected, results for each hearing test are described above.

Abnormal values: Whenever the vibrations of a tuning fork are not felt or heard, or when the vibrations are perceived differently on one side of the body than on the other side. Abnormal values for specific hearing tests are described above.

Risk factors: None.

Pain/discomfort: None.

Cost: There is usually no charge when the test is part of a routine office examination.

Accuracy and significance: The tests are about 90 percent accurate and are of major value in helping to identify the part of the body that might have nerve problems. Then, too, the combination of all the tuning-fork tests is of great significance in arriving at the cause of ear problems. The Teal test is of value in recognizing malingerers.

24-HOUR AMBULATORY BLOOD PRESSURE MONITORING, see *Blood Pressure*

24-HOUR AMBULATORY ELECTROENCEPHALOGRAM MONITORING, see *Electroencephalogram*

24-HOUR ESOPHAGEAL pH MONITORING, see *Gastroesophageal Reflux*

TWO-STEP TB (TUBERCULIN), see *Skin Reaction*

TYMPANOMETRY

Tympanometry is a test to measure the functioning of the eardrum. Under controlled pressures, tones of different frequency are applied to the external ear (the outer ear canal, which leads to the eardrum) and are monitored by a microphone as differences in pressure are administered. A small plug containing three tiny tubes is inserted into the ear canal, and the pressure as a response to sound is recorded on a graph. The test is twice as effective as direct examination of the ear with an otoscope (looking into the ear) for detecting middle-ear infection (otitis media).

When performed: Primarily in infants and schoolchildren who are not prone to cooperate when being examined directly for otitis media; whenever there is suspicion of middle-ear infection in patients who will not allow direct examination, particularly when a patient has repeated ear infections; when aspiration of the middle-ear chamber (deliberately putting a hole in the eardrum to obtain material for diagnosis) is not possible; whenever allergy is suspected as a cause of ear problems; in children with cleft palates, both before and after repair of the defect.

Normal values: From 10 to 40 millimhos (mmho), depending on the frequency of the tone and pressure applied.

Abnormal values: No matter what the frequency of the tone, the detected mmho is usually reduced in half when there is middle-ear infection or fluid (usually pus) in the middle-ear chamber.

Risk factors: None.

Pain/discomfort: None.

Cost: From $25 to $50.

Accuracy and significance: The test is 90 percent accurate in helping to diagnose infection of the middle ear (the passage from the ear to the back of the nose). It is also significant in diagnosing ear disease in uncooperative children.

TYPE A–TYPE B HEPATITIS, see *Hepatitis*

TYPE A–TYPE B PERSONALITY, see *Jenkins Activity Survey*

TYPHOID FEVER, see *Agglutination*

TYPHUS, see *Agglutination*

TYPING AND CROSS-MATCHING (Blood Grouping)

Typing and cross-matching are performed to determine a person's blood type. Blood may be typed according to the common A, B, AB, and O groups (called the ABO system); the Rh positive and Rh negative groups (called the Rh system, which now has many additional subgroups); the MNS's system; or the Kell system. There are nearly 100 known blood group systems at present. Typing is essentially an **Agglutination** procedure to search for certain antibodies in the blood.

When a transfusion is prescribed by a doctor (usually after severe blood loss or during surgery), knowledge of the type of blood of both the donor and the recipient is not enough. Donor blood may be labeled as the same type as that of the patient, but the two must be specifically cross-matched (mixed) to prevent an incompatible transfusion, which causes hemolysis (destruction of the red blood cells) and can be fatal. Most commonly, the donor's red blood cells (which contain the antigens, or agglutinating-precipitating factor) are tested for any possible reaction to the patient's serum (which contains the antibodies or response to agglutinating-precipitating factor). At times, the blood may also be tested for sickle cells prior to transfusion. Because of the number and variety of blood type groups and subgroups, the test is one of the first to be performed in disputed **Parentage** cases.

When performed: The test is performed whenever a blood transfusion is prescribed. A patient about to have surgery will often have his blood typed and cross-matched with potential donors well ahead of time. It is also performed in disputed **Parentage** cases.

Normal values: There should be no evidence of agglutination or hemolysis when the blood of the donor and the recipient are mixed.

Abnormal values: Any evidence of agglutination when the two different blood samples are mixed indicates incompatibility.

Risk factors: Negligible (see general risk factors for blood testing).

Pain/discomfort: Minimal (see general pain/discomfort factors for blood testing).

Cost: From $5 to $10 for the basic ABO system; when Rh grouping is added, there is usually an additional charge of $5 to $7. When subgroup types are identified, the fee ranges from $10 to $200 or more, depending on the number of different subgroups identified. When a patient's blood is matched to donor blood for transfusion, the charge is $35 to $50 for the first pint; $5 to $10 for each additional pint of blood tested.

Accuracy and significance: Blood typing is 98 percent accurate in identifying blood groups. Its particular significance, in addition to helping identify parentage, is in the matching of blood for transfusion. Every pint of blood used in a transfusion must precisely match the patient's blood. Even though two bloods might belong to the same ABO system and/or Rh system, they could still pertain to different subgroups. Imprecise matching of donor and recipient blood can bring on a transfusion reaction, which might prove fatal.

TYROSINEMIA, see *Aminoaciduria*

TZANCK SMEAR

Until recently, the usual test for **Herpes** has been to isolate the virus from a "blister-like" lesion after specific antibodies have been detected in the patient's blood. But culturing and isolating the virus can take several days, and other, newer forms of testing, such as the use of enzymes and/or fluorescent staining, can, at times, be misleading. Although the Tzanck test was first published in medical journals in 1947, it is only recently being reintroduced as a rapid means of detecting the herpes virus in pregnant women prior to delivery, in patients with immunodeficiency conditions, in medical personnel, and in others where time is of the essence in arriving at a diagnosis. To perform the test, a suspect blister is opened—usually with the point of a scalpel—and then the center of the blister area is scraped with the edge of the scalpel blade. A glass slide is pressed against the raw surface, and the residue on the glass slide is stained and examined under the microscope. Certain fairly distinct cells, when present, are considered to indicate the herpes virus as the cause of the condition.

When performed: In particular, on a woman about to give birth where there is a suspicion of herpes; the test can help the doctor decide whether the woman should deliver normally or by cesarean section—to protect the baby from direct contact with genital herpes lesions. To help differentiate herpes from other blisterlike lesions. On patients whose immune system is so defective that an infection could be fatal.

Normal values: No evidence of the unique cells that are usually present in a herpes lesion.

Abnormal values: The presence of the special cells seemingly unique to a herpes infection.

Risk factors: Very little for the patient; the scraping of the lesion rarely even causes bleeding. There can, however, be a risk of transmitting the disease to others, notably the medical personnel performing, or otherwise involved in, the test.

Pain/discomfort: Very little; usually, the blisters themselves are more uncomfortable than the scraping of them.

Cost: Since the test only takes a few minutes, when performed in the doctor's office, the charge ranges from $10 to $50, depending mostly on the doctor's specialty (status). If performed in a hospital, or if the specimen must be sent to a laboratory, the cost averages from $50 to $100.

Accuracy and significance: Although there is some disagreement among physicians, it does appear that the test is at least 80 percent accurate. Much depends on use of the proper technique in obtaining the specimen for staining (tests on the crusts of the blisters were much less accurate) and where the blisters are located (those around the mouth give more positive results than genital lesions). If a patient has had outbreaks of blisters in the past, the test is much more accurate. Its significance is in its lower cost and faster results.

U

UCG, see *Pregnancy*

ULCER, see *Gastrin*

ULTRASOUND

Ultrasound is a diagnostic technique that uses sound waves to create a "picture" of certain areas of the body. The technique is similar to an X-ray, but without any of the dangers of radiation exposure (although the absolute safety of ultrasound is also being questioned). High-frequency sound waves (above the range of human hearing) are directed toward a body organ or cavity. The sound echoes back from the selected organ or tissue to form the "picture." The procedure is performed with a transducer (a microphonelike instrument that emits sounds and also detects the echo), which is touched to the body over the area to be studied. Before the transducer is used, a coating of mineral oil is applied to the skin to prevent any air from coming between the body and the instrument. The results may be reproduced in graphic form (resembling an electrocardiograph record) or as shadow illustrations; the latter are especially important for determining the exact location of the fetus during pregnancy (see **Amniocentesis**). The **Echocardiogram** also uses ultrasound as a measuring technique.

At times, sound waves that are reflected back from moving objects (such as the heartbeat or blood flow through an artery or vein) show a change in frequency with changes in the speed of movement. This is called the "Doppler effect," and measurement is known as Doppler ultrasonography. Such tests are particularly valuable in discerning the heartbeat of the fetus and in measuring the arterial blood flow to and in the brain as a means of detecting and even preventing stroke. In cases of suspected deep-vein thrombosis (see **Plethysmography**), the tests can sometimes ascertain whether blood is easily flowing through the vein or is blocked by a clot.

With recent developments in ultrasound techniques, the illustrations produced can, in many instances, achieve results similar to **Computerized Tomography** without the hazards of X-ray and at a lower cost. For example, ultrasound scanning can show up a mass in the abdomen (liver, gallbladder, spleen, pancreas, kidney); of even greater value, it can show if the mass is cystic (containing fluid, such as an abscess) or solid (tumor). Lesions only an inch in size can be detected by ultrasonography. An echoencephalogram (brain scan by ultrasound) can show if there are any tumors or other masses (clots or hemorrhages) in the brain. An eye sonogram can reveal pathology inside the eye when there is no other way of seeing inside (see **Fundoscopy**). The thyroid, prostate, and lymph glands may also be tested with ultrasound. An ultrasound scanner is portable and can be brought to the bedside of a patient too ill to move. And now it is possible to have a visual qualitative representation of abnormal heart and blood vessel sounds and murmurs (sometimes called bruits) by using ultrasound to perform spectral bruits analysis; this can be especially valuable when measuring blood flow in the carotid arteries.

When ultrasound detectors are combined with **Endoscopy**, the probes that emit and then detect the sound waves can be placed inside or adjacent to the body organ being studied. This allows examination of the wall of the intestines and the inside of the heart and aorta, as well as closer visualization of many other organs. Ultrasound is also becoming an objective test for prostate gland problems.

Some doctors have applied ultrasound testing for breast evaluation, especially when there is a question as to whether a breast mass is either solid or cystic. This technique is said to be far more precise than mammography (see **Radiography**), in that it can detect the difference in a mass less than three-eighths of an inch in size. The cost runs from $75 to $125.

The most recent application of ultrasound is to detect fetal heart problems, such as congenital defects, in the third month of pregnancy. This test can be quite important to pregnant women who have certain diseases such as diabetes or to those who have abused drugs or alcohol, thus provoking physical abnormalities in the fetus.

When performed: After head or abdominal injury; whenever a mass is suspected in the head or abdomen; whenever there is undiagnosed pain in the abdomen (ultrasound can at times substitute for exploratory surgery); with heart disease, when the heartbeat can be observed in its entirety (to test heart valve function); to determine if there is any growth in a body organ; to diagnose prostate disease; to help locate deep-vein thrombosis; to reduce any risks that may accompany amniocentesis by helping to locate the exact position of the fetus and placenta; to detect ectopic pregnancy (in which the fetus is outside of the uterus).

Normal values: Body organs should appear normal in size and location and show no evidence of pathology.

Abnormal values: As with several other tests, interpretation depends primarily on the physician's experience rather than on established standards.

Risk factors: Although most physicians and health-monitoring agencies claim there are no risks attributed to sound waves, there have been reports of potential hazards. While one study attributes the possibility of birth defects and low birth weight when used during pregnancy, another study says no ill effects were found in 10,000 mothers and their children exposed to ultrasound while pregnant. As with all medical tests, the risks—either real or possible—must be weighed against the need for the information to be derived.

Pain/discomfort: None.

Cost: Ultrasound simply to delineate the position of the fetus is $35 to $50. When this procedure precedes amniocentesis, the cost is $125 to $200. Ultrasound survey of the abdomen is $100 to $200; when various organs are surveyed (thyroid, kidney, liver, gallbladder, etc.), the fee is $100 to $200. When extremities are studied (for thrombosis), the fee is $100 to $150; when the carotid arteries, which carry blood to the brain, are examined by ultrasound, the fee is $100 to $300.

Accuracy and significance: Many doctors find ultrasound to be an excellent, safe, noninvasive means of detecting organ pathology. Various studies have shown that ultrasound is 80 to 98 percent accurate in detecting internal pathology. The test is extremely valuable in outlining the fetus during pregnancy and helping to detect potential abnormalities. Accuracy problems have been attributed to the quality of interpretation; it is only as good as the technician and physician employing the technique.

UNDERWATER WEIGHING, see *Anthropometric Measurements*

UPPER-BOWEL X-RAY, see *Radiography*

UPPER GI SERIES, see *Radiography*

UREA, see *Urea Nitrogen*

UREA CLEARANCE, see *Creatinine*

UREA NITROGEN (Blood Urea Nitrogen, BUN)

Urea is produced primarily in the liver and is the main nitrogen end product of protein metabolism; it is eliminated by the kidneys into the urine. Normally, there is very little urea in the blood. When kidney function is impaired by disease, the normal excretion of urea may be decreased, and urea nitrogen in the blood (BUN) is therefore increased. Urea nitrogen varies with dietary protein intake. Blood is collected from a vein, and the serum is examined. Urea nitrogen may also be measured in the urine.

A somewhat similar test, called nonprotein nitrogen (NPN), measures all the nitrogen end products in the blood in addition to urea. The NPN is not considered as accurate as the BUN. In fact, many doctors do not consider the BUN alone to be an accurate indicator of kidney function, although it is probably the most commonly ordered kidney test.

When performed: When kidney disease is suspected; when there is an indication that urine production is blocked; when the patient displays mental confusion or disorientation; with evidence of increased pituitary activity (acromegaly); with heart failure; after excessive vomiting, diarrhea, or sweating.

Normal values: BUN normally ranges from 10 to 20 mg per 100 ml of blood. Urine urea is measured over a specific period of time and compared with blood urea to determine normal values.

Abnormal values: BUN is increased (over 30 mg per 100 ml) in kidney disease, fever, starvation (increased breakdown of body protein), internal bleeding, and with the taking of a number of drugs, including certain antibiotics, thiazides (diuretics), methyldopa, salicylates, and chloral hydrate. BUN is decreased in liver disease and with increased pituitary activity. At times, urine urea secretion will be low even if BUN is normal; this is an indication of kidney disease.

Risk factors: Negligible (see general risk factors for blood testing).

Pain/discomfort: Minimal (see general pain/discomfort factors for blood testing).

Cost: $3 to $24. The test is usually included in **Comprehensive Multiple Test Screening** panels, which range from $7 to $42.

Some doctors consider the NPN test outmoded, and it is possible that a health insurance company or government-sponsored medical program will not reimburse the doctor or patient for the cost of the test.

Accuracy and significance: As abnormal values occur in such a variety of conditions, the test serves merely as a rough screening test for kidney disease. It is not considered of enough significance to help in arriving at a specific diagnosis; about 60 percent accurate.

URETHRAL OBSTRUCTION, see *Urine Flow Rate*

URIC ACID

Uric acid is an end product of the body's protein metabolism. The amount varies with certain diseases as well as with ingestion of foods such as sweetbreads, liver, anchovies, and sardines. Blood is collected from a vein, and the serum is examined for uric acid levels. A 24-hour urine specimen may be collected for measuring uric acid excretion by the kidneys.

When performed: Primarily when there is suspicion of gout; to aid in the diagnosis of leukemia, toxemia of pregnancy, glycogen storage disease, Lesch-Nyhan syndrome (an inherited form of mental retardation), and other conditions where there is destruction of the body's cells.

Normal values: Normal serum uric acid ranges from 2 to 8 mg per 100 ml. Women and children usually have slightly lower values.

Abnormal values: Higher-than-normal values are usually found with gout, leukemia, heart disease, toxemia of pregnancy, pneumonia, severe kidney damage (which decreases excretion), glycogen storage disease, and Lesch-Nyhan syndrome. Eating certain foods and taking ascorbic acid, salicylates (such as aspirin), theophylline, or thiazides (diuretics) can also increase values. Lower-than-normal values are usually found in patients taking coumarin products (anticoagulants) and piperazine (worm medicine).

Risk factors: Negligible (see general risk factors for blood testing).

Pain/discomfort: Minimal (see general pain/discomfort factors for blood testing).

Cost: From $4 to $34. Usually included in **Comprehensive Multiple Test Screening** panels, which range from $7 to $42.

Accuracy and significance: Although this is the basic screening test for gout, it is not significant enough to allow a specific diagnosis of the disease. Furthermore, there are so many foods and drugs that can raise and lower blood uric acid levels that the test is generally repeated several times once the patient is on a special diet and no longer taking medication that interferes with the test. About 70 percent accurate.

URINALYSIS, see Urine Examination

URINARY BLADDER, see Cystometry

URINARY 17-KETOSTEROIDS (17-KS), see Cortisol

URINARY TRACT CALCULUS

When a stone, or calculus (plural: calculi), appears anywhere in the urinary tract (from kidney to bladder), it is essential to analyze the stone to identify its composition. If the primary ingredient of a kidney stone can be determined (identification is possible only in about half of all cases), proper treatment can be started much sooner. Stones may come from eating an excessive amount of food high in **Calcium** and **Oxalates,** metabolic problems, dehydration, excessive vitamin D intake, excessive bed rest, **Parathyroid** gland problems, and many other conditions. Nephrocalcinosis (stone formation limited to the kidney) is sometimes visualized by X-ray examination, but in most instances, diagnosis is made by identification of the type of crystals in the urine.

When performed: When abdominal, back, or groin pain cannot be diagnosed; when there is evidence of blood in the urine; when the amount of urine is decreased.

Normal values: Normally, no crystals should be seen in a microscopic examination of freshly passed urine (at times, certain proteins may crystalize when the urine has cooled to room temperature).

Abnormal values: Pathological crystals have uniquely identifiable shapes and colors. Those that can reflect disease include calcium oxalate (the most common), calcium phosphate, uric acid (not always due to gout), cystine (see **Aminoaciduria**), and tyrosine (usually associated with liver disease). The presence of urinary tract stones more often represents a metabolic or inherited disease rather than kidney pathology.

Risk factors: None.
Pain/discomfort: None.
Cost: From $20 to $40.

Accuracy and significance: Analysis of a kidney stone is 98 percent accurate in revealing the stone's chemical makeup. The test is significant in that once the stone's chemical composition is identified, appropriate therapy can be given and preventive measures undertaken.

URINE CONCENTRATION, see *Mosenthal*

URINE CULTURE, see *Culture*

URINE EXAMINATION

Many urine tests are described under the names of the blood tests that usually accompany them (see, for example, **Albumin/Globulin, Glucose**, and **Phenykletonuria**). Urine is one of many waste products that indicate the general health of the body in addition to being a specific measure of kidney function. A routine, or screening, urine examination usually consists of tests for specific gravity (concentration of solids), protein (albumin), and sugar (glucose); microscopic examination for bacteria, parasites, chemical crystals, and casts (solid matter made up of bacteria, blood cells, pus, protein, etc.); and examination for acid or alkaline reaction, color, odor, and transparency. Many doctors feel the test for protein in the urine is the best single indicator of kidney disease. A new procedure is the nitrite test, which can give a rapid indication of bacterial infection anywhere in the urinary tract.

The Addis count is a test of urine sediment to determine the amount of protein and the number of red blood cells, white blood cells, casts and epithelial cells in a 12-hour urine specimen. The Addis count is elevated in kidney disease.

Approximately 2 ounces (50 ml) of urine is collected, preferably from an early morning specimen, which contains materials excreted by the kidneys during the night and will usually be of less volume (more concentrated, higher in specific gravity). If the patient drinks an excessive amount of fluids, the amount of urine will increase automatically and the specific gravity will be reduced (see **Mosenthal**). Today, most urine tests are performed by dipping a multi–chemically coated paper in the urine, allowing up to 10 separate urine examinations to be performed simultaneously.

A recent, much more rapid way of detecting bacteria and pus cells in the urine is the leukocyte esterase test; it is positive when the urine contains specific **White Blood Cell** chemicals not usually found in typical urinary tract infections and can be an early warning sign of a more severe kidney problem. It can also help explain the cause of painful urination when there is a concurrent vaginal infection.

When performed: As a routine screening test to determine kidney function; when liver disease is suspected; as a measure of any disorder of the urinary, cardiovascular and metabolic systems.

Normal values: Urine should range in color from yellow to light amber and should be clear or transparent. It is normal for early morning urine to have a spicy odor and to be slightly acid. On microscopic examination, an occasional red or white blood cell may be seen; the appearance of a few casts after strenuous exercise is still considered normal. Normal specific gravity ranges from 1.010 to 1.025, with a reading toward the higher limit in an early morning specimen.

Abnormal values: With liver disease, certain anemias, melanoma (a form of skin cancer), and excessive intake of vitamins, the urine may have a greenish or brownish tint. A reddish or brownish tint usually indicates the presence of blood.

Whenever the urine is not clear or transparent, more often than not it contains pus, bacteria, blood, and/or chemical crystals. **Gonorrhea** usually causes long, thin, whitish shreds to appear in the urine.

Urine that has an ammonia odor is almost always indicative of some disease condition that causes excessive urine to be retained in the bladder. A sweet or fruity odor is indicative of a dangerous stage of diabetes mellitus.

While the urine normally has a very slight acid reaction, the degree of acidity may increase with kidney disease, heart disease, and diarrhea (from any cause). An alkaline reaction may be seen with certain anemias or various infections and after prolonged vomiting.

Risk factors: None.

Pain/discomfort: None.

Cost: A "routine" urinalysis usually consists of observing the color of the urine and testing for **pH**, specific gravity (see **Mosenthal**), protein (usually albumin; see **Albumin/Globulin**), and sugar **(Glucose)** and may include a microscopic search for crystals, casts, blood cells, and parasites. This can cost from $3 to $22. Some doctors and laboratories also test for **Bilirubin** and **Urobilinogen, Ketones,** and blood and may perform the nitrite tests for infection; a microscopic examination is done only if the nitrite test is positive. The cost for one or more additional tests may be included in the "routine" urinalysis fee, or an additional fee of $5 to $10 may be charged for each and every extra test. If urine is cultured to identify a microorganism, the fee is from $20 to $30. An Addis count runs from $10 to $25.

Accuracy and significance: Urine examination is one of the simplest and most effective ways to help diagnose a variety of diseases. Even though it is not a diagnostic test for specific diseases, it is probably the most significant medical test for general health screening. Overall, it is considered 90 percent accurate.

URINE FLOW RATE

The uroflow meter is an electronic device that records the pressure (force), amount, and time required to pass urine. The test is used to determine if any partial obstruction exists in or at the entrance to the urethra (the duct that carries urine from the bladder to outside the body). Reduced flow is most commonly seen in men with prostate problems (an enlarged prostate gland pushes up against the urethra and narrows its diameter). Urine flow is also reduced with old infection, bladder tumors, polyps, urinary tract stones, and nerve diseases that are reflected in lack of normal bladder function.

After drinking at least a quart of liquid four hours before the test, the patient voids (urinates) into a funnel attached to the uroflow meter. Because many patients find it difficult to urinate on command, privacy must be offered to achieve accurate results.

When performed: When a patient complains of pain or difficulty in urinating (getting started, maintaining an even flow) or of frequent urination (usually in very small amounts); when prostatic disease is suspected; following urethral infections, especially gonorrhea; with certain nerve conditions (multiple sclerosis); before and after any surgery in the bladder and urethral area (such as prostate operations).

Normal values: The normal rate is 20 ml per second at maximum flow.

Abnormal values: A rate of less than 10 ml per second is considered abnormal. If the urine flow rate pressure has been measured previously, any relative decrease in that pressure indicates some partial obstruction of the urethra. A decreased amount, or prolonged time for urinating, also indicates obstruction.

Risk factors: None.

Pain/discomfort: None.

Cost: From $15 to $40.

Accuracy and significance: The test is primarily a measure of urinary difficulty before treatment and provides a graphic record of the rate of urine flow after treatment. As such, the test merely confirms a doctor's observations.

URINE TEMPERATURE, see Body Temperature

UROBILINOGEN

Urobilinogen comes from **Bilirubin** (a yellow pigment found in bile and after the normal breakdown of red blood cells). The urine normally contains small amounts of urobilinogen, but in certain disease conditions (anemias, liver damage, some infections), the urobilinogen level in the urine increases. Maximum excretion of urobilinogen usually occurs between 1:00 and 3:00 in the afternoon. A 2-hour specimen or a 24-hour sample may be required for examination. The test is also performed on feces.

When performed: When there is suspicion of gallbladder or biliary tract obstruction; with blood or liver problems.

Normal values: One Erlich unit per 100 ml is considered normal in a 2-hour sample of urine, preferably collected between 1:00 and 3:00 p.m. In a 24-hour sample, excretion of 1 to 4 mg is within the normal range.

Abnormal values: Increased amounts of urobilinogen are found with liver damage and hemolytic anemia. Ingestion of salicylates (such as aspirin) will cause the results of the test to be falsely elevated. Decreased urobilinogen is found in obstructive jaundice. Ingestion of antibiotics may cause the results to be falsely lowered.

Risk factors: None.

Pain/discomfort: None.

Cost: While this test is usually part of a routine urine examination, it can be performed separately to establish a record of the exact amount of urobilinogen. In such cases, the fee for quantitative measurements is $9 to $30.

Accuracy and significance: The test is primarily used as confirmation when particular anemias are suspected. It is also used to help distinguish between obstructive jaundice (gallstone) and nonobstructive jaundice (liver disease). The test is of no great significance. It is less than 70 percent accurate, even when performed along with the **Bilirubin** test as it should be.

UROGRAM, see "Pyelography," in *Radiography*

URTICARIA, see *Allergy*

UTERINE IRRIGATION, see *Dilatation and Curettage*

V

VAGINAL pH, see *pH*

VAGINITIS, see *Wet Mount*

VAGINOSCOPY, see *Endoscopy*

VAN DEN BERGH REACTION, see *Bilirubin*

VANILLYMANDELIC ACID, see *Catecholamines*

VAPOR PRESSURE OSMOMETRY, see *Sweat*

VARICOSE VEIN INCOMPETENCY, see *Tourniquet Test for Varicose Veins*

VASCULAR ENDOSCOPY, see *Endoscopy*

VASECTOMY ASSURANCE, see *Semen*

VASOACTIVE INTESTINAL POLYPEPTIDE, see *Cancer*

VASOPRESSIN

Vasopressin is a hormone produced in the hypothalamus area of the brain (the part of the brain that translates such stimuli as light, sound, pain, body reactions to the time of day, body positions—especially discomfort—and virtually any emotional excitation into physical, nerve, or hormonal action). It is also known as the antidiuretic hormone (ADH) because it seems to work with the kidney to prevent the body from excreting fluids as urine. In other words, the more vasopressin produced, the more water the body retains, even to the point of edema. When excessive vasopressin is secreted for no reason that can be ascertained, the condition is known as the syndrome of inappropriate antidiuretic hormone secretion (SIADH). On rare occasions, certain cancers, injuries, and drugs will increase vasopressin production; more frequently, however, it is emotional upset, apprehension, and anger that cause the increase. In turn, the body shows its retention of water through puffiness in the feet and ankles and especially in the face and under the eyes.

Another vasopressin-related disease is diabetes insipidus, in which the patients drink liquids almost incessantly (a condition called polydipsia) while at the same time suffering from polyuria (a condition forcing patients to urinate so constantly they excrete about 10 quarts a day). In this case, either there is insufficient vasopressin, or the kidneys simply do not react to its presence. With diabetes insipidus, the urine's specific gravity, or the amount of solid matter it contains, is very low (see **Mosenthal**).

Normally, if a patient takes diuretic drugs, the amount of vasopressin in the body increases as a reaction to the water loss. In addition, the **Osmolality** of the blood helps to control the production of vasopressin. (Generally, the osmolality test and vasopressin test are performed concurrently.) Vasopressin is tested from a blood sample, usually obtained from a vein. It should be measured before and after the patient drinks large quantities of fluid for several days; it should also be measured after the patient has been deprived of liquids for a prolonged period of time. At times, a patient is given an intravenous salt solution to gauge its effect on vasopressin production.

An interesting observation concerning one form of vasopressin is that when the drug was given to patients, their memories improved markedly and the cognitive benefits lasted for a month following treatment.

When performed: To help diagnose diabetes insipidus; to help diagnose persistent edema; to measure the intensity of the effect of certain emotions on the body; to ascertain the diuretic effect of certain drugs, especially lithium; after head injuries; to help diagnose some types of kidney disease. (Also see **Pituitary Function**.)

Normal values: From 1 to 5 pg per ml; when osmolality is measured, the amount of vasopressin should correspond to the osmolality value (e.g., when osmolality is low, vasopressin levels should be about 1 or 2 pg per ml; when osmolality is high—as with water loss—vasopressin levels should be close to 10 pg per ml).

Abnormal values: A vasopressin level that does not accord with the osmolality level (a vasopressin level of 1 to 2 pg per ml when a patient is dehydrated and the osmolality level is high); no evidence of vasopressin with diabetes insipidus; an extremely elevated vasopressin level as a reaction to stress.

Risk factors: Negligible (see general risk factors for blood testing).

Pain/discomfort: Minimal (see general pain/discomfort for blood testing).

Cost: From $50 to $80 for each test; approximately $125 if two or three vasopressin test samples are collected and frozen after forcing and withholding fluids and then submitted for testing at the same time.

Accuracy and significance: This is a difficult test to perform. If the blood is not properly collected, stored, and transported to the laboratory, errors are common. In addition, vasopressin secretion is easily influenced by the patient's position (standing, sitting, or lying down), the patient's dietary habits, and perhaps most important, the patient's emotional state at the time of blood collection. All such observations must be noted. In general, this is not a very accurate test (about 60 percent); most often, its significance is corroborated by other tests.

VCG, see *Vectorcardiogram*

VDRL, see *Syphilis*

VECTORCARDIOGRAM (VCG)

Sometimes called spatial or three-dimensional electrocardiography, the vectorcardiogram is a somewhat refined version of the standard **Electrocardiogram** (ECG). The VCG shows heart muscle activity or heart damage from two different points in the heart at the same time, thus giving an indication of the *direction* of heart muscle activity as well as its force (contraction and relaxation). The ECG records only the force of heart muscle and from only one location at a time. In the VCG, electrodes are attached to at least four body surfaces (compared with two in the ECG). The electrodes are connected to a measuring instrument with an oscilloscope or cathode-ray tube (similar to a television picture tube), which produces a moving "loop" configuration (in the ECG, a line graph on paper is produced). The loop may be observed directly on the oscilloscope, or it may be fed into a computer so that a permanent image can be recorded for analysis at a later time. The image will show the size, shape, and direction of heart muscle activity.

When performed: The VCG is most commonly used to teach physicians how to understand and interpret the ECG; it is also employed when the ECG shows no obvious heart abnormalities but the patient's symptoms indicate a heart problem. Should two or more heart problems be suspected and the ECG show only one, the VCG may reveal the others. It can also aid in determining the extent of heart pathology.

Normal values: There are no standards that can be used for correlation (as exist for the ECG); interpretation of the VCG is based on the doctor's experience with the test.

Abnormal values: By knowing the placement of the electrodes for a particular recording, the physician can determine any abnormalities in the loop formations.

Risk factors: None.

Pain/discomfort: None.

Cost: From $50 to $200.

Accuracy and significance: Most physicians consider this test only about 50 percent accurate—less accurate than a standard ECG. Its significance is in its application when no other heart-function test coincides with a patient's symptoms.

VEIN PRESSURE, see *Blood Pressure*

VEIN SCAN, see *Nuclear Scanning*

VEIN THROMBOSIS, see *Plethysmography*

VENEREAL DISEASE RESEARCH LABORATORY, see *Syphilis*

VENEREAL DISEASES

(This term is no longer used; tests employed to aid in the identification of what are now called sexually transmitted diseases include: **Acquired Immunodeficiency Syndrome, Chlamydia Identification, Cytomegalovirus, Frei, Gonorrhea, Hepatitis, Herpes, Syphilis,** and the **TORCH** group.)

VENOUS BLOOD PRESSURE, see *Blood Pressure*

VENTILATION, see *Pulmonary Function*
VENTILATION SCAN, see *Nuclear Scanning*
VERTIGO, see *Caloric*
VIRAL HEPATITIS, see *Hepatitis*
VIRAL PNEUMONIA, see *Agglutination*

VIRUS DISEASE

Viruses cause more disease than any other group of microorganisms. In the past, when doctors had difficulty in arriving at a specific diagnosis, the final decision as to the cause of the illness was usually: "It must be a virus." Now, however, when specific virus-caused diseases are suspected, there are myriad tests that can pinpoint the particular causative organism—or at least identify which of the closely related groups of viruses that attack certain areas of the body (e.g., rhinoviruses, which cause colds, a running nose, or a sore throat; or enteroviruses, which cause meningitis, poliomyelitis, heart muscle inflammation, and pleuritis) is the culprit. Most important, there are now tests to distinguish between a bacterial infection and a viral infection, which is of considerable clinical significance in treating patients with pneumonia, diarrhea, or meningeal symptoms. While antibiotic drugs have no direct effect on virus-caused infections, new antiviral drugs are becoming available. Specifically, there are drugs to treat herpes simplex encephalitis, certain virus-caused eye conditions, and some types of influenza.

The usual way to diagnose a specific virus-caused condition is through serological testing (examining the blood, most often taken from a vein, for specific antibodies to the suspected virus). The way these tests work is described under **Agglutination** and **Complement Fixation**; each test usually takes one week to perform. While many of the new techniques offer faster results—some in one day—basically, they are only more sophisticated versions of agglutination processes. In almost all diagnostic evaluations for viral diseases, at least two different blood serum examinations must be made from two to three weeks apart. In most instances, antibodies are not evident for at least one week after the virus infects the individual; confirmation of infection comes weeks later when a dramatic increase in the antibody level is seen following testing of the second specimen. However, some doctors accept a single test as evidence of disease if it reveals an unusually high titer (reflection of an abnormally large number of antibodies) against a specific virus. Also, when testing pregnant women for **Rubella** (German measles) immunity, any trace of rubella antibodies is considered to mean that the woman once had that disease and will not pass it on to her baby. For a more precise diagnosis, specific viruses can also be cultured once isolated from body specimens such as sputum, feces, urine, and eye secretions.

Viruses are closely related, but each variation within a group can cause different symptoms and signs. As examples, see **Herpes** and **Hepatitis**. Tests are now available for several viral groups, as well as for individual viral diseases. A few examples include:

Adenovirus
This virus causes nose, throat, lung, and gastrointestinal diseases.

Arbovirus group
These viruses cause encephalitis, eye, and bladder diseases.
Chicken pox (varicella)
The test for this virus helps differentiate among diseases producing rashes.
Coxsackie groups
There are two distinct groups. Within group A, there are 23 known types; within group B, there are 6 known types. They cause lung disease, paralytic types of illness, and a heart disease in newborn infants that imitates congenital defects.
Cytomegalovirus
Echovirus/Enterovirus
Both belong to the same group and can cause poliomyelitis, meningitis, heart and lung conditions, diarrhea, and other gastrointestinal symptoms.
Hepatitis
Herpes
Influenza and parainfluenza (flu)
Influenza of the lungs is usually designated Type A, B, or C; A and B are the most familiar. Type C is a very mild form of the "flu." Parainfluenza, a lung disease generally limited to very young children, is divided into Types 1, 2, 3, and 4.
Lymphocytic choriomeningitis
Another form of meningitis.
Measles (rubeola)
The test for this virus can distinguish between it and German measles (rubella) in pregnant women and newborn infants. The virus can, however, also cause encephalitis.
Mononucleosis
Mumps (parotitis)
This virus causes infection and swelling of the salivary glands, as well as swelling and possible sterility of the testicles.
Reovirus
At times, this is considered part of the echovirus group. The *r* stands for "respiratory," the *e* for "enteric" (gastrointestinal), and the *o* for "organs." This virus causes pneumonia and diarrhea, especially in children.
Retroviruses
A family of viruses associated with **Acquired Immunodeficiency Syndrome** and, more recently, with schizophrenia.
Rotavirus
The cause of gastroenteritis in children.
Rubella (German measles)
If the mother has German measles during pregnancy, it can cause congenital malformations in newborn infants. The viral disease tests are especially useful in determining whether or not a particular rash indicates German measles. It is extremely difficult to make a specific diagnosis clinically (merely by the appearance of the rash), as so many diseases produce similar skin

eruptions. Furthermore, the absence of rubella antibodies in a newborn infant does not rule out the possibility of the disease; antibodies may not have formed at that point. When there is doubt, culture and isolation of the specific virus must be attempted.

Of course, erroneous results are always possible. A false-negative report may be given if: the specimen was taken at the wrong time, it was stored or delivered to the laboratory improperly, the wrong antigens were used in the testing process, or some contaminants obscured the presence of the antibody. A false-positive test can occur if: there is contamination, more than one virus is present, or there are cross-reacting related antigens.

Syncytial
The cause of pneumonialike disease in young children.

The most common viral disease tests are listed separately. As with any illness, the test results must be correlated with the evident pathology and the patient's history, signs, and symptoms.

VISCERAL LARVA MIGRANS, see *Toxocariasis*

VISION, see *Visual Acuity*

VISUAL ACUITY

Tests of visual acuity (or vision) measure the ability of each eye to perceive the size and shape of an object clearly at standard distances. The tests also measure the ability of both eyes, working together, to discern the distance and depth of objects and their relationship to one another (which object is nearer or farther away), called stereopsis, or depth perception.

The most common vision test uses the Snellen chart: the patient reads a series of unrelated letters or numbers of various sizes at a distance of 20 feet; for those who cannot read, the letter **E** is used in different sizes and positions (**E,ɯ,ɯ**). A person with normal vision will easily designate a letter ⅜ inch high from 20 feet away; such visual acuity is recorded as 20/20. The largest letter on the Snellen chart is 3½ inches high; if this is the only letter that a patient can read at a distance of 20 feet, the visual acuity is recorded as 20/200 (reflecting the fact that someone with normal vision could read that letter 200 feet away). The legal definition of blindness is 20/200 vision or worse with the use of the most efficient corrective lens. Normal visual acuity is called emmetropia; a vision defect that can be corrected by the use of lenses is called ametropia.

Myopia, or nearsightedness, is a form of ametropia characterized by difficulty in seeing objects clearly at a distance (usually 20 feet) but being able to read or see objects close up. In hyperopia, sometimes called hypermetropia or farsightedness, patients can see objects clearly at a distance but have difficulty with reading or close work. In presbyopia, usually considered a form of hyperopia as a result of normal aging, the lens of the eye can no longer accommodate (change shape) to focus well on both near and far objects. With astigmatism, the eye cannot focus properly in certain planes. For example, a person might be able to distinguish all the numbers on a clock except those that are on a line from 11 to 5. Anisometropia is characterized by a difference in visual acuity of the two eyes. This can become a serious problem in children if the eye with the worse vision is not used (amblyopia). Failure to use one eye (sometimes called "lazy eye") can cause **Strabismus,** where the eye no longer focuses on an object and strays outward or inward (cross-eyes). In aphakia, the lens of the eye is absent.

The standard method of vision testing is to have the patient read an eye chart, using trial lenses of different strengths (called refraction) at a distance of 20 feet. Retinoscopy is a much more objective way to test vision, especially with children; it measures the precise way light focuses on the retina in the back of the eye. There are also electronic devices (used mostly by schools, industry, and motor vehicle departments) that can detect most vision problems within minutes. (The Snellen wall chart is best for myopia, but it can easily miss other forms of ametropia.) For more accurate visual acuity testing of patients under 20 years of age whose pupillary muscles are difficult to relax, many doctors use a cyclopegic drug to dilate (relax) those pupillary muscles so that the eye cannot accommodate, or react to light. A simple test for visual acuity involves looking at an object through a pinhole opening. If the object seems much clearer through the pinhole, professional vision testing is indicated.

Note: The most recent test of visual acuity is performed with the Amsler grid. When looking at what resembles a piece of graph paper, using one eye at a time, all the lines—both horizontal and vertical—should appear clear, continuous, and straight. Failure to see all the lines as they are could indicate a condition called macular degeneration (involving the retina and usually limited to elderly individuals); if this test is performed weekly, detection of the disease within the first few weeks of its existence greatly reduces the chance of a permanent disability. Looking at a flagpole, telephone pole, or the edge of a door to see if the line is straight and complete is a similar test.

Measurement of visual acuity is only one of many different ways to test the eyes. For other, more specific tests, see **Color Blindness, Fluorescein Eye Stain, Fundoscopy, Pupillary Reflex, Schirmer's, Strabismus, Tonometry,** and **Visual Field.**

When performed: Whenever there is difficulty in seeing clearly; as a screening test to detect vision problems before they become serious; as a way of following the course of various diseases such as diabetes; as part of testing candidates for certain occupations (flying).

Normal values: Although 20/20 vision (ability to see a standard-sized letter at 20 feet) is considered normal, up to 20/40 vision without the aid of glasses is still considered satisfactory (a driver's license is usually permitted with this vision). Normally, an individual who can see clearly at 20 feet also can read tiny print at a distance of 14 inches. When two objects are in line, a patient with normal vision can discern their relative depth (which one is in front and which one is in back).

Abnormal values: Indications of impaired vision include the inability to read at least 20/40-size letters at a distance of 20 feet (some people may be uncomfortable without 20/20 vision), the inability to read small print at a distance of 14 inches or less, and the inability to perceive the relative depth of objects. Poor visual acuity may be inherited, or it may be caused by bodily disease, by many drugs and poisons, and of course, by problems of the eye itself such as glaucoma, cataract, eye muscle weakness, and any trauma to or around the eye.

Risk factors: None.
Pain/discomfort: None.
Cost: Generally, there is no additional charge for tests of visual acuity when they are part of a routine eye examination.
Accuracy and significance: Most tests for visual acuity, when selected to match the patient's age, are 90 percent accurate and extremely significant when the result is the restoration of a patient's vision to normal.

In 1984, a new eye chart was introduced that has been reported to be more accurate than the standard Snellen chart. Using circles and bars of different contrasts, it allows visual acuity measurements under varying light conditions and, unlike the Snellen, better determines the ability to see while driving (some people show 20/20 vision with the Snellen chart yet cannot see well enough to drive).

VISUAL FIELD

Central visual field measurements test the eye's ability to see objects over a wide area (peripheral vision) while looking at a specific point. For example, when an individual looks straight ahead, he should still be aware of any object directly at his side. In most instances, an instrument called a perimeter is used to obtain exact measurements (perimetry) of just how far the eye can distinguish objects above, below, and to the side (called field of vision). Perimetry is usually performed after screening tests indicate a visual field defect.

By charting the visual field for each eye, the physician can diagnose various diseases of the brain, the nerves, and the retina. Blind spots (scotoma) can indicate disease; but the eye also has a normal blind spot (where the optic nerve enters the brain). Locating this specific area can verify the test's accuracy as well as detect patients who are faking vision problems. Hemianopia (inability to see the entire visual field) usually indicates a nerve or brain problem.

The simplest way to test visual field is for the doctor and patient to sit three feet apart and each look at the other's nose while the doctor moves his finger above, below, and to the side; both should see the fingertip at the same places. The physician may also mark the patient's visual margins on a tangent screen (a black felt sheet with circles on it) for a permanent record.

When performed: As a routine screening test in any eye examination; when there is suspicion of a brain lesion or an eye defect that cannot be corrected with glasses (such as glaucoma); when inherited eye disease is suspected; in instances of hysteria.

Normal values: The eye, looking directly ahead at a point, should be able to perceive a small (3 mm) spot (it may be a dot on the end of a stick or a tiny light) at an almost 90° angle to the side (away from the nose, toward the temple area of the head). The field of vision normally extends downward past the top of the cheek to an angle of about 65° and upward to an angle of no more than 45°. When looking straight ahead, the eye should also see anything not blocked by the nose. The normal blind spot (which has no visual receptors) is the point where the eye will not see the test spot when looking straight ahead. The patient's perceptions are recorded on a standard visual field chart.

Abnormal values: Any reduction in visual field is indicative of disease. The reduction may be in one direction only, or it may affect the overall field of vision in equal proportions (as with glaucoma or inherited degenerative retinitis). Most abnormalities of the visual field show specific patterns that aid in the diagnosis of a number of eye and brain lesions. Patients can have a markedly diminished field of vision and still have normal **Visual Acuity.**

Risk factors: None.

Pain/discomfort: None.

Cost: There is usually no charge for visual field tests when they are part of a routine eye examination.

Accuracy and significance: The test is 95 percent accurate in revealing the extent of a patient's peripheral vision. When performed regularly, the test allows the doctor to detect glaucoma and nerve and brain disorders at the earliest possible moment.

VISUAL MOTOR PERCEPTION

The Bender Gestalt test of visual motor perception measures how well a child perceives an object and how well he can draw or copy that object. Years of experience have shown that the test not only is an indicator of intelligence (as a predictor of achievement in school, see **Intelligence Quotient**) but also can help diagnose brain injury and mental retardation in children from 5 to 10 years of age.

The child is shown nine geometric and abstract designs and is asked to make a copy of each. The child's response is evaluated for distortions, incompleteness, rotation, or inaccuracies and is scored according to standard values. The age of the child, the time it takes to complete the drawing, and the overall accuracy of the reproduction are taken into account.

When performed: When there is a question of learning ability, especially in a young child about to start school; to assess the possibility of brain damage or mental retardation at the time a child is entering school.

Normal values: The older the child, the less deviation there should be from the original drawing. At the age of 5, the child may introduce at least a dozen inaccuracies in copying the drawings. The number of inaccuracies normally decreases to two or fewer by the time the child reaches 10 years of age.

Abnormal values: With brain injury, the child not only makes a great many more errors in copying but introduces many more distortions and has greater problems with integration of shapes. With mental retardation, the child shows no special area of error; the errors are spread uniformly over the test measurements but are markedly increased for the child's age.

Risk factors: None.

Pain/discomfort: None.

Cost: From $25 to $50, depending on the time required.

Accuracy and significance: When combined with other evaluations of a child's learning ability, the test helps to distinguish mental retardation from brain damage; alone, it is considered to be 60 percent accurate.

VITAL CAPACITY, see *Pulmonary Function*

VITAMIN A, see *Retinol*

VITAMIN B$_1$, see *Thiamin*

VITAMIN B₂, see *Riboflavin*

VITAMIN B₃, see *Niacin*

VITAMIN B₆, see *Pyridoxine*

VITAMIN B₁₂, see *Schilling*

VITAMIN C, see *Ascorbic Acid*

VITAMIN D

Vitamin D, which exists in several different forms, is essential to proper development of bones and teeth and proper utilization of calcium in the body. It is found in large amounts in fish (especially fish oils), egg yolks, and butter. Deficiency of vitamin D can cause rickets and osteomalacia (softening of bones, accompanied by pain and muscular weakness). Tooth decay can be caused by too little vitamin D. Excessive intake of vitamin D can cause nausea, loss of appetite, slow growth, and headaches. Any one of the many forms of vitamin D can be measured in the blood. The 25 hydroxyvitamin D level test is considered a good measure of vitamin D intake, whether the vitamin comes from the diet or from sunlight; this form of vitamin D is also used to help evaluate the effectiveness of vitamin D therapy.

The **Alkaline Phosphatase** test is performed to confirm the severity (possible bone involvement) of vitamin D deficiency. Blood is taken from a vein, and the serum is examined.

When performed: To diagnose rickets and other bone or teeth abnormalities; to monitor drugs being taken by patients with kidney problems; to help diagnose disorders of mineral metabolism.

Normal values: From 10 to 75 ng per ml. Alkaline phosphatase levels range from 2 to 4.5 Bodansky units per 100 ml of serum in adults. The normal range in children is 5 to 15 Bodansky units per 100 ml of serum.

Abnormal values: Decreased amounts of vitamin D are found with malabsorption; with dietary deficiencies; in some thyroid conditions; in a number of patients who have taken antiepileptic medications for prolonged periods; in normal pregnancy. Although an increased amount of vitamin D usually reflects an intoxication from an excessive amount of the vitamin, it can also indicate **Parathyroid** disease.

Values for serum alkaline phosphatase may be increased in vitamin D deficiency and many other conditions (Paget's disease, cancer, hyperparathyroidism, osteogenic sarcoma). An excessive amount of vitamin D can cause decreased alkaline phosphatase values.

Risk factors: Negligible (see general risk factors for blood testing).
Pain/discomfort: Minimal (see general pain/discomfort factors for blood testing).
Cost: From $50 to $100.
Accuracy and significance: The test is not quite precise, as even a short exposure to sunlight can alter blood values. The test assumes significance when a specific cause of bone disease is difficult to diagnose; about 70 percent accurate.

VITAMIN E, see *Tocopherols*

VITAMIN K, see *Prothrombin Time*
VLM, see *Toxocariasis*
VMA, see *Catecholamines*
VOICE, see *Hearing Function*

W

WALDENSTROM'S MACROGLOBULINEMIA, see *Macroglobulin*
WASSERMANN, see *Complement Fixation; Syphilis*
WATER PROVOCATION, see *Tonometry*
WATSON-SCHWARTZ, see *Porphyrins*
WBC, see *White Blood Cell*
WEBER, see *Tuning Fork*
WECHSLER, see *Intelligence Quotient*
WEIL-FELIX, see *Agglutination*
WESTERGREN, see *Sedimentation Rate*
WESTERN BLOT, see *Acquired Immunodeficiency Syndrome*

WET MOUNT

This test is considered the most important diagnostic procedure to detect the cause of vaginitis or vaginal discharge and is often called the saline wet mount test, because it uses a saline (salt) solution. A cotton-tipped stick is dipped in saline and then mixed with a bit of vaginal discharge; it is examined immediately under the microscope for one of the three most common causes of vaginitis: trichomoniasis, a tiny parasite; candidiasis, a fungus; or hemophilus vaginalis, a bacterium that induces certain specific cell shapes. In some instances, a woman's sex partner's urine is also examined to make certain that she is not being constantly reinfected (sometimes called a "Ping-Pong" infection) as a consequence of sexual activity.

When performed: When a woman complains of a vaginal discharge or experiences itching, rash, or swelling in the genital area.
Normal values: No evidence of parasites, fungus, or other than normal bacteria.
Abnormal values: Visible evidence of a specific cause of vaginitis.
Risk factors: None.
Pain/discomfort: None.

Cost: Usually, there is no charge when the test is part of a routine physical examination. When performed by a commercial laboratory, the fee is $5 to $20.

Accuracy and significance: The test is 95 percent accurate when it is properly performed. It is particularly significant when the source of the infection turns out to be the sexual partner, allowing for complete cure.

WHISPER, see *Hearing Function*

WHITAKER, see "Pyelography," in *Radiography*

WHITE BLOOD CELL (Leukocyte, WBC)

The five different types of white blood cells (see **Blood Cell Differential**) are formed and stored in the bone marrow, thymus, lymph glands, and spleen. They are particularly important in fighting infections. The amount of certain kinds of white blood cells usually increases with infection or inflammation in the body, and these blood cells help destroy the causative agents. The white blood cell count is the total of the five kinds of white cells.

A drop of blood from the fingertip, heel, or earlobe (or blood drawn for other tests) is examined. White blood cells are also searched for in spinal fluid, urine, joint fluid, and mucus. The cells may be counted manually under a microscope, but most often they are counted electronically. (With modern equipment, the cells can be viewed on a TV screen and counted automatically.)

The Christmas tree test determines if the white blood cells are performing their function of killing bacteria. A tiny amount of blood is placed on a glass slide stained with a dye. Dead bacteria show up red; live bacteria, green (thus, the name *Christmas tree*). Normally, the slide shows very little green color; a lack of red-colored cells indicates the patient's inability to fight infections. The test takes only a few hours (older, similar tests take days).

The leukocyte adherence inhibition test, in which a specific antigen (see **Agglutination**) is added to white blood cells and prevents their normal adherence, has been used to help diagnose cancer of the pancreas (see **Pancreas Function**) and prostate.

When performed: When infection is suspected; in toxic reactions to certain drugs (sulfa drugs and other antibiotics, analgesics); in toxic reactions to chemicals or poisons (arsenic); in blood disorders, especially leukemias.

Normal values: There should be 5,000 to 10,000 white blood cells per cubic millimeter (cu mm). Children may have higher values.

Abnormal values: The total white blood cell count increases temporarily with most bacterial infections, blood disorders, emotional stress, hemorrhage, rheumatic fever, and burns. A white blood cell count may be falsely elevated when patients feel tense or embarrassed as a result of undergoing an examination. The white blood cell count decreases following ingestion of certain drugs or chemicals, after X-ray treatments, with malaria, typhoid, brucellosis, certain forms of leukemia, and virus and rickettsial infections. The count also decreases when the body produces autoimmune antibody globulins that stop white blood cell production.

Risk factors: Negligible (see general risk factors for blood testing).

Pain/discomfort: Minimal (see general pain/discomfort factors for blood testing).

Cost: From $3 to $20; most laboratories include a **Blood Cell Differential** as part of the test. The white blood cell count alone is usually included in **Comprehensive Multiple Test Screening** panels, which range from $7 to $42.

Accuracy and significance: The test is 90 percent accurate in determining bacterial infection and such blood disorders as leukemia, providing the many extraneous factors that can affect the white blood cell count are considered. The test assumes a special significance when used to aid in diagnosing those diseases caused by viruses. Although blood cell counting is fairly accurate, recent evidence indicates that when the blood cells are counted by automated machines, the results can show false lower-than-normal amounts. Thus, it is important to know when a blood cell count is performed by automated machines.

WHITE BLOOD CELL DIFFERENTIAL, see *Blood Cell Differential*

WHOOPING COUGH, see *Agglutination*

WIDEL, see *Agglutination*

WINTROBE, see *Sedimentation Rate*

WIRT STEREOPSIS, see *Strabismus*

WOOD ALCOHOL, see *Methanol*

WORM, see *Feces Examination*

WORTH FOUR-DOT, see *Strabismus*

X

XEROMAMMOGRAPHY, see *Radiography*

X-RAY, see *Radiography*

XYLOSE BREATH, see *Lactose Tolerance*

XYLOSE TOLERANCE

The xylose tolerance test ascertains if the intestines absorb nutrients and medications properly. After fasting for at least eight hours, the patient is given a dose of from 5 to 25 g of D-xylose (a form of sugar in water); too large a dose can cause nausea and diarrhea. All urine excreted over the next five hours is collected and then tested for D-xylose, which is usually excreted unchanged. The test normally is not performed when the patient is known to have kidney disease; but if necessary then, the level of the sugar can be determined in the blood. At times, antibiotic drugs are given a day or two before the test in order to reduce intestinal bacteria, which can interfere with absorption.

A somewhat related test for malabsorption is the measurement of indican in the urine. It is a reflection of protein breakdown in the intestines and can help indicate how well the bowels are performing—in both absorption and transit movement. It can also reflect bacterial overgrowth in the intestinal tract. Normally, a very small amount of indican is found in urine, but amounts greater than 100 mg per 100 ml are considered a sign of disease and, when found, usually lead to **Serotonin** and bile acid breath testing (see **Nuclear Scanning**).

When performed: Primarily when there is suspicion of liver or pancreas disease, causing a decreased amount of digestive enzyme secretion; when there is unexplained weight loss; when there is suspicion of parasitic diseases; when toxic conditions that affect the intestinal lining (celiac disease, tropical sprue) are suspected; following surgery on the intestines; in certain anemias; when patients take large amounts of drugs such as alcohol, certain antibiotics, and mineral oil. (Also see **Malnutrition**.)

Normal values: When 5 g of D-xylose are given, the urine should show at least 1.5 g; when 25 g of D-xylose are given, the urine should show more than 3 g. Blood should show at least 20 mg per 100 ml five hours after a 25 g dose.

Abnormal values: D-xylose values are decreased when there is malabsorption in the small intestine. When patients have kidney disease or low thyroid activity, there may be normal absorption by the intestine but decreased urine values. Values may decrease as a patient gets older, but this is not necessarily indicative of disease.

Risk factors: Negligible (see general risk factors for blood testing).

Pain/discomfort: Minimal (see general pain/discomfort factors for blood testing).

Cost: From $20 to $25 whether on blood or urine. An indican test is $36.

Accuracy and significance: The test is of value as a means of determining how well the small intestine absorbs nutrients. Generally, however, it does not indicate a specific diagnosis; about 50 percent accurate.

Y

YERSINIA DISEASE, see *Agglutination*

Z

ZETA SEDIMENTATION RATIO, see *Sedimentation Rate*

ZINC

A deficiency of zinc, one of the trace elements (a mineral needed in the body in only minute amounts), has been associated with a number of disease conditions; in fact, in virtually all illnesses, blood zinc levels are usually decreased. Zinc is essential to certain enzyme functioning and to the prevention or treatment of certain developmental abnormalities such as hypogonadism and growth retardation. One specific dwarfism condition can be corrected by adding zinc to the diet. On a normal diet, the average adult takes in approximately 10 to 15 mg of zinc per day. Oysters, herring, and whole grains are good dietary sources of zinc. Since zinc is necessary to produce testosterone and the testes are known to contain the largest amount of zinc in the body, the "old wives' tale" of oysters being an excellent treatment for male impotence would seem to have some basis in fact.

Blood serum, plasma, urine, and even hair are examined for zinc levels. For confirmation of a specific zinc deficiency problem, supplementary zinc is prescribed and the patient is clinically observed for reversal of symptoms.

When performed: When symptoms of abnormalities in taste and smell suggest a zinc deficiency; with prostate disease.

Normal values: Normally, the level of zinc found in blood serum is 90 to 110 mcg per 100 ml; 0.5 mg per day is excreted in the urine.

Abnormal values: Lower-than-normal values of zinc are found in alcoholism, during pregnancy, after a heart attack, after surgery when there is poor wound healing, in liver disease, infections, cancers, prostate problems, sickle-cell disease, and for a few hours after eating. Certain hormones may also lower zinc levels.

Higher-than-normal levels of zinc are found in patients who inherit a tendency toward hyperzincemia and also in certain metal workers (usually from breathing zinc fumes); an excess amount of zinc can cause drowsiness, dizziness, and muscular incoordination.

Risk factors: Negligible (see general risk factors for blood testing).

Pain/discomfort: Minimal (see general pain/discomfort factors for blood testing).

Cost: From $15 to $25.

Accuracy and significance: Since little of the body's zinc supply can be measured in the blood or urine, the test is not noted for its precision. It can be of help, however, when other diagnostic tests fail to reveal the cause of illness; about 50 percent accurate.

ZOLLINGER-ELLISON SYNDROME, see *Gastrin*
ZUNG SELF-RATING DEPRESSION SCALE, see *Depression*

MEASUREMENTS: EQUIVALENCY CHART
MASS OR SOLID SUBSTANCE MEASUREMENTS

kg	kilogram	1,000 g; 2 pounds, 3 ounces; 2.2 lb.; 35.27 oz.
g	gram	1,000 mg; 0.035 oz.; 1/30 oz. (28.35 g = 1 oz.); 15½ grains (weight of a paper clip)
mg	milligram	1,000 μg; 0.001 g; 0.000035 oz.; 1/65 grain (2 particles of table salt)
μg, mcg	microgram	1,000 ng; 1/1,000,000 g (one-millionth of a gram)
ng	nanogram	1,000 pg; 1/1,000,000,000 g (one-billionth of a gram)*
pg	picogram	1/1,000,000,000,000 g (one-trillionth of a gram)**

*Drugs such as LSD and amphetamines can cause a toxic or even fatal reaction in such small doses that they are measured in nanograms. Cardiac glycosides (such as Digoxin and Digitoxin) and other drugs that produce a therapeutic effect in very small amounts are also measured in nanograms; in some patients, a toxic overdose can be caused by a rise of only one nanogram in the blood.

**Many hormone tests are reported in picograms.

LIQUID MEASUREMENTS

L	liter	1,000 ml; 1.06 qt.; 1 qt., 2oz.; 33.81 oz.
dl	deciliter	100 ml; 3.4 oz. (gradually replacing 100 ml in reported test values)
ml	milliliter	.001 L; 1/1,000 L (one-thousandth of a liter); (5 ml = 1 teaspoon; 30 ml = 1 oz.)*
μl	microliter	1/1,000,000 L (one-millionth of a liter)
mol	mole	amount of substance in a solution; with the adoption of the International System units of test reporting (IU), this term is replacing many older test result reports such as "mg per 100 ml" measurements
mmol	millimole	1/1,000 of a mole
mEq	milliequivalent	1/1,000 equivalence of chemical combining capacity or substance; number of grams of a substance in 1 ml of solution

*At times, cc (cubic centimeter) is used inaccurately for, or interchangeably with, ml; cc is more properly a measure of area than of volume or quantity of liquid.

ABOUT THE AUTHORS

Cathey (Catherine Larkum) Pinckney was a regular book reviewer for "Parade of Books," a weekly column distributed by King Features Syndicate. Trained in psychology and microbiology (New York University, Syracuse University, The New School for Social Research), she is health and medical editor for Vector TV Consumer News, a program prepared for cable TV stations throughout the United States that reports on health, food, and other related consumer matters.

Dr. Edward R. Pinckney's academic positions have included: chairman of the Department of Preventive Medicine and director of the Comprehensive Medical Clinic at Northwestern University College of Medicine, Chicago; lecturer, School of Public Health, University of California, Berkeley; and associate clinical professor of medicine at Loma Linda College of Medicine, Los Angeles. He is a regular book reviewer for the American Association for the Advancement of Science. Dr. Pinckney also has additional graduate degrees in law (LL.B.) and public health (M.P.H.) and is certified as a specialist (Diplomate) in Preventive Medicine and Public Health by the American Board of Preventive Medicine. In 1970, he was requested to prepare comprehensive information, and to testify directly, for two U.S. Senate committees on the cost and quality of medical care and on problems in the drug industry. He was a consultant to the California Assembly Committee on Malpractice.

Among the many professional organizations with which he is affiliated, Dr. Pinckney is a Fellow of the American College of Physicians, a Fellow of the American Association for the Advancement of Science, and a Fellow of the American College of Preventive Medicine, on whose Committee on Policy and Legislation he once served.

Dr. Pinckney has also authored: *You Can Prevent Illness* and *How to Make the Most of Your Doctor and Medicine*. Other writing included a regular health column in *Blue Print for Health*, the magazine of the Blue Cross Association; multiple contributions for Encyclopedia International; 134 screenplays for postgraduate medical teaching films distributed by Encyclopaedia Britannica Films; and more than 100 scientific articles in professional medical journals. Editorial positions have included: associate editor of *The Journal of the American Medical Association*; editor of *The New Physician* (received the 1960 American Medical Writers' Association Honor Award in Journalism for this editorship); executive editor of *Trauma* (a medical journal for the legal profession); and associate editor of *Physician's Management*.

Dr. and Mrs. Pinckney together have authored: *Medical Encyclopedia of Common Illnesses, The Fallacy of Freud and Psychoanalysis, The Cholesterol Controversy*, and *Do-It-Yourself Medical Testing* (also from Facts On File).

For many years, they wrote the syndicated daily newspaper medical column "Mirror of Your Mind," distributed to 110 U.S. and foreign newspapers by King Features

Syndicate. They have also coauthored articles in *The Saturday Review*, *Media & Consumer* (where they were contributing editors), *Consumer Newsletter*, and various newspapers.

The Pinckneys live in Beverly Hills, California.